DIABETES

DIABETES

The Comprehensive Self-Management Handbook

DIABETES EDUCATION CENTER

NASSAU HOSPITAL, MINEOLA, N.Y.

John F. Aloia, M.D., F.A.C.P.
Director

Patricia Donohue-Porter, R.N., M.S.N.
Clinical Nurse Specialist

Laurie Schlussel, R.D., M.A.
Nutritionist

DOUBLEDAY & COMPANY, INC.

GARDEN CITY, NEW YORK

1984

NOTICE

Medicine is ever-changing. As new experiences broaden our knowledge, changes in treatment and drug therapy are required. The editors and the publisher of this work have made efforts to ensure that the drug dosage schedules herein are accurate and in accord with the accepted standards at the time of publication. Readers are advised to check the product information sheet included in the package of each drug they plan to administer to be certain that changes have not been made in the recommended dose or in the contraindications for administration. This recommendation is of particular importance in regard to new drugs.

Line Drawings by Phillip Jones

Library of Congress Cataloging in Publication Data
Aloia, John F.
Diabetes, the comprehensive self-management handbook.
Includes index.
1. Diabetes—Treatment—Handbooks, manuals, etc.
2. Diabetics—Care and treatment—Handbooks, manuals,
etc. 3. Self-care, Health—Handbooks, manuals, etc.
I. Donohue-Porter, Patricia. II. Schlussel, Laurie.
III. Diabetes Education Center (Mineola, N.Y.)
IV. Title.
[DNLM: 1. Diabetes mellitus—Popular works. WK 850 A453d]
·RC660.A574 1984 616.4′6205
ISBN 0-385-18292-9
Library of Congress Catalog Card Number 82-45392

*To our patients in
the Diabetes Education Center,
the most important members of the Diabetes team,
who have added to our clinical experiences,
warmed our hearts and demonstrated the
true meaning of self-management*

PREFACE

This book represents the outcome of a decade's effort to establish a comprehensive educational program for people with diabetes mellitus. This effort culminated in the establishment of the Nassau Hospital Diabetes Education Center. The Center provides a thirty-five-hour curriculum in self-management of diabetes. Instruction is provided by a team comprised of a clinical nurse specialist, nutritionist and physician. The team approach to diabetes is stressed, with the patient recognized as the most important member of the team.

Diabetes may not be curable at present, but it can be controlled. "Control" is a word that you will find used frequently, and in several different ways, in this book. Through proper self-management, your blood glucose can be controlled. As a result of blood glucose control, the complications of diabetes may be minimized ("controlling" diabetes). "Self-control" is another important way this term is used. Without self-control, the obese diabetic person will never lose weight and the insulin-dependent diabetic will continually have marked rises and drops in blood glucose levels. The complications of diabetes will then inevitably develop.

This book provides the information required for self-management. But knowledge and behavior are separate entities. Self-control is needed to choose the action that your intellect tells you is correct. Unfortunately, it is possible to know all there is to be known about diabetes and yet behave incorrectly. The insulin-dependent diabetic person must replace the function of a normal pancreas with conscious attention to diet and activity. He must also measure his own blood glucose and adjust his insulin dosage. Obviously a great deal of self-control is necessary to carry out a self-management program to control diabetes.

This requirement is further compounded by the fact that a major goal of good control is prevention of complications in the future. Moderate elevations in blood glucose do not result in feeling ill; indeed, those who are very well controlled are frequently on the brink of hypoglycemia. It is difficult to perform certain tasks without feedback. For example, an elevated blood glucose may not be causing you pain or discomfort. Yet, to prevent an elevated blood glucose, you must exert self-control in many areas of your life.

The first step in controlling diabetes is to avoid denying that you have a chronic illness. Denial is an acceptable way to deal with a fleeting or minor problem. Diabetes is not such a problem; it will not go away. Denial of diabetes will lead to illness; acceptance of having diabetes can lead to its control. The second step involves motivation: you must want to control diabetes. This book provides the third step, which is education. You should know as much about diabetes as you are capable of learning. We realize that this book contains more information than many will consider desirable, but it is meant to be comprehensive. It is written for the individual who selects ideal self-management. The last step involves remotivation and reeducation. We all slip back into old habits and forget what we learned. Always remember that you are the one with diabetes. Other members of the team may be helpful, but you will make all the important choices that affect the outcome of having diabetes.

The philosophy of this book may be regarded as progressive, emphasizing your role in achieving control. There is abundant evidence, now, that the long-term complications of diabetes are due to the elevation of blood glucose. There is strong evidence both in animal research and in human studies that keeping the blood glucose as close to normal as possible will delay the long-term complications. This possibility of preventing the complications of diabetes has led to the development of home blood glucose monitoring and insulin infusion pumps. It has also led to the recommendation of a diet that is low in cholesterol with an appropriate ratio of polyunsaturated to saturated fats and a higher fiber content. It has intensified our efforts to encourage exercise, discourage cigarette smoking and aggressively lower high blood pressure with medication.

Implicit in this approach is that the informed diabetic individual continuously chooses health over illness. He selects the behavior that keeps his blood glucose as normal as possible and prevents the accelerated development of atherosclerosis. The uninformed and unmotivated individual with diabetes chooses illness. The modern individual who espouses the philosophy of self-control emerges from the life crisis of having diabetes as a stronger person with sufficient self-control to affect the outcome of his diabetes.

Finally, how should this book be used? It is not written to provide minimal information that is required when diabetes is first diagnosed. Rather, it should be used as a textbook would be used in a course. It must be studied, not read like a novel. All the information should be mastered. Other members of the health-care team should be consulted to answer questions that may arise. This book should be consulted when memory fails and should be periodically re-studied. It provides the knowledge to choose healthy behavior. It will enable you to control diabetes.

ACKNOWLEDGMENTS

The Diabetes Education Center was originally partially supported by grants from the Center for Disease Control and the New York State Department of Health as a Diabetes Control Program. It is with great appreciation that we acknowledge the following patients and professionals. Many of their suggestions helped make this book possible.

We thank you: David Adamovitch, Ed.D., John Ascenzio, Henry Balboa, D.P.M., Elizabeth Brennan, Ruth Cusack, Ph.D., Vincent DiScala, M.D., Geraldine Donohue, R.N., Kathleen Dooney, R.N., Mary Greaney, Cynthia Gross, Linda Growl, Michael Klotz, Marina Lazaro-Moore, Beatrice Leahrman, David Lyon, M.D., James McCorkel, Ph.D., Mary Beth McNiery, R.D., John Michel, Sharon Pearl, Philip Rasulo, M.D., Lynne Sampson-Chimon, R.D., Kathy Sawitsky, Burton Sultan, M.D., Ashok Vaswani, M.D.

We would also like to thank our families for their support during the writing of this book.

A special thank-you goes to Lois Swawite for typing the manuscript.

We are also grateful for the editorial assistance of Jean Anne Vincent and Doreen DeFlorio of Doubleday.

CONTENTS

DIABETES

1

Introduction to Diabetes

Although this book is aimed at educating you about diabetes, it is important that you have a general idea of how your body works. If you understand how the body works normally, you will have a better understanding of the consequences of abnormal body function. The beginning of this chapter will briefly review some important aspects of biology. Your body is composed of millions of cells, the smallest units of living matter. Cells of the same type make up tissues; an organ is composed of several types of tissues and performs a special function. Examples of organs are the heart, lungs and kidneys. A system is a group of organs that perform similar functions or work together to perform one complex function. The body systems work together like instruments in an orchestra so that the entire body functions properly. The nervous system and the endocrine system work together to coordinate body systems. If you are unfamiliar with biology, it would be useful to study "How Your Body Works" at the end of this book.

BODY SYSTEMS AND THEIR FUNCTIONS

System	Function
Respiratory	Exchanges oxygen and carbon dioxide between the lungs and bloodstream
Circulatory	Delivers oxygen and nutrients to all areas; removes wastes from tissues
Gastrointestinal	Processes food, allowing it to be used as nutrients or excreted as wastes

Urinary	Eliminates water, salt and waste products
Nervous	Regulates internal processes of the body, including thoughts; interacts with environment
Endocrine	Integrates the body's biochemical activities
Reproductive	Continues the species
Musculoskeletal	Provides a framework for locomotion

As you read this chapter, you should marvel at the complexity of the human body. The way that all of its different activities are continuously changing and yet remain coordinated is truly amazing. Although continuous changes occur in this remarkable human machine, its internal environment remains relatively unchanged. The internal environment is kept ideal so that the human machine functions optimally. The numerous checks and balances that maintain the body's internal environment are referred to as homeostasis. When your body functions optimally, you are said to be "healthy." If homeostasis fails, the internal environment of the body becomes altered. Ideal conditions are no longer maintained. When this occurs, a disease of metabolism is said to be present.

Diabetes mellitus is a disorder of carbohydrate, protein and fat metabolism. This is caused by a relative or absolute lack of insulin. Let us now look more closely at the meaning of metabolism.

Metabolism is the process in which food is broken down and used for energy. Food provides the energy needed for your body to work. Since food is really the tissues (or organs) of other living beings (plants and animals), much of it is in complex form. However, in order to enter cells, food must be broken down into simple building blocks. For example, starches, proteins and fats must be broken down to glucose, amino acids and free fatty acids. The process of digestion involves breaking down food in the gastrointestinal tract to a simpler form. When nutrients become small enough, they are then absorbed into the gastrointestinal cells and then into the bloodstream. They are carried by the blood to other body cells, where they are used for growth, repair and the production of energy. Nutrients can also be stored for later use when food is not available. Nutrients are converted into their more complex forms when they are stored (starches, proteins and fats).

THE ENERGY CYCLE

Food provides fuel for the body in the form of carbohydrates (glucose), proteins (amino acids), and fats (fatty acids). These fuels can be changed to energy in the cell through the Krebs cycle, which is like a nuclear power plant that creates energy. The Krebs cycle helps to form ATP (adenosine triphosphate). ATP provides the energy necessary for the function of all body cells. It provides energy not only for basic functions but also for activity such as exercise. Glucose must enter the cell in order for this energy cycle to take place. Once in the cell, glucose is used like fuel. It mixes with the oxygen you breathe from the air. The glucose and oxygen produce carbon dioxide, water and energy. The energy is used to do work, but the carbon dioxide and water must be eliminated through the lungs and kidneys.

CARBOHYDRATE METABOLISM

Carbohydrates may be found in simple or complex forms. The major simple sugar in the blood is known as glucose. Complex carbohydrates (starches) are changed into simple forms in the intestine. Carbohydrates are also stored as a starch called glycogen. Let us now look at normal carbohydrate metabolism. Usually, the blood glucose level stays within a fairly narrow range (glucose homeostasis). After meals, the blood glucose may rise slightly. Insulin is then secreted and allows the glucose to be used. The blood glucose then returns to the level present before eating.

Glucose is used for immediate energy needs. If there is no immediate need for glucose, insulin will help to store it for future use. Glucose is stored in muscles and the liver as glycogen. Glycogenolysis is the process whereby glycogen is broken down into glucose and released into the circulation. If more glucose is absorbed than is needed for cellular energy, insulin will cause it to be stored as fat. Continuous ingestion of any fuel (carbohydrate, protein or fat) in excess of the body's need will lead to obesity. This key point, of supply and demand of energy (balance), should help you understand the nutrition basics presented later in the book.

In summary, there are two basic aspects of carbohydrate metabolism: the provision of energy for immediate cell use and the storage of excess energy for use in the future.

PROTEIN METABOLISM

Proteins are another form of fuel available from your diet. When proteins enter the intestine, they are broken down into smaller molecules known as amino acids. Insulin helps the body use amino acids. Amino acids are combined to build muscle proteins. They can also be changed to glucose in the liver (this is

called gluconeogenesis or the synthesis of new glucose). The continuous secretion of small amounts of insulin ("basal insulin") prevents excessive gluconeogenesis in the liver. If insulin is totally absent from the body, gluconeogenesis raises the blood glucose even if you have not eaten.

FAT METABOLISM

Your body can also use fats for fuel. Fats can be metabolized to fatty acids
and glycerol. In the presence of insulin, excess fat can be stored in adipose (fat)
cells as a reserve fuel. Only a small amount of fat is broken down into glucose.
It is primarily used as a fuel directly in the form of fatty acids or stored as a
potential fuel in the fat cells. Insulin allows the proper storage of fat and prevents
the release of free fatty acids from fat into the blood. Insulin helps to store fatty
acids as triglycerides in the liver. The production of ketones, by-products of
fatty acids, by the liver is controlled by insulin. In order to fully understand
diabetes as a metabolic disorder, let us review the role of the endocrine system.

THE ENDOCRINE SYSTEM AND DIABETES

The endocrine system controls body processes according to messages it receives from the nervous system and from various substances in the blood. It
sends messages from one part of the body to another by releasing hormones
into the blood. A hormone is a chemical that is carried by the bloodstream to
another part of the body where it acts to control rates of chemical reactions.
Endocrine glands produce, store and secrete (release) hormones. Individual
hormones (chemical messengers) must be recognized by cell receptors before
they can bind with the cell membrane. After the hormone attaches to the cell
membrane, it is able to work.

The pancreas is an endocrine gland. There are small areas within the pancreas
called the islets of Langerhans. The islets contain three types of cells which
produce different hormones. The beta cells produce insulin, the alpha cells
produce glucagon and the delta cells produce somatostatin. Somatostatin decreases the secretion of growth hormone, insulin and glucagon. As another
function, the pancreas produces digestive enzymes.

INSULIN

About 20 to 40 units of insulin are produced each day in the beta cells of the
normal human pancreas. The first product made by the beta cells is proinsulin,

a chain of 81 amino acids. The chain of amino acids is broken into two separate pieces, insulin and connecting peptide (C-peptide). Both pieces are stored in the beta cell to be released in response to stimulation. The C-peptide does not affect blood glucose levels. Yet it is known that when an insulin molecule is released, a C-peptide molecule is also released. Because of this, the C-peptide molecule can be measured in the blood to determine the ability of the beta cell to release insulin. Insulin may also be measured in the blood.

Insulin is released from the beta cells in several phases. When the blood glucose rises, there is an immediate release of insulin lasting for 10 to 15 minutes. The second phase is a gradual release of insulin that continues as long as blood glucose is elevated. This second phase also involves the synthesis (formation) of additional insulin. The beta cell must produce more insulin to keep up with the demand.

The storage of insulin in the beta cells helps to provide for the proper balance of blood glucose. The non-diabetic person always has insulin available in storage. Precisely the right amount of insulin is released into the blood when needed. In this way, blood glucose is closely regulated. Each normal pancreas has approximately 100,000 islets of Langerhans and each islet contains between 80 and 100 beta cells. These cells can measure blood glucose every ten seconds within a highly sensitive range. Within one and a half minutes, normal beta cells can deliver any amount of insulin necessary to regulate the blood glucose. Imagine the difficulty of trying to simulate this exquisite system by a single injection of insulin.

How does insulin act to regulate the blood glucose? It moves the glucose into the cell to be used for energy. At this point, the example of an automobile may help in understanding the energy cycle. A car's motor can be compared to a cell in the body. Fuel for the automobile can be compared to blood glucose. In attempting to start a car, you can't get the fuel into the engine without turning the key. Consider insulin as the key to using your body's fuels properly. Remember that insulin also regulates blood glucose by controlling the amount of glucose entering the blood from the liver.

CONTRAINSULIN HORMONES

Counterregulatory hormones act in an opposite or antagonistic way to insulin. They include glucagon, epinephrine, cortisol and growth hormone. After you eat, insulin is released to lower your blood glucose. Glucagon is also present and prevents your blood glucose from going too low. Glucagon raises blood glucose by increasing glycogenolysis in the liver. Glycogenolysis, as you will recall, is the process whereby glycogen (the storage form of glucose in the liver) is broken down into glucose and released into the blood. Glucagon also increases liver gluconeogenesis (the formation of new glucose from amino acids). If blood glucose is low, glucagon is secreted and returns blood glucose into the normal range.

The brain needs a constant supply of glucose to use as its fuel. When blood glucose is low, it sends out signals to release hormones from various endocrine glands. Epinephrine from the adrenal glands is also released during hypoglycemia. Epinephrine, too, stimulates glycogenolysis and gluconeogenesis. Glucagon and epinephrine are the primary contrainsulin hormones. Over a long time, cortisol from the adrenal glands and growth hormone from the pituitary gland act in concert with glucagon and epinephrine to prevent hypoglycemia.

CARBOHYDRATE HOMEOSTASIS

As you can imagine, blood glucose levels are influenced by many factors, including whether you are fasting or have just eaten. The secretion of insulin or glucagon is affected by the amount of the various body fuels present in the blood. These two hormones are secreted in just the right amounts on a minute-to-minute basis, and counteract each other. The result is that blood glucose stays in a fairly narrow range. A small amount of insulin is always secreted to prevent gluconeogenesis from being excessive. This is true even during fasting. Insulin prevents blood glucose levels from becoming too high. If blood glucose levels decrease too much, glucagon and epinephrine are secreted and raise blood glucose by increasing glycogenolysis and gluconeogenesis. In diabetes, carbohydrate, protein and fat homeostasis is disturbed because of the lack of insulin.

Diabetes mellitus may be defined as a chronic disorder of carbohydrate homeostasis caused by a lack (or ineffectiveness) of insulin. This definition is an oversimplification. Protein and fat metabolism is also affected by the lack of insulin, and glucagon is usually present in excess. Hyperglycemia (a high blood glucose) is the hallmark of diabetes.

As a result of the low insulin levels (and high glucagon levels), gluconeogenesis and glycogenolysis are not properly controlled. Blood glucose will be elevated even when you are fasting. In addition, the lack of insulin secretion after eating will result in further increases in blood glucose after meals (postprandial hyperglycemia). Over a period of time, the high glucose levels result in complications in the circulatory and nervous systems as well as the eyes and kidneys.

HISTORY OF DIABETES

Diabetes has been recognized by man for thousands of years. It was written about in the Ebers Papyrus as early as 1500 B.C. Ancient physicians thought of diabetes as a disease of the kidneys rather than the pancreas. The symptom of increased urination led to this idea. Arateus, in A.D. 2, described the disease using the Greek word *diabetes*, "to run through a siphon." Again, urination in large amounts helped to give the disease its name. The honeylike composition of the urine was described in writings of the sixth century, and the Latin word *mellitus*, "honey," was used later.

In the nineteenth century, the German scientist Paul Langerhans described clusters of cells in the pancreas. These cells now bear his name, the islets of Langerhans. Late in the nineteenth century, two other German scientists, Joseph von Mering and Oskar Minkowski, discovered that removal of the pancreas from animals produced diabetes. It was later discovered that if the islet cells were not destroyed, the animals did not become diabetic. Working in the United States, E. L. Opie discovered that islet cells of the pancreas were damaged in humans who had diabetes.

All this previous information led to the discovery of insulin by Frederick G. Banting and Charles H. Best of Canada in 1921. They isolated islet cell tissue from animals and injected an extract into diabetic animals. The result was a drop in blood glucose levels. This important contribution is, of course, highly valued and has saved the lives of millions of diabetic persons. Yet diabetes has not been cured by the discovery of insulin. As you continue reading, the reason for this will become more clear. In order to understand fully how diabetes affects the human body, it is necessary first to look at fuel homeostasis in diabetes.

FUEL HOMEOSTASIS IN DIABETES

Insulin controls the metabolism and storage of nutrients. If you do not have enough insulin working for you, you are not able to store body fuels for later use. You are not able to adequately use glucose derived from food. Without insulin, excessive glucose is produced by the liver (gluconeogenesis and glycogenolysis). Less glucose is used by muscle and fat cells, and glucose storage becomes less efficient. Thus blood glucose rises. The lack of insulin causes amino acids to be changed to glucose (gluconeogenesis). With a lack of insulin, amino acids are released more rapidly from muscles and travel to the liver to undergo gluconeogenesis. Fats are broken down rapidly and there is an increase in the release of free fatty acids. Free fatty acids are quickly converted to ketones. These are drastic effects. As these changes occur, some symptoms of diabetes appear.

WHAT CAUSES THE SYMPTOMS OF DIABETES?

The absence of insulin in diabetes causes changes to occur in the energy cycle. Blood glucose rises. Early symptoms may include fatigue and weakness.

You can't obtain energy from food and may have extreme hunger (polyphagia). You may overeat without weight gain because food is not being utilized properly.

As glucose accumulates in the blood, it is filtered through the kidneys. Although glucose is usually retained by the kidneys as a useful substance, any excess is excreted. The kidneys will usually return all glucose to the blood unless the blood glucose exceeds 160–180 milligrams per deciliter (mg./dl.). This level is known as the "renal threshold." Above this level, glucose is usually excreted into the urine (glycosuria). As glucose is excreted, water is also lost.

Each body cell is surrounded by a cell membrane that separates the inside of the cell from its liquid environment. The cell membrane is semipermeable. Water can enter and leave the cell freely, but other substances may not be able to pass through the membrane. This characteristic of the cell membrane enables the body to maintain an exact balance on either side of the membrane. This balance is vital to life. If the concentration of particles (such as glucose) outside the cell increases, water moves out of the cell to restore the chemical balance. This process is known as osmosis. The excess volume of water is excreted by the kidneys. A major sign of diabetes is urination in large amounts (polyuria). With the loss of excess water, extreme thirst (polydipsia) may develop. These three symptoms, polyphagia (extreme hunger), polydipsia (extreme thirst) and polyuria (large amounts of urination), form the classic triad of diabetes symptoms.

For certain individuals, weight loss may be another symptom. The body is unable to use nutrients. The glucose necessary for energy production does not enter the cells and is lost in the urine. Because cells do not have enough glucose for fuel, another fuel source is used: fat. Fat breakdown results in the overproduction of ketones. The ketones cause life-threatening acidosis. This is called diabetic ketoacidosis. Symptoms of diabetic ketoacidosis include increased thirst, increased urination, weakness, abdominal pain, generalized aches, nausea, vomiting, headaches, heavy breathing and loss of consciousness.

The symptoms noted above are danger signs of diabetes. Be aware of these symptoms and share your knowledge with people who do not have diabetes. Today, over 10 million Americans have diabetes. Diabetes affects more women than men and is more common over the age of forty. Because a diabetic individual is diagnosed every sixty seconds, the American Diabetes Association has compiled the following warning symptoms of diabetes. For the insulin-dependent ("juvenile") diabetic, the acronym CAUTION is used to keep in mind the following symptoms: *C*onstant urination, *A*bnormal thirst, *U*nusual hunger, *T*he rapid loss of weight, *I*rritability, *O*bvious weakness and fatigue, *N*ausea and vomiting.

For the person with non-insulin-dependent diabetes, the word "diabetes" is used as an acronym: *D*rowsiness, *I*tching, *A* family history of diabetes, *B*lurred vision, *E*xcessive weight, *T*ingling, numbness, pain in the extremities, *E*asy fatigue, Skin infections and slow healing of cuts and scratches, especially on the feet.

CLASSIFICATION OF DIABETES

In the past, some confusing terms were used to describe diabetes mellitus. Such terms as "old age diabetes," "juvenile diabetes," "sugar diabetes," "mild diabetes" and "brittle diabetes" were common. To avoid this confusion, in 1979 the National Diabetes Data Group proposed a reclassification of diabetes mellitus. New terms are now used to describe two distinct types of diabetes.

Type I is insulin-dependent diabetes mellitus (IDDM). There is a lack of insulin and markedly decreased or absent beta cell function of the pancreas. Insulin must be injected daily or diabetic ketoacidosis will develop. This type of diabetes was formerly called juvenile diabetes. Its onset is usually in youth but insulin-dependent diabetes may occur at any age.

Type II, non-insulin-dependent diabetes mellitus (NIDDM), was formerly known as adult-onset or maturity-onset diabetes. The pancreas is able to produce more insulin than in Type I diabetes. Although these patients may inject insulin to prevent hyperglycemia, they do not develop diabetic ketoacidosis if they omit insulin. The insulin deficiency in Type II thin individuals is not as severe as in Type I; this results in hyperglycemia but not ketoacidosis. Most Type II individuals are obese and do not have a deficiency of insulin. Instead, their obesity makes their insulin less effective; they are resistant to the effect of insulin (insulin resistance). Think of this classification in terms of insulin production: Type I individuals produce almost no insulin, Type II thin individuals produce a decreased amount of insulin and Type II obese individuals produce a normal (or even greater than normal) amount of insulin but are insulin-resistant. In the Type II obese person, hyperglycemia occurs because obesity prevents the insulin from working effectively. The warning signs for each type are important to remember because Type II diabetic persons can become Type I.

Other classifications that are used include "impaired glucose tolerance" and "gestational diabetes." Impaired glucose tolerance refers to the situation in which blood glucose is normal during fasting but rises to higher than normal after drinking glucose during a glucose-tolerance test. If you fit into this category, you would be instructed to lose weight, if necessary, or maintain your ideal body weight. You would also be advised to have future blood glucose determinations and to be alert to warning signs of diabetes. Impaired glucose tolerance may or may not lead to overt diabetes. Gestational diabetes refers to the classification that was formerly known as diabetes during pregnancy. Hyperglycemia, here, has its onset or recognition during pregnancy. Gestational diabetes usually disappears after childbirth, but approximately 30 percent of such women have permanent diabetes within 5 to 10 years.

Two other statistical risk categories have also been developed. The classification of "previous abnormality of glucose tolerance" describes individuals who previously had hyperglycemia. For example, if you were overweight with a high blood glucose and you lost weight which resulted in normal glucose tolerance, you would fit into this classification. Of course, individuals in this category are cautioned to maintain their ideal body weight. Another classification, "potential abnormality of glucose tolerance," refers to individuals who are at risk for the development of diabetes. Siblings or identical twins of diabetic individuals are examples of people who are at risk for the development of insulin-dependent diabetes. An example of an individual at risk for the development of non-insulin-dependent diabetes is any first-degree relative of a non-insulin-dependent diabetic individual. You will find other examples of persons in this classification throughout this book. These classifications allow your doctor to categorize you and further evaluate you. They are most helpful in aiding researchers in collecting data regarding diabetes. They do not involve any other treatment except general health recommendations such as weight maintenance.

Many of the new classifications set up by the NIH Workgroup are for the protection of the patient. The word "diabetes" has been omitted from certain categories to safeguard employment and insurance rights. The interpretation of the laboratory tests for the detection of diabetes is intended to prevent the overdiagnosis of diabetes. Although the cutoff point has been designated at 140 mg./dl., strict blood glucose control demands levels below 140 mg./dl.

THE ETIOLOGY OF DIABETES

Etiology refers to the cause of a disease. There are many factors involved in the development of diabetes. Although both insulin-dependent and non-insulin-dependent diabetes are characterized by total or partial lack of insulin, these two types of diabetes have different causes. In this section the causes of diabetes will be examined according to the type of diabetes. Diabetes can be caused by other diseases or conditions. The occurrence of diabetes may be secondary to other causes such as pancreatic disease, other endocrine diseases, drug administration or the use of hormones that elevate blood glucose.

CAUSES OF IDDM

The major areas now being examined as possible causes of insulin-dependent diabetes mellitus are related to autoimmunity and viruses. Immunological factors may be responsible for the development of insulin-dependent diabetes. Your immune system helps to protect you from foreign substances (like bacteria) by producing antibodies that destroy the foreign substances. Antibodies to islet cell tissues have been found in recently diagnosed diabetics. They are called autoantibodies because they develop in response to one's own organs, not to a foreign substance. The production of these antibodies may be triggered by a viral infection of the pancreas. There have been more new cases of diabetes after epidemics of certain viruses. Destruction of beta cells has been demonstrated following particular virus infections in mice. Of course, many of the viruses being examined now occur in many individuals without diabetes.

Recently histocompatibility locus antigens (HLA) have been thought to be a clue to the development of insulin-dependent diabetes. These are specific cell antigens that are genetic markers. Certain HLA antigens have been found more frequently in insulin-dependent diabetics. Yet many people have these HLA antigens and do not develop diabetes. Although insulin-dependent diabetes may be inherited, another factor in the environment (such as the presence of viruses) must also be present.

CAUSES OF NIDDM

Non-insulin-dependent diabetes mellitus is not caused by viruses or antibodies. Obesity and heredity are the major factors that may cause its development. If one identical twin develops non-insulin-dependent diabetes, there is almost a 100 percent chance that the other twin will develop the disease. Close relatives of persons with non-insulin-dependent diabetes have a 20–30 percent risk of developing this form of the disease. Obesity has long been recognized as a cause of non-insulin-dependent diabetes. Obesity causes insulin resistance. This results in a slight elevation in blood glucose and increased production of insulin. In a non-diabetic person, the pancreas produces enough insulin to keep blood glucose normal. However, a diabetic person who has inherited a defect in the pancreas may be manufacturing more insulin than a non-diabetic person but the insulin is insufficient to maintain normal blood glucose. The resistance to insulin in obesity is now known to be due to a decrease in insulin receptors. In order to understand more fully this concept of obesity and insulin resistance, let us look at insulin receptors in more detail.

You have already learned that water passes in and out of cells through osmosis. Other substances, besides water, have to enter and leave the cell. Cell receptors are responsible for allowing specific substances, such as hormones, to cross the cell membrane. For insulin to work it must bind to specific receptors on the cell membrane. When a hormone binds with a receptor, the cell recognizes the hormone, in this case insulin. With this binding, the hormone begins the work of controlling chemical reactions. Insulin receptors are found on fat, liver, and muscle cells as well as some other cells. Insulin must attach to these receptors before glucose can enter the cell.

In certain cases, such as obesity, the number of insulin receptors on a cell may be decreased. With fewer cell receptors insulin will work less effectively. "Affinity" is the term used for the active binding that takes place between insulin and the receptor. The receptor attracts the hormone. Affinity is also decreased in Type II obesity-related NIDDM. Proper use of diet and exercise can increase the number and affinity of cell receptors. Patients with diabetes also may have abnormal responses within the cell ("post-receptor defect"). This is an intense area of current research. Insulin resistance is a feature of obesity-related non-insulin-dependent diabetes and will be further described in Chapter 7. For a review of the differences between Type I and Type II diabetes, see Table 1.

TABLE 1
DIFFERENCES BETWEEN TYPE I & II DIABETES

| | TYPE I Diabetes | TYPE II Diabetes | |
		THIN	OBESE
Amt. Insulin Produced	very little or none	low or very little	high
Usual Weight	thin	thin	fat
Insulin Needed	always	usually	sometimes
Autoantibodies	yes	no	no
Insulin Receptors Decreased	rarely	rarely	always
Ketoacidosis	yes	no	no

DETECTION OF DIABETES

We have discussed possible causes of diabetes, but how is diabetes actually identified? Diabetes is never diagnosed on the basis of urine tests. Blood tests must be taken to detect the presence of excess blood glucose. There are many tests in use to determine blood glucose levels. In 1979, the National Diabetes Data Group of the National Institute of Health published standards for diagnosing diabetes mellitus. In non-pregnant adults, one of the following must be present in order for the diagnosis to be made: obvious symptoms of diabetes such as polyuria, polydipsia or polyphagia with a blood glucose greater than 140 mg./dl., or if symptoms are not present a fasting blood glucose (FBS) of 140 mg./dl. (venous plasma) or greater on more than one occasion. If the FBS is elevated, an oral glucose tolerance test (OGTT) is not required. Elevated plasma glucose levels during an OGTT that are above 200 mg./dl. at the two-hour time *and* at some other point between the zero hour and two hours are considered to represent abnormal glucose tolerance.

These various blood tests may seem confusing. First, let us examine what type of blood is being tested. Usually the blood used for laboratory tests is plasma. Plasma carries glucose in the blood, and because of this, whole blood values are usually 15 percent lower than plasma values. Glucose levels in blood drawn from a capillary, such as at the fingertip, are 20–30 mg./dl. higher than in venous blood. (Capillary blood is a mixture of arterial and venous blood and it has a higher concentration of glucose.) Capillary blood testing has now assumed importance because of self-monitoring. This is further described in Chapter 3.

A type of test frequently performed is a fasting blood sugar (FBS). This blood specimen is taken while you are in a fasting state, not having eaten overnight. A postprandial glucose test is a blood glucose level drawn 1–2 hours after eating a carbohydrate-containing meal. This test determines how well your body metabolizes carbohydrate.

If fasting hyperglycemia is not present, the next test that may be ordered is the oral glucose tolerance test. The present recommendation is to give 75 gm. of glucose to an adult who has been fasting overnight. All medications which may affect glucose tolerance (the ability of the body to handle glucose) must be omitted, if possible, before the test. The individual follows a high-carbohydrate diet for three days prior to the test. During the test, blood samples are drawn at various intervals. There is generally little value to performing an oral glucose tolerance test. In patients with fasting hyperglycemia, the test may raise blood glucose to dangerous levels. If the fasting glucose is normal, generally very little is gained by the knowledge that impaired glucose tolerance is present. Too many oral glucose tolerance tests are performed.

A relatively new lab test is the hemoglobin A_{1C} level. Hemoglobin A_{1C} has been called a ''sugar-coated'' hemoglobin. It is also known as glycosylated hemoglobin. This test is used to monitor blood glucose levels over a prolonged time. Hemoglobin is found in the red blood cells. The hemoglobin A_{1C} is a measurement of the hemoglobin which has been found to be elevated in diabetic persons. Glucose molecules join the hemoglobin molecule. When the blood glucose rises, it causes an increase in the A_{1C} part of the hemoglobin. Since the red cells live for 120 days, this test can measure diabetes control over a prolonged period. It reflects the average of the blood glucose that red blood cells have been exposed to over time.

THE IMPORTANCE OF DIABETES CONTROL

Why is it so essential that your blood glucose be under control and not be allowed to remain elevated? Good control of blood glucose will prevent or delay the complications of diabetes. A normal state of blood glucose control is known as euglycemia, or normoglycemia. In the past, patients were not encouraged to achieve normal blood glucose because of the danger of causing hypoglycemia. It is essential that blood glucose be as close to normal as possible without causing hypoglycemia. The remainder of this book offers guidance in the areas of diabetes self-management.

Diabetes has been recognized by man for thousands of years. It is a disease of metabolism in which insulin is either absent or unable to work effectively. Glucose builds up in the blood (hyperglycemia), causing a variety of symptoms. There are two different types of diabetes. The Type I insulin-dependent person has no pancreatic beta cell function and must inject insulin daily. The Type II thin non-insulin-dependent person may take insulin and have some insulin deficiency. The Type II obese non-insulin-dependent individual usually has excess insulin but is insulin-resistant. Other people may be classified as having impaired glucose tolerance, gestational diabetes or potential abnormality of glucose tolerance, based on criteria set by the National Diabetes Data Group. Causes of diabetes are varied. The insulin-dependent form may be related to autoimmunity and viruses. Heredity and obesity are major factors causing NIDDM. Diabetes is diagnosed with a blood test. The oral glucose tolerance test is seldom useful. A new test, the hemoglobin A_{1C}, is now being used to monitor blood glucose levels over a prolonged time period.

2

Introduction to Nutrition

In today's society, the daily decision of choosing what to eat has truly become a science. There are so many changes in the food supply, the environment and individual lifestyles. It seems difficult to choose a meal plan (the type and amount of food you eat) necessary to promote health without knowing the basics of nutrition.

There are over 50 nutrients the body needs for health. Throughout this chapter we will explore nutrients (substances necessary for growth, maintenance and repair of the body) that are "fuelers" and those that are "non-fuelers." The fuelers provide calories. They include protein, carbohydrate, fat and alcohol. The non-fuelers help body processes function in a normal fashion. These include vitamins, minerals and fiber. You will read what happens to each nutrient once it enters your gastrointestinal system. This chapter is devoted to helping you learn how to appropriately evaluate the way you eat so you can be sure you are supplying your body with adequate nutrition. We hope you will see that this chapter is for everyone in your family. No longer is the diabetic person special because he has to eat different foods. Food for the diabetic person is the same as a healthy meal plan needed by the whole family.

CARBOHYDRATES

Carbohydrates are used to provide energy. Foods that contain carbohydrates will also provide vitamins, minerals and fiber. Each type of carbohydrate provides 4 calories per gram. To give you an idea of what a gram is, a small packet of sugar weighs approximately 5 grams. Therefore, the packet of sugar would contain 20 calories (4 calories × 5 grams = 20 calories). A carbohydrate is composed of the chemicals carbon, hydrogen and oxygen. There are two different types of carbohydrates—simple and complex.

SIMPLE CARBOHYDRATES (SUGARS)

Simple sugars include the monosaccharides and disaccharides. The monosaccharides have the simplest carbohydrate structure. They are the chemical building blocks for more complex carbohydrates. They include the sugars glucose, fructose and galactose.

The monosaccharide glucose is extremely important in body metabolism. Glucose is the major source of cellular energy. It is required by every part of your body. Many of the body cells can use either glucose or fat for their fuel, but the brain relies on glucose as its fuel. If glucose from dietary carbohydrates is unavailable, the body will act quickly to call on its carbohydrate reserves to protect the brain.

The disaccharides are made of two monosaccharide units. Thus, fructose combined with glucose is sucrose. Sucrose is found in table sugar, cane and beet sugar, candy, cakes and fruit. Glucose combined with glucose is maltose. Maltose is the carbohydrate found in beer and ale. Glucose plus galactose forms lactose. This is the simple sugar found in milk and milk products. In order for the disaccharides to be utilized by the body, they must first be broken down (metabolized) to their respective monosaccharides. Both the disaccharides and the monosaccharides are absorbed rapidly. Absorption of simple carbohydrates from the small intestine into the blood usually occurs within 15 to 20 minutes after eating. Since simple sugars are absorbed rapidly, they can raise your blood glucose quickly. Foods containing simple sugars include jam, jelly, cake, candy, ice cream, soda and many other similar items.

Just about every fruit you can think of is a combination of fructose and glucose. You will recall that this combination makes sucrose. Therefore, it is practically impossible for you to get a sugar-free diet. Does this mean, however, that if you have diabetes, you should not be eating fruit? Of course not. You should, in fact, be eating fruit rather than candy or cake. The primary reason for this is that fruit is more nutritious (a nutritious food provides more nutrients than a non-nutritious food) than candy or cake. Milk and milk products must also be included in your meal plan even though they contain the simple carbohydrate lactose. People in all age groups should try to consume some milk products daily.

COMPLEX CARBOHYDRATES

The next type of carbohydrates consists of the starches, or polysaccharides. Polysaccharides are composed of many glucose molecules linked together in a long chain. These long chains must eventually be broken down into glucose.

This occurs through the process of digestion. Some of the foods that contain complex carbohydrates are potatoes, bread and macaroni. Digesting complex carbohydrates takes longer than digesting simple carbohydrates because it takes the body longer to break the long glucose chains. The starches can begin to raise the blood glucose 15 to 30 minutes after you eat them. They are also used by the body for energy. If they are not needed for energy, they will be converted to glycogen or fat. Recently, complex carbohydrates have been shown to help insulin work more efficiently. They make the body tissues more sensitive to insulin's action. This is true both for the insulin supplied by injection and for the insulin made by the pancreas. In the past, complex carbohydrates were restricted in diets for people with diabetes. Today, this limitation is considered unnecessary, and will be discussed further in Chapter 8. The goal of a healthy, nutritious meal plan is to provide adequate nutrition without allowing blood glucose levels to rise above normal levels. Therefore, carbohydrates are important for health. Rather than restrict carbohydrates, your goal should be to combine adequate insulin and exercise with a healthy diet to keep blood glucose normal. Simple and complex carbohydrates have the same function of providing energy. Both provide 4 calories per gram and act to raise your blood glucose levels. However, they are absorbed into the bloodstream at different speeds.

In order for you to prevent marked increases in your blood glucose level, you must know which foods contain simple or complex carbohydrates. To identify foods that contain simple or complex carbohydrates, think of where the food originates. Take sherbet, for example. Sherbet is made of a variety of ingredients, but its primary component is cane sugar. Sherbet is considered a simple sugar. Cheesecake usually contains cane sugar, therefore the carbohydrate is considered simple. Cinnamon raisin bread, however, contains mainly flour, which is made from wheat. Wheat is a complex carbohydrate. Therefore the primary carbohydrate is complex. The following are examples of a few foods containing simple and complex carbohydrates.

EXAMPLES OF FOODS CONTAINING CARBOHYDRATES

Simple Carbohydrates	Complex Carbohydrates
cheesecake	whole-wheat English muffin
Jell-O	sweet potato
sherbet	matzoh
Oreo cookie	sesame-seed stick
malted	wheat thins
plum pie	rye toast

FATS

Let's move on to the next type of nutrient that provides calories, the fats. By definition, a fat is a concentrated source of energy, supplying 9 calories per gram. Fats also provide an essential fatty acid called linoleic acid. It is essential because it cannot be made by the body and must be consumed in food. Linoleic acid is necessary to maintain smooth skin and healthy hair. Fats aid in the transport of the fat-soluble vitamins and surround your vital organs to help protect them from physical shock. Fat also serves as your body insulator. Only a small amount of the fat you eat can be converted to glucose. Therefore, the role of fat in raising blood glucose levels is not significant unless the total caloric intake is high.

Fats provide more than twice the amount of calories as carbohydrates. To help you visualize a gram of fat, think of a teaspoon of oil that you may use on a salad. This amount of oil weighs approximately 4.5 grams. The caloric content of the oil is 40.5 calories (4.5×9 calories per gram $= 40.5$ calories). Therefore, if you put a tablespoon of olive oil (3 teaspoons $= 1$ tablespoon, so $40.5 \times 3 = 121.5$ calories) on your tossed salad, you are adding an additional 121.5 calories to a food that started out calorie-free.

Fats are composed of fatty acids and glycerol. There are three different categories of fatty acids. All fatty acids are made of carbon and hydrogen molecules linked together. A fatty acid with one bond between molecules is saturated. The presence of two or more double bonds is a polyunsaturated fat, while a monounsaturated fat has one double bond. (The presence of a double bond means more hydrogen molecules can be added to the fatty acid.)

Cholesterol is a fatlike substance. Cholesterol in the blood comes from two sources. Exogenous cholesterol is obtained from food you eat; endogenous cholesterol is made in your liver. A certain amount of cholesterol is essential for life. It is needed for the production of sex hormones, vitamin D and bile acids. In addition, cholesterol is an essential part of all cells. Fats are stored in the body as triglycerides. Triglycerides may appear in the blood after being formed from dietary fat and carbohydrate.

Fats in food can be divided into two distinct groups: "logical" fat sources and "hidden" fat sources. The logical sources are foods that you would naturally think of as containing fat. These include foods such as margarine, oil, butter and salad dressings. In addition, fats that you can see on food are logical fat sources. These include the white, thin marbling in meat, the fat around a piece of steak and the fat underneath chicken skin. A hidden fat source may not be visible on food. Therefore, you may not realize that the food contains fat. Some examples of this are commercially prepared baked goods like muffins, creamed soups, potato chips, ice cream, cheese, nuts and avocados.

Digestion of fats is a slow process that takes longer than digestion of carbohydrates. Remember, fats have to be broken down to basic components, and this process takes time. You must control your intake of fat because of its caloric value and its effect on blood glucose levels. Fat intake must also be controlled in order to prevent heart disease.

PROTEINS

The next fueler to be discussed consists of proteins. Proteins are structural components of all plants and animals. They build and maintain body tissues and regulate body functions such as growth and repair. They form essential body substances such as hormones, enzymes, antibodies and genes. Proteins are formed by the joining of smaller substances called amino acids into longer chains. Amino acids are the building blocks of protein. Twenty amino acids have been identified. However, only eight are known to be essential to life. The body cannot manufacture them, so they must be obtained through food. All foods contain various essential amino acids. However, foods differ in their capability of promoting growth. In general, animal proteins (except collagen-type proteins like gelatin) contain a complete set of eight essential amino acids. These foods include dairy products, beef, poultry and fish. Vegetable sources of protein are designated as incomplete proteins since they have smaller amounts of one or more essential amino acids. These include peas, beans, seeds, nuts and whole grains.

Proteins provide 4 calories per gram; they are similar, in this respect, to carbohydrates. However, most protein-containing foods also contain fat, which provides 9 calories per gram. Digestion of proteins usually takes longer than digestion of other nutrients. The body must break down the proteins into the small amino acids so they may be absorbed. It can take an hour for the blood glucose to rise after the ingestion of proteins.

Your caloric intake must be adequate, and all essential amino acids must be present in the proper amounts, in order for proteins to be used for body growth and repair. If these conditions are not met, then amino acids will be converted to glucose for energy use. Glucose will be stored as glycogen or fat if it is not needed for energy.

You may find it helpful in meal planning to be able to identify the different nutrients in food. To do this, think about where the food comes from. For example, chicken is an animal source. It will, therefore, have a certain amount of protein and fat as the major nutrients. Corned beef also comes from an animal and will provide fat and protein. Rice, however, comes from a plant and is a complex carbohydrate. Salad dressing contains oil, which is a fat source. Here are some examples of the major nutrients in foods.

SOME NUTRIENTS IN FOODS

Food	*Main Nutrients*
salmon	protein and fat
rice with butter	complex carbohydrate and fat
pastrami	protein and fat
peas	complex carbohydrate
clams	protein and fat
popcorn	complex carbohydrate
roast beef	protein and fat

Remember, proteins and carbohydrates have only 4 calories per gram, but fats have 9. So any food that has fat in it will have more calories than foods without fat. Therefore, animal products usually have more calories than food containing complex carbohydrates.

ALCOHOL

The next fueler is alcohol. Alcohol provides 7 calories per gram. Just think: that's almost as much as the amount of calories per gram supplied by fat! Different types of alcohol are absorbed at different rates. Distilled liquors are absorbed more quickly than wine, which is absorbed faster than beer. The absorption rate is also affected by the presence of food in the stomach. Alcohol is metabolized in the liver without the aid of insulin. It is metabolized as a fat, not as a carbohydrate.

Alcohol can have different effects on your blood glucose level. If you have eaten, alcohol will cause your blood glucose to rise due to the breakdown of glycogen in the liver. However, if you have not eaten, and you drink alcohol and take insulin or oral agents, alcohol can cause the reverse to happen. It can cause hypoglycemia. This occurs because alcohol stops the process of gluconeogenesis. Alcohol can also make you confused, so that you are unable to recognize the symptoms of hypoglycemia as they begin to develop. Therefore, if you drink alcohol and take medication for diabetes, you must be careful to avoid hypoglycemic episodes. You can refer to Chapter 10 for further details.

Alcohol may have another effect on the body. A moderate intake of two ounces of alcohol per day is associated with higher HDL (high-density lipoprotein) levels compared to heavy drinking or non-drinking. The elevated HDL level may be a protective factor in preventing coronary heart disease (see Chapter 17). Additional research is needed to determine whether there is a beneficial effect of moderate alcohol intake in people with diabetes.*

If you are going to drink alcohol, there are a number of guidelines you can follow. Be aware of the calories that come from alcohol. You can calculate the calories by knowing the following formula: $0.8 \times$ the proof $\times$ the ounces $=$ calories. The proof of the alcoholic beverage is double the percentage of alcohol by volume. Therefore, a 4-ounce glass of dry wine with 12 percent alcohol would provide 77 calories, or $0.8 \times 24 \times 4 = 77$. Nutrition labeling is not required on alcoholic beverages, so you must pay attention to the proof of the beverage. You can cook with alcohol because the alcohol evaporates at high temperatures and along with it go the calories. Cooking with alcohol provides you with flavor for food.

It may help you to know the general caloric content of common alcoholic beverages. For example, each can of beer contains approximately 150 calories. Each 3-ounce glass of dry white wine contains approximately 80 calories, and 1.5 ounces of a distilled liquor will provide anywhere from 90 to 110 calories. The decision to include alcoholic beverages in your meal plan should be discussed with your doctor. Then consult a nutritionist to learn how to fit alcohol into your meal plan. Remember that alcohol can provide a substantial amount of calories, which may cause you to gain weight.

If you are following the Exchange System, remember to count alcohol as a fat exchange. You will learn about this in Chapter 8. Deduct one fat exchange for every 45 calories in the beverage. Each 3-ounce serving of wine is equivalent to 1.5 fat exchanges. Each 12-ounce can of beer is equivalent to 3 fat exchanges, and each 1.5 ounces of distilled liquor is equivalent to 2.5 fat exchanges. Your caloric allotment for the day should be planned so that alcoholic beverages do not contribute to weight gain. Excessive alcohol intake can also cause you to eat more food or to forget to eat. If you eat more, remember that your blood glucose may rise because of the extra calories. If you forget to eat, remember that you run the added risk of hypoglycemia.

The types of alcoholic beverages to choose should be dry in nature; that is, dry wines and plain liquors. Avoid sweet wines or cordials. It is preferable to choose alcoholic beverages that provide the fewest calories. If you can switch from a glass of wine to a wine spritzer or from regular beer to light beer, you eliminate a substantial amount of calories. If you have a mixed drink, remember that you will be adding calories. For example, a screwdriver will have extra calories from orange juice. The calories of a fruit exchange from the orange

---

* Also, some people who drink may find alcohol raises their serum triglyceride level. Since high triglycerides may play some role in atherosclerosis, for these people drinking is inadvisable.

juice must also be included. Switching to rum and Tab from rum and Coke saves calories. There are a variety of refreshing non-alcoholic drinks that you can have. These include a tall glass of Perrier with a twist of lime, club soda with a twist of lemon or any diet beverage that you may desire. Alcoholic beverages are pleasant to drink, and may add a special gaiety to events, but should be consumed in moderation.

FIBER

The next sections of this chapter will discuss fiber and other nutrients that do not provide calories. The role of fiber in diabetes is exciting and has provided many persons with new foods to eat. Fiber has also contributed to increased control of blood glucose levels. Plant fibers are portions of plants that are not digested or absorbed by the intestine. They are usually structural components of the cell wall. Fibers provide fuel as well as perform other special functions for plants. In humans, plant fibers aid in improving the mechanical action of digestion, absorption and the breakdown of nutrients.

Many years ago it was observed that people in rural African tribes had a lower incidence of diabetes because they consumed a diet that was high in fiber. Persons living in a Westernized culture had a higher incidence of diabetes, perhaps in part because they had a reduced intake of fiber-containing foods. While this hypothesis was based merely on several observations, it has led to much subsequent research. We are now at the point where definite recommendations can be made as to how to increase the fiber content of your meal plan. Dietary fiber may play a role in preventing cardiovascular diseases, colonic cancer and diverticulosis.

There are several different types of fibers. They include cellulose, hemicellulose, lignins, pectins, gums and storage polysaccharides such as guar. They each exert a certain effect on the gastrointestinal system depending on their ability to bind water. Cellulose is the most widely distributed fiber in the plant cell wall. It makes up 25 percent of all plant fiber and is found in grains, fruits and vegetables. Hemicellulose is a structural part of the cell wall. It makes up 50 to 70 percent of the structure of grains and vegetables. Lignins are not carbohydrates, but they are structural components of the plant cell walls and are resistant to digestion. The lignin content of plants is about 10 percent of the total plant fiber of grains, vegetables and fruits. Pectin is also a structural fiber. It comprises 40 percent of the plant fiber of fruit. Pectins are completely digested in the large intestine. Gums serve other specialized functions in the plant. Specifically they act at the site of injury in plants. Guar is a storage polysaccharide. It is stored in the plant for future use as energy. Guar is used in the food industry in foods such as ice cream, sauces, salad dressings and frozen foods.

Fiber can be divided into two groups: the "insoluble" fibers include cellulose, lignin and hemicellulose. These fibers are found primarily in whole grains—wheat and bran. Insoluble fibers cause food to pass through the stomach, small intestine and colon rapidly. They are incompletely digested in the colon and act to increase fecal bulk. The "soluble" fibers are those that can be dissolved in water. They include guar, pectin and gums. Small amounts of each of these fibers are found in most foods. The soluble fibers cause food to move slowly through the small intestine.

Soluble fibers play the most significant role in diabetes by lowering the blood glucose levels in both Type I and Type II diabetes. When carbohydrates are eaten with certain plant fibers, less hyperglycemia results than if the carbohydrate had been ingested without fiber. Fiber reduces the rise in blood glucose and insulin levels that occur after meals. In addition, after you increase your fiber intake, it may become apparent that your insulin dose may need to be reduced to avoid hypoglycemia.

Patients have been placed on high-carbohydrate, high-fiber diets to determine the effect of fiber on blood glucose control. In these diets carbohydrates make up 50 to 70 percent of the total calories ingested. Some patients can discontinue their use of oral agents as a result of this dietary change. In addition, some of the Type II persons taking insulin are able to reduce their insulin dosage. Insulin-dependent (Type I) patients are also able to reduce the amount of insulin they need each day. So the use of high-carbohydrate, high-fiber meal plans may be advantageous whether you have Type I or Type II diabetes. High-carbohydrate, high-fiber diets will not aggravate your blood glucose control. Some patients do report gastrointestinal symptoms such as abdominal gas, which may last a short time.

By now you may be asking yourself what types of foods contain fiber and how you can incorporate them into your meal plan. Fiber-containing foods include whole-wheat bread and whole-wheat macaroni, brown rice, raw fruits and vegetables, whole-wheat cereals, beans, legumes, nuts and seeds. These are your best choices and you should begin to consume some every day. Strive for 25–30 grams of plant fiber per 1,000 calories, daily. If you are dependent on insulin, you must beware of hypoglycemic episodes. Therefore, when changing your meal plan from one that was low in fiber to one that is high in fiber, proceed very slowly. Initially, you may eliminate all sources of white bread. This would mean that you change to whole-wheat English muffins, whole-wheat bagels and whole-wheat, rye or pumpernickel bread. The same would hold true for macaroni. Reduce your intake of plain macaroni and switch to whole-wheat macaroni, which may be obtained in health-food stores. Consuming raw fruits or raw vegetables at each meal is also something that you can do. Whole-grain cereals such as all-bran and 100% bran or oatmeal can be eaten rather than other cereals without fiber. The end results should be that you (a) eat more legumes, potatoes and other types of vegetables, (b) eat more whole-grain breads and cereals on a daily basis and (c) consume fresh fruits or vegetables at each meal. A list of foods that are good fiber sources is given in the "More Useful Information" section at the end of this book. You will find that the use of fiber-containing foods can make your meal plan more exciting and very tasty. These foods are well worth trying. Many recipes have been developed using fiber foods, which can add zest to any meal plan.

THE VITAMINS

Vitamins are organic (compounds containing carbon) substances needed by the body in small amounts. They are constituents of all foods and are essential for life. Most vitamins cannot be made inside the body. Therefore you must obtain them in food. Vitamins act in the body as enzymes or coenzymes (substances that control chemical reactions). Enzymes help to release energy from food for use by the body. They also help in the process whereby food undergoes chemical change during digestion and absorption. Vitamins are divided into two groups: fat-soluble and water-soluble.

The fat-soluble vitamins are soluble (dissolve) only in a fatty substance. A fat-soluble vitamin cannot be dissolved in water (the way oil cannot be dissolved in vinegar) or blood. If you eat more than the daily requirement of fat-soluble vitamins, the excess is stored in the liver. The fat-soluble vitamins include A, D, E and K. The vitamins can be eaten in food, but vitamin K is also made by the intestinal bacteria and vitamin D may be made by exposure of the skin to sunlight.

Water-soluble vitamins can be dissolved in water, and most of them are not stored in the body. Therefore, a certain amount of each water-soluble vitamin is required daily. These vitamins are eliminated from the body through the kidneys. The water-soluble vitamins include all of the B vitamins and vitamin C. There is no benefit to taking larger doses of the water-soluble vitamins because most of the excess will simply be eliminated from the body through the urine.

Many people take vitamins in the form of a pill. This form of vitamin is chemically exactly the same as that which you obtain in food. In other words, the body does not recognize the chemical nature of the vitamin pill as being different from that of the vitamin in food. The extra use of vitamins is not generally warranted, especially if your diet contains a variety of foods. If you remain healthy, you will probably not become vitamin-deficient. Vitamin supplements (added amounts of vitamins) may be needed by infants, pregnant women, the elderly, alcoholics, persons with some illnesses or those on a diet of fewer than 1,000 calories per day.

THE MINERALS

The minerals are micronutrients that are essential for good health and growth. They are also required in the body in small amounts. Minerals are needed for functions that affect the skeleton and soft tissues of the body. They are also responsible for regulating body systems such as the heartbeat, blood clotting and blood pressure, and they act in the transmission of nerve impulses. The charts that follow will give you an idea of the names of vitamins and minerals, their food sources and their function in the body.

Fat-soluble Vitamins	*Food Source*	*Function*
Vitamin A	Liver, eggs, milk, fortified margarine, butter, spinach, sweet potatoes, carrots	Normal vision in dim light after exposure to bright light; smooth, moist skin
Vitamin D	Liver, eggs, fish oils, fortified margarine, milk	Aids in bone-calcification process; helps utilize calcium and phosphorus appropriately
Vitamin E	Milk, egg yolks, seeds, oils	Prevents rancidity of fats
Vitamin K	Eggs, milk, spinach, carrots, peas	Aids in blood coagulation

Water-soluble Vitamins		
Thiamine (B_1)	Whole-grain cereals, rice, beef, lamb, pork, poultry, peas, legumes	Involved in enzyme systems that help break down foodstuffs
Riboflavin (B_2)	Whole-grain cereals, rice, beef, lamb, pork, poultry, peas, legumes, milk	Involved in enzyme systems that help break down foodstuffs
Pyridoxine (B_6)	Cheese, egg yolks, beef, lamb, chicken, pork, potatoes, spinach, peas, beans, carrots	Involved in the breakdown of protein-containing foods
Niacin	Beef, pork, fish, eggs, milk, cheese, potatoes, liver, peanuts, legumes, flour	Aids in the release of energy from protein, carbohydrates and fats

Fat-soluble

Vitamins	Food Source	Function
Folic acid (folacin)	Green leafy vegetables, liver, kidney	Assists in formation of and part of the structure of hemoglobin; needed for genetic code (RNA and DNA)
Vitamin B$_{12}$	Beef, milk, cheese, eggs, some fish (no plant source)	Normal development and maintenance of nervous tissue
Ascorbic acid (vitamin C)	Citrus fruits, green leafy vegetables, tomatoes	Formation of the body cement or collagen tissue; maintains healthy gums; helps maintain strong blood vessels and capillaries

Minerals

Calcium	Milk, tofu, yogurt, salmon, cheese, oysters	Bone and tooth formation; needed for blood clotting and transmission of nerve impulses
Phosphorus	Meat, poultry, fish, eggs, cereal products	Needed for bone calcification; aids in obtaining energy from carbohydrates, proteins and fats
Magnesium	Rice, soybeans, fish, grains, milk	Involved in energy expenditure; promotes conduction of nerve impulses
Zinc	Oysters, whole-wheat cereals, liver, beef	Part of many enzyme systems involved in protein breakdown needed for insulin action
Iodine	Lobster, shrimp, oysters, saltwater fish, iodized salt	Part of thyroid hormone
Iron	Liver, beef, dried fruit	Aids in formation of hemoglobin
Potassium	Bananas, tomatoes, watermelon; a variety in all foods	Involved in releasing energy from glycogen; helps glucose enter body cells; plays a role i muscle contractions

Minerals	Food Source	Function
Sodium	Processed and convenience foods, brine foods such as pickles and sauerkraut, olives, spices with salt, cold cuts and smoked fish	Helps in glucose absorption; aids in transmitting nerve impulses; osmotic pressure

THE DIETARY GOALS

This section will help you to evaluate your food choices and understand that the meal plan for diabetic persons is no different from the meal plan for people without diabetes. You will recall that the first part of this chapter was devoted to major nutrients: carbohydrates, proteins, fats, vitamins and minerals. Now we must try to answer the question asked in the beginning of this chapter; that is, how do you decide what to eat? In 1977, Senator George McGovern and his Senate Select Committee on Nutrition developed the Dietary Goals for the United States. These goals were developed for many reasons. Much epidemiological (the study of environmental factors affecting disease) evidence linked the way Americans eat with disease states. Health professionals and the media were presenting conflicting views of nutrition and health. Americans were confused as to what were the best food choices to keep them healthy. The dietary goals met with much controversy, and many health professionals did not agree with them. They felt that not enough evidence was available to support the guidelines. Since that time, however, another document, in a simplified form, was developed. It is entitled "Nutrition and Your Health: Dietary Guidelines for Americans." It may be obtained from the Superintendent of Documents, Washington, DC. The dietary guidelines were developed to help you make informed choices regarding food. They are useful whether or not you have diabetes. The purpose of the guidelines is to get the correct balance of vitamins, minerals and fiber without consuming an excess of salt or calories from sugar and fat. The guidelines promote good, healthy eating habits based on moderation and variety. As each dietary guideline is discussed, try to think of how you may achieve it.

1. *Eat a variety of foods.* There is no one food that can supply you with all the nutrients that you need each day. Remember, there are over fifty nutrients that your body requires for good health. Therefore, you must eat a variety of foods in order for you to receive all the trace minerals and vitamins. A variety of foods includes vegetables, fruits, whole-grain breads and cereals, milk, cheese, yogurt, meat, poultry, fish, eggs, beans and peas.

2. *Maintain ideal body weight.* For the person without diabetes, obesity causes many problems. It can lead to hypertension and heart disease, and can be a contributing factor in causing non-insulin-dependent diabetes.

3. *Avoid too much saturated fat and cholesterol.* As you proceed through this book, particularly the chapter on cardiovascular disease, you will learn that diets that contain a majority of calories from fat, particularly saturated fat, can lead to an increase in your blood cholesterol level. This can be a risk factor for coronary heart disease. People in the United States have diets high in saturated fat and cholesterol (and high blood cholesterol levels).

4. *Eat food with adequate starch and fiber.* At the beginning of this chapter we reviewed foods containing complex carbohydrates which are better to eat than foods containing simple carbohydrates, for many foods containing simple carbohydrates provide nothing more than calories. You can obtain many nutrients from foods containing complex carbohydrates. You have also read about the role that fiber plays in diabetes and digestion. Therefore, choose foods that are good sources of fiber and starch, such as whole-grain breads, cereals, fruits, vegetables, peas and beans.

5. *Avoid too much sugar.* This may be obvious for the person with diabetes, since foods with simple sugars raise the blood glucose. In addition, foods that contain sugars can contribute excess calories and lead to obesity. Another reason to avoid excess sugars is that sugar has been cited as one of the major causes of dental caries. You can choose fresh fruits rather than those canned in sugar. Eliminate brown and white sugar, as well as honey. Consume fewer foods containing sugar, such as soft drinks, ice cream, cakes and candies.

6. *Avoid too much sodium.* Large intakes of sodium, either naturally occurring in food or added to food, may be a factor in the development of hypertension. High blood pressure, or hypertension, is the leading cause of stroke and heart disease today. Hypertension also contributes to diabetic eye and kidney disease. You can avoid extra sodium by cooking without added salt. You can develop a taste for foods without salt by experimenting with spices. Also, you can limit your intake of salty foods.

7. *If you drink alcohol, do so in moderation.* Alcohol tends to lower your blood glucose in a hazardous manner. From a caloric point of view, alcohol provides 7 calories per gram, which in excess can contribute to obesity.

THE RECOMMENDED DIETARY ALLOWANCES

The Recommended Dietary Allowances, or the RDAs, were first developed in 1943 by the Food and Nutrition Board of the Nutrition Research Council. The Food and Nutrition Board was composed of a group of scientists whose task was to evaluate the dietary intake of large groups of people and then provide a rational guide for practical nutrition. The RDAs are updated approximately every five years, and in 1980 the ninth edition was published. The present RDAs list levels of intake of seventeen essential nutrients, considered in the judgment of the Committee on Dietary Allowances of the Food and Nutrition Board, on the basis of available scientific knowledge, to be adequate to meet the known nutritional needs of practically all healthy persons.

The RDAs recommend an average daily amount of calories and each nutrient that a group of persons should consume. The RDAs are estimated values and are designed to exceed the needs of most individuals in order to ensure that all nutrient requirements are met by all persons. They are recommended goals for healthy people without a special illness. The RDAs were not designed for you to evaluate your individual food intake. The RDAs provide the amount of nutrients for several different age groups and they also distinguish between the sexes.

There is an RDA for your caloric intake and the amount of protein you should consume each day. In addition, there is an RDA for ten vitamins and six minerals. The vitamins include A, D, E, C, thiamine (B_1), riboflavin (B_2), niacin, pyridoxine (B_6), folic acid (folacin) and B_{12}. The minerals include calcium, phosphorus, magnesium, iron, zinc and iodine. In addition, the 1980 RDAs provide an estimated safe and adequate daily dietary intake of additional vitamins and minerals. The vitamins include K, biotin and panthothenic acid. The minerals include copper, manganese, fluoride, chromium, selenium, molybdenum, sodium, potassium and chloride. The RDAs are listed in the "More Useful Information" section at the end of this book.

THE UNITED STATES RECOMMENDED DAILY ALLOWANCES

The United States RDAs were developed by the Food and Drug Administration for nutrition labeling. These values are different from the RDAs. These are approximate amounts of protein, vitamins and minerals needed to keep Americans older than four years of age healthy. Special U.S. RDAs have been developed for children under four and pregnant and lactating women. You will find the U.S. RDAs for nutrients on the nutrition label. The label lists the U.S.

RDA by percentage. In other words, the label may state that a food contains 20 percent of the Recommended Daily Allowance of niacin and 15 percent of vitamin C. The U.S. RDAs are not considered a satisfactory guide for planning an adequate diet since the values may be high for some nutrients while lower for others. You can use the U.S. RDAs to compare products and to find foods that are good sources of particular nutrients.

As you read and listen to various media sources, you will constantly be exposed to nutritional myths and fads. From what you have already read, we hope you will be able to evaluate future nutritional fads. Read on to find out about several that exist today.

FOOD FADDISM

Food faddism and food cults have been popular in this country. One of their claims is that particular foods play specific roles in curing diseases. Some food faddists also advocate eliminating specific foods from the diet because they are harmful. Or they place special emphasis on so-called natural foods. Food fads place a false promise of better health on special foods, claiming that they can prevent or cure diseases. There is no scientific evidence that one or two specific foods can prevent or cure disease. Therefore, be leery of any food company that claims to manufacture a food that can improve or cure symptoms of a disease. A good rule is to avoid food fads and health-food crazes.

ORGANICALLY GROWN FOODS

The use of organically grown foods seemed to increase in the late sixties and early seventies and perhaps has now fallen by the wayside. An organically grown food is presumably a food that is grown without the use of additional chemicals for fertilizing or processing. It is interesting to note here that there is no federal agency which certifies whether or not foods were processed without additional chemicals. The phrase "organically grown" does imply something mysterious. It is somewhat deceiving to term a food organically grown, since all food is organic. There have been some claims that organically grown foods are superior to non-organically grown foods. There is no scientific basis for this. In fact, if plants are grown in soil that does not have additional fertilizer, it is likely that the crop size will be smaller rather than that the quality of the product will be deficient. Organically grown foods do not taste better and they may or may not be safe. Additives and pesticides used today in agriculture are regulated by law. Finally, organically grown foods usually cost more than non-organically grown foods.

NATURAL FOODS

"Natural" foods have received much popular attention. By definition, natural foods are those that remain in their original state with minimal refining and processing. Examples of these include fruits, vegetables, honey, flour and some cereals. The claim that a food is "natural" is quite misleading. There is no standard definition for natural food. You may think natural foods provide more nutrients than a food that is not natural. This is untrue. However, sugar is a natural food coming from a natural plant, and sugar does not provide extra nutrients. Therefore, it would be wise for you to look twice at a package labeled as a "natural" food product.

MEGAVITAMIN THERAPY

Megavitamin therapy is treatment with a vitamin or vitamins far above the RDA. Megavitamins may be used for a variety of reasons, presumably to compensate for vitamin deficiencies. There are several ways that a vitamin deficiency may occur. These include inadequate ingestion, absorption, utilization or increased excretion or increased need. As you will read, in only one of these conditions are massive doses of vitamins indicated. Inadequate ingestion of a vitamin means that you are not eating a sufficient amount of the vitamin. To solve this problem, you must simply increase your intake of the nutrient to meet the RDA level. Massive doses of vitamins are not required. Inadequate absorption of the vitamin may occur in individuals suffering from structural or functional damage in the digestive tract. In malabsorption syndromes the underlying medical problem must be treated in order to correct the vitamin deficiency. Inadequate vitamin metabolism may occur as a result of a physical problem present at birth (congenital) or acquired later in life. In the case of such congenital problems, massive amounts of vitamins may be required. These are rare disorders in ill children. A doctor would diagnose the specific disease and recommend appropriate treatment. Increased excretion or increased need for vitamins may occur during various periods of your life. Here again, the solution is to supply moderately increased amounts of the vitamin rather than massive doses.

Excessive* amounts of vitamins can cause a variety of health problems. Large amounts of vitamin A can result in decreased appetite, growth retardation in children, an enlarged liver, dry skin, bone and joint pain and hair loss. An excess

---

* Generally, a large amount is considered more than 5 to 10 times the RDA. However, it is important to realize that this is very individual. The amount of a vitamin supplement that can be hazardous may vary from person to person.

of vitamin D may result in loss of appetite, nausea, vague aches, tissue calcification, kidney stones, kidney failure and death. A large intake of vitamin E leads to nausea, headaches, blurred vision and decreased sexual functioning. Increased niacin or nicotinic acid may lead to flushing, itching, liver damage, high blood glucose levels, elevated uric acid levels and jaundice. Large amounts of vitamin C can cause adverse effects on growing bones, kidney problems, diarrhea and gout. Vitamin C also destroys some vitamin B_{12} in food, which can lead to a B_{12} deficiency. Vitamin C excess causes rebound scurvy in infants of mothers who took large doses of ascorbic acid during pregnancy. Scurvy is a disease caused by inadequate intake of vitamin C. Finally, excess vitamin C can cause a false negative urine test with Tes-Tape, a false positive urine test with Clinitest and a false negative test for blood in the stool, thus preventing accurate diagnosis of gastrointestinal bleeding. You can now understand that an excessive intake of vitamins is not without hazard.

VITAMINS B_{15} AND B_{17}

Vitamins B_{15} and B_{17} have become popular items. Unfortunately, neither is a vitamin. A vitamin is needed in small quantities and a lack of it must cause a deficiency state. A lack of these chemicals does not cause a deficiency state. Vitamin B_{15} has been hailed as a cure for many illnesses, including cancer, alcoholism, hepatitis, heart disease, diabetes and glaucoma. In reality, B_{15}, also known as pangamate, pangamic acid, Aangamik or Caldiomate, is really a mixture of a variety of chemicals. The amount and the type of chemicals used depends on the manufacturer. The FDA has called B_{15} a non-identifiable substance which has no scientific evidence of being useful in nutrition or medicine. Those who purchased this product have wasted their money on a useless product.

Vitamin B_{17} is Laetrile, or amygdalin. It is found in kernels of apricots and peaches, bitter almonds and apple seeds. Amygdalin is actually 6 percent cyanide by weight and thus causes mild cyanide poisoning when ingested. There has been no scientific evidence to support the claim that B_{17} prevents, cures or controls cancer.

NUTRITION QUACKS

Nutrition quacks (those who claim to be nutritionists but have had no education in the field) are abundant. These people usually have various educational backgrounds (including doctorates in medicine) and numerous impressive titles, but little or no training in nutrition. Often they have received some type of nutrition certificate by paying a fee.

A bonafide nutritionist or dietitian has had years of training in nutrition. A nutritionist cannot buy his or her registered dietitian title. It must be earned through hard work. It is unfortunate that nutrition quacks exist, as they detract from the reputation of an ethical, knowledgeable profession and often confuse and worry the general population. Always ask the nutritionist you are working with about his or her educational background. Be on the lookout for nutrition quacks who promise to alleviate diseases that doctors cannot cure. Nutrition quacks often place great emphasis on one specific nutrient or food to cure a problem. They feel that foods that are not natural as well as foods that contain additives are bad. Finally, nutrition quacks often claim they are victims of the FDA and the medical community and criticize medically accepted procedures. Be careful of those who give you easy solutions to difficult problems.

HAIR ANALYSIS

Many people have recently visited hair-analysis clinics to determine their nutritional status. Those interested in obtaining a hair analysis go to a special laboratory where a sample of hair is taken to determine vitamin and mineral stores. Or a hair sample may be mailed to the laboratory. A computer printout of the vitamins or minerals which are allegedly deficient is received. Here again, you must question what the analysis will determine. It is impossible to determine your vitamin status from your hair because the vitamins are located in the root underneath your scalp. You cannot detect your mineral status either, unless toxic levels of some metals are present.

You can have an analysis of your hair to determine its cosmetic condition. You can also determine the presence of toxic levels of some metals or minerals in your hair, but you cannot get an assessment of your vitamin or mineral status as it relates to your health. In addition, to date there have been no accepted normal ranges for minerals or vitamins for the hair. Even if an analysis were to show the presence or absence of nutrients, standard normal values have not been determined. Hair analysis is an unscientific approach to nutrition and provides unreliable and possibly dangerous advice.

VEGETARIAN MEAL PLANS

A vegetarian meal plan is described in this section only because it differs from the usual Western meal plan. It is considered a healthy way to eat if foods are consumed wisely. Some people with diabetes may want to follow a vegetarian meal plan, which may be safe if a variety of foods are eaten. Nutrient intake must be adequate to meet the demands of growth and good health. Foods have a variety of different nutrients, and no one food can supply them all. Therefore, you must choose a mixed diet. There are three different types of vegetarian meal plans you can follow. A lacto-ovo-vegetarian meal plan is one in which meat, poultry and fish are excluded but dairy products and eggs are allowed. A vegan diet is one in which all meat and dairy products are excluded from the diet. There are also lactovegetarian diets in which milk and milk products are allowed but eggs and other meat products are excluded.

The vegetarian diet may have advantages for the person with diabetes. First of all, it is low in fat, thus reducing the risk of heart disease. It may facilitate weight loss because you eat foods that increase the volume of the diet yet decrease the caloric content. You will also be eating foods that contain more fiber. Therefore, you may have a slower rise in blood glucose. You will be able to eat most of the nutrients you need for health as long as you have enough time to preplan your meals. Some nutrients may be somewhat deficient in the meal plan of a vegetarian. This includes vitamin B_{12}, which can only be obtained from animal products. You can use a vitamin supplement or purchase B_{12}-fortified foods. If you are excluding milk or milk products from your meal plan, then calcium, riboflavin and vitamin D may also be deficient. Again, there are vitamin and mineral supplements available for these nutrients.

How can you receive all the protein that your body needs if you are eating only foods from plants? Remember that every food, whether it is from an animal or plant source, has essential amino acids; foods simply differ in the amount of amino acids they contain. Plants simply do not provide as good an assortment of amino acids as animal products. Therefore, in the same meal, you can combine foods which are adequate in one or more amino acids with foods that contain the other amino acids. This is called protein complementarity. You can mix plant proteins in a variety of ways to ensure protein complementarity. You can combine grains with seeds, grains with beans, or grains with dairy products. Make sure you consult your nutritionist or doctor prior to embarking on a vegetarian meal plan. Remember to allow for extra time for advance planning to obtain an adequate nutrient intake.

The major nutrients and how they affect your body and blood glucose level have been discussed. Remember that the major nutrients—carbohydrates, proteins and fats—can all be used for energy and an excess can be stored as fat. Vitamins and minerals do not provide calories but are essential for life. Fiber has become an important component in the meal plans of persons with diabetes. Evaluate your meal plan on the basis of the dietary goals. You no longer need to feel discriminated against in the way you eat because you should be eating in a way that is healthy for you and your family. This is suggested in the Dietary Goals for the United States. The most important goal of your meal plan is to attain adequate nutrition while keeping your blood glucose at the proper level.

3
Self-Testing

Self-testing of blood glucose is now practical and should be learned by all individuals with diabetes. Urine glucose and acetone are also measured by many patients. In this chapter, measurements of both urine and blood will be discussed.

Although we will discuss both methods of testing, we do believe that urine testing is archaic. Any person with diabetes who is committed to obtaining optimum blood glucose values should learn to perform blood glucose testing.

URINE TESTING

Urine testing is not as accurate as blood testing. Urine glucose is only a reflection of blood glucose. Nevertheless, if you are testing your urine for glucose and acetone, it is necessary that you do it properly. The significance of urine test results, collection of specimens, testing schedules, record keeping and tips on how to avoid pitfalls in urine testing will now be given.

Glucose appears in the urine only when blood glucose is elevated. The kidneys can no longer reabsorb excess glucose when the blood glucose is between 160 and 180 mg./dl., so glycosuria appears. This point is known as the renal threshold for glucose. The renal threshold may change in conditions like pregnancy or kidney disease. Some diabetic persons are able to reabsorb glucose through the kidneys even when blood glucose is high. These people have a "high renal threshold" for glucose. Here, urine tests may be negative for glucose although blood glucose may be elevated. Some people have a low renal threshold; urine glucose may be present at a point lower than the 160–180 mg./dl. blood level.

How do you determine your renal threshold and the accuracy of urine test results? To determine your own renal threshold, compare urine tests taken at the same time that your blood specimen is drawn. If you have an elevated blood glucose and a negative urine test, you may have a high renal threshold.

If urine glucose tests are only a reflection of blood glucose levels, why do we continue to test urine? At the present time, this may be the only testing method known that is practical for certain people. It is a simple, inexpensive and easily accomplished technique. It is a useful way to detect acetonuria. However, blood testing is the preferred method to determine glucose control.

The first urine specimen you check in the morning should be double-voided rather than single-voided. A single-voided specimen means that you collect and test the urine that you have just voided. A double-voided specimen refers to the procedure of emptying your bladder completely and then in 15 or 20 minutes collecting a second urine specimen for testing. This specimen reflects the glucose level at the time of collection, rather than the glucose that has been previously stored in the bladder. For example, if you sleep from 10:00 at night to 7:00 the next morning, that urine has been stored in the bladder overnight. It will not as accurately reflect the glucose reading of urine you collect from a second-voided specimen. Instead, it reflects the sum of all urine tests over that time period, not what your blood or urine glucose is at the time of the test. Thus, if your blood glucose was about 300 mg./dl. from 10 P.M. to midnight, 250 mg. from midnight to 4 A.M., 150 mg. at 6 A.M. and 50 mg. at 8 A.M., your 8 A.M. single-void reading may be elevated but you may be having symptoms of hypoglycemia.

Timing Schedules for Urine Testing

The more you test your urine, the more information you receive about your diabetes. If you take insulin, it is best to test four times a day, prior to every meal and at bedtime. If this is not possible, you will have to adjust to the best testing schedule for your lifestyle. If you take a split dose of insulin (an insulin dose in the morning and another prior to your evening meal), it is necessary to test before your evening meal as well as in the morning. In this way, you can see the effects of both insulin injections. If you do not take insulin, you may wish to test your urine when you are fasting or two hours after a large meal.

Urine Testing for Glucose

There are several urine tests for glucose available. The Clinitest Two Drop Method and Five Drop Method are copper-reducing procedures. These give a most accurate estimate of the percentage of glucose in the urine. The percentage refers to the number of grams of glucose spilled out in every 100 milliliters of urine. For example, a 1 percent reading shows that one gram of glucose is being lost in every 100 milliliters of urine. The amount of urine passed in a 24-hour period can far exceed 1,500 ml. With one gram of glucose spilling out in every 100 ml. of urine, much urine glucose can be lost over a period of 24 hours. When glucose is lost from the body, so are calories.

Clinitest tablets display, by color changes, the amount of glucose present in the urine. The most accurate test is the Clinitest Two Drop Method. Prior to beginning any testing, wash your hands thoroughly and organize your materials. Follow the directions exactly as they are given on the test bottle or package insert.

Clinitest Two Drop Method

Assemble these materials: a clean, dry container for urine, a clean, dry test tube, Clinitest tablets, a clock or watch with a second hand, an eye dropper, a container of water, the Clinitest Two Drop Method chart.

Instructions:

1. Wash your hands thoroughly before beginning.
2. Collect the urine sample in a clean, dry container.
3. Withdraw the urine from the container into the eye dropper.
4. With the dropper in the upright position, squeeze two drops of urine into the clean, dry test tube.
5. Rinse the dropper with water.
6. Fill the dropper with water and slowly add ten drops of water into the test tube.
7. Shake one Clinitest tablet out from the container into the container lid. Do not touch the Clinitest tablet. (Use tweezers, if available, to take the Clinitest tablet from the bottle.)
8. Drop the tablet from the lid into the test tube. Recap the bottle immediately.
9. Now observe the test tube while the reaction takes place. Do not shake the test tube. The test tube may become very hot. Place it in a holder without touching the bottom of the tube. Avoid eye contact with the open top of the tube.
10. After the boiling has stopped, wait 15 seconds and then shake the tube gently.
11. Now compare the color of the liquid in the tube with the nearest color on the Two Drop Method chart.
12. Record your results as 0%, trace, ½%, 1%, 2%, 3% or 5%.

The use of the color chart for the Clinitest Two Drop Method is absolutely necessary when performing this procedure. The Clinitest tablet is the same for both the Clinitest Five Drop Method and the Two Drop Method of testing, but the color chart is not. The color chart for the Clinitest Two Drop Method will reflect the percentage of urine glucose up to 5 percent. The Clinitest Five Drop Method will only show a urine glucose reading of up to 2 percent. To avoid confusion, remember that the Clinitest Two Drop Method procedure is used with the Clinitest Two Drop chart only.

Clinitest Five Drop Method

The Clinitest Five Drop Method has been used by many people. If you are testing with the Clinitest Five Drop Method, complete the procedure as described above. The procedure is identical except for two steps. You will use five drops of urine rather than two drops of urine to complete this procedure accurately. The Clinitest Five Drop Method chart is used to compare color results.

Stick Methods

Tes-Tape and various kinds of sticks (Clinistix and Diastix) are also used to determine urine glucose. On one end of the stick there is a block containing an enzyme, glucose oxidase, which reacts with urine glucose and produces a change in color. These sticks are convenient to use because they need only be moistened by urine in order for a reaction to occur. They must be kept away from moisture in order to retain their accuracy.

Tes-Tape (Eli Lilly and Company)

Assemble the necessary equipment: a clean, dry container for urine, Tes-Tape, a clock or watch with a second hand, the color chart on the back of the Tes-Tape dispenser.
Instructions:

1. Wash your hands thoroughly before beginning.
2. Collect the urine sample in a clean, dry container.
3. Withdraw approximately 1½ inches of Tes-Tape. Do not touch the edge of the tape that will be dipped in the urine.
4. Dip the tape in the urine. Remove it immediately.

5. Begin timing immediately for exactly 60 seconds.
6. Do not place the tape on any surface. Hold it in the air and do not blot it with a paper towel.
7. Exactly one minute after the tape has been wet, compare the darkest area on the Tes-Tape with the color chart on the dispenser. Always read the darkest area for your results. It may be helpful to hold the Tes-Tape against a white background, such as a paper towel or tissue. This will help you to read the results accurately.
8. Record your results as 0%, $\frac{1}{10}$%, $\frac{1}{4}$%, $\frac{1}{2}$% or 2%.

Diastix 5 (Ames Company)

Assemble the necessary equipment: a clean, dry container for urine, Diastix, a clock or watch with a second hand, the Diastix color chart on the bottle.
Instructions:

1. Wash your hands thoroughly before beginning.
2. Collect the urine sample in a clean, dry container.
3. Take a Diastix strip out of the bottle. Hold the strip away from the test end. Recap the bottle immediately.
4. Dip the strip into the urine. Remove it immediately.
5. Begin timing immediately for 60 seconds. Hold the strip in your hand during this time and do not touch the test area.
6. Compare the color of the test area with the color chart.
7. Record your results as normal, $\frac{1}{10}$%, $\frac{1}{4}$%, $\frac{1}{2}$%, 1%, 2%, 5% or more.

Recording Your Results

Accuracy is important, but your test is only half completed if you neglect to record your results. If you test four times a day and show varied results, it will be impossible for you to remember them without keeping a record. Percentages will soon be the only way to determine urine test results, as pluses become phased out of product packaging. As you can see from Table 2, a ½ percent reading equals 1+ using the Clinitest Five Drop Method, 2+ using Diastix and 3+ using Tes-Tape. To avoid such confusion, report your urine tests in percentages and never record in colors. Colors vary from one test method to another.

Record keeping should be simple. It is not necessary to use a complex set of notes. In a simple notebook, record each date, time and urine test result. See

TABLE 2
RECORD YOUR URINE TEST RESULTS IN PERCENTAGES

PRODUCT	NEGATIVE	$^1/_{10}$%	¼%	½%	¾%	1%	2%	3%	5%
Clinitest 2 drop	0		tr	½%		1%	2%	3%	5%
Clinitest 5 drop	0		tr	+	+ +	+ + +	+ + + +		
Diastix	0	tr	+	+ +		+ + +	+ + + +		
Tes-Tape	0		+	+ +	+ + +		+ + + +		

+ = PLUS
% = PERCENTAGE
tr = TRACE

For greater accuracy, record test results as percentages

TABLE 3

URINE-GLUCOSE/ACETONE					INSULIN DOSE	COMMENTS
DATE	TIME					
	BEFORE BREAKFAST	BEFORE LUNCH	BEFORE DINNER	BEDTIME		
Urine Glucose / Acetone						
BLOOD GLUCOSE						

Table 3. Notice if increases in negatives or positives occur. Try to correlate this with your activity, diet, exercise or medical regimen. Bring these records with you when you visit your doctor or nurse and ask them to review the records with you.

Testing for Ketones (Acetone)

Ketones are products of fat breakdown. They appear in the blood and are excreted in the urine when glucose is not being used for fuel. Ketones can be measured in the urine as acetone. When glucose is not available for energy, fat is broken down. Starvation ketosis occurs with many diets that do not supply enough carbohydrates. The breakdown of fat for fuel may also occur in diabetes when, because of a lack of insulin, food is not used properly for energy. The burning of fats for fuel is a danger signal. If acetone begins to appear and accumulate in the bloodstream, diabetic ketoacidosis may occur. You will be able to detect this condition by testing your urine for acetone. Test your urine for acetone whenever your blood glucose is above 250 mg./dl., when urine glucose results are above 2% and whenever you are ill. Become familiar with this procedure and have materials at home to test with, if necessary.

How to Test for Ketones (Acetone)
Ketostix (Ames Company)

Assemble the necessary equipment: a clean, dry container for urine, Ketostix, a clock or watch with a second hand, the color chart for Ketostix.
Instructions:

1. Wash your hands thoroughly before beginning.
2. Collect the urine specimen in a clean, dry container.
3. Remove a Ketostix from the container. Hold the strip away from the test end. Recap the bottle immediately.
4. Dip the strip into the urine. Remove it immediately.
5. Begin timing immediately for 15 seconds. Hold the strip during this time.
6. Compare the color of the test area with the color chart.
7. Record your results as negative, small, moderate or large. This refers to the amount of acetone present in this urine sample.

Acetest (Ames Company)

Assemble the necessary equipment: a clean, dry container for urine, Acetest tablets, an eye dropper, a clock or watch with a second hand, the Acetest color chart, a paper towel.
Instructions:

1. Wash your hands thoroughly before beginning.
2. Collect the urine sample in a clean, dry container.

3. Shake one Acetest tablet out from the container into the container lid. (Use tweezers, if available, to take the Acetest tablet from the bottle.)
4. Drop the tablet from the lid onto the paper towel.
5. Using the eye dropper, place one drop of urine onto the Acetest tablet.
6. Begin timing immediately for 30 seconds.
7. Compare the color of the Acetest tablet with the colors on the Acetest chart.
8. Record your results as small, moderate or large. This refers to the amount of acetone present in the urine.

Some test strips measure both urine glucose and urine acetone. A description of two of these test methods follows.

Ketodiastix 5

Ketodiastix provides a convenient test that combines both urine glucose and urine acetone testing. This test is performed in the same manner as other "stix" tests. The timing is different for the urine glucose and the urine acetone. Urine acetone readings are checked after 15 seconds; urine glucose readings are checked after 60 seconds. Both colors are compared with the Ketodiastix color chart. The Ketodiastix is a convenient but more costly method of urine testing. Having two tests on one stick increases the price. This method may be used for special occasions, such as when traveling.

Chemstrip uGK (Bio-Dynamics)

This urine glucose and urine acetone test is performed in a similar manner. After the strip is dipped into the urine, wait 2 minutes to compare the colors with the scale on the bottle. Both colors should be compared simultaneously. You will have to estimate your reading when the color of the glucose patch does not precisely match a color on the bottle but falls somewhere between two colors.

Pitfalls in Urine Testing

There are certain pitfalls in urine-testing procedures. One important factor is *correct timing*. If a procedure demands a particular amount of time, follow that time exactly. Do not estimate; instead use a watch with a second hand or test in front of a clock with a second hand. Even counting out loud as the seconds pass is more accurate than estimating. Use the *correct color chart* that corresponds exactly with the test you are now using. Change your color charts frequently when you buy new test materials. When using the Clinitest Two Drop Method versus the Five Drop Method, it is essential that you use the correct color chart. Use the *correct materials* for your individual lifestyle. You will then be able to test your urine regularly. If you use the Clinitest Five Drop Method at home but find it cumbersome when you are on vacation, switch to Diastix while away. Vary, if necessary, your urine test methods but continue to test every day.

It is important to care for urine test supplies. Store them away from humidity. The bathroom may not be the best place, because humidity and moisture can affect the materials. Store them in a cool, dark place. When you open a bottle of test materials recap the bottle immediately. Clinitest and Acetest tablets are made of corrosive materials. Do not touch these tablets. Either shake the tablet into the cap of the bottle or use tweezers to take the tablet out of the bottle. Check pills for discoloration or deterioration. Clinitest tablets will change color from off white with a few blue specks to dark blue with darker blue spots. Diastix will turn to a greener shade when deteriorating. The yellow shade of Tes-Tape will turn brown. Ketostix, which are off white, will turn brown. Do not use the test materials if color change has occurred, even if this happens before the expiration date. Never use test materials if they have expired. Check their expiration dates often. Old testing materials may not always change color but may change your test results. Soap and dirt will interfere with your results, so wash your test tube, eye dropper and urine container with soap and water. Rinse them thoroughly after use. You can check the accuracy of Clinitest, Diastix and Tes-Tape by using one teaspoon of regular cola mixed with one-third cup of water. This should give you positive test results. Urinalysis control strips are available from the Ames Company. Certain safety precautions should be used with test materials in your home. The Clinitest tablets are corrosive and poisonous and may cause burns if you touch them with wet fingers. Run cold water on any burn that occurs but remember to avoid touching the Clinitest tablets directly. Childproof your Clinitest bottles; keep them away from young children or confused adults. Call your doctor or emergency room for immediate advice if Clinitest tablets are swallowed. Do not try to induce vomiting if Clinitest tablets have been swallowed. Encourage the person who swallowed them to drink large amounts of water or milk and seek help immediately.

Drug Interactions

Ask your doctor or pharmacist if other medications you are taking may interfere with urine tests. You may need to switch to a different urine test when taking medications such as vitamin C or aspirin, which can cause misleading urine test results. Large amounts of vitamin C in the urine may give a low

TABLE 4

TEST VEXERS
HERE'S HOW SOME SUBSTANCES CAN AFFECT YOUR URINE TESTS.

SUBSTANCES AFFECTING URINE *GLUCOSE* TESTS	Possible Effects (by test)			
	DIASTIX 5	CLINISTIX	TES-TAPE	CLINITEST
Sugars other than glucose				
Galactose	No effect	No effect	No effect	Reacts positive
Lactose	No effect	No effect	No effect	Reacts positive
Levulose (fructose)	No effect	No effect	No effect	Reacts positive
Maltose	No effect	No effect	No effect	Reacts positive
Drugs				
Salicylates ASA	No effect	No effect	No effect	No effect
Ascorbic Acid (Vitamin C)	Large amount may give low reading	May cause false (−)	Large amount may interfere with color formation	Large amount may cause false (+)
L-Dopa	Large concentration may cause false (−)	Large concentration may cause false (−)	No effect	No effect
Cephalosporins (Kelfin, etc.) Certain antibiotics	No effect	No effect	No effect	May cause false (+)
Pyridium	Masks color reactions	No effect	No effect	No effect

Adapted with permission from D. Guthrie,
- "Use Those Urine Tests," *Diabetes Forecast,* July–Aug. 1980.

glucose reading when urine is tested with Diastix. Large amounts of vitamin C may give a high glucose reading when using Clinitest. These would be called false negatives or positives. A false negative is a urine test reading that shows no glucose present when it really is present. A false positive shows a positive glucose reading when no glucose is present. This is caused by the chemical

TABLE 5
ADVANTAGES/DISADVANTAGES OF
URINE TESTING MATERIALS

TEST	ADVANTAGES	DISADVANTAGES
Clinitest	color changes easy to read	false positive may occur
	less expensive	less convenient
	accurate at 5% level	
	no false negatives	
Diastix 5	color changes easy to read	more expensive
	convenient	may under read high glucose
	no false positives	some false negatives seen
Tes-Tape	most convenient	difficulty in interpreting color shades
	less expensive	under reads 2%

reaction of certain drugs with urine test materials. Check Table 4 for further information regarding drug interactions.

The "pass-through phenomenon" occurs with the use of Clinitest tablets and refers to a complete color change seen during the reaction. All colors of the reaction are seen, including bright orange, but at the *end* of the reaction the color change reverts to blue. If you did not watch this reaction you would think that your test was negative. Rather, a "pass-through phenomenon" signals that the glucose reading is higher than the highest number on the color charts, a different situation than the "negative" reading. See Table 5 for a review of advantages and disadvantages of urine tests for glucose.

Evaluation of Urine Test Results

A final comment concerning urine-testing techniques involves a most important aspect of diabetes self-management. The urine-testing technique itself, the accuracy with which you perform it and the results which you obtain are of no value if you do not evaluate the results. Try to identify the cause of elevated urine glucose readings. Avoid becoming overinvolved in the constant checking of urine test results. At times you may have an unexplained spillage of glucose into the urine. Many people find this frustrating. Even with the greatest effort, you may not attain the degree of control that a normal pancreas provides. You must accept having as nearly perfect control as possible. Closely monitor your urine test results and correct your management program in the future to prevent glycosuria. Review urine tests on a biweekly basis, and also look at your results over a one- to three-month period.

A philosophy of the past emphasized that it was better to have some urine glucose spillage rather than to have all negative urine test results. This was to reduce the risk of hypoglycemia; by having ½ percent readings you would be "safely" hyperglycemic. In order to attain good control you must have as many negative urine glucose readings as possible without having hypoglycemic reactions. This may be a difficult goal to attain but, when reached, it is one that will help you stay in control of your diabetes.

In conclusion, some people still use urine testing to monitor diabetes. However, urine glucose is only a reflection of blood glucose. Therefore, it is not as accurate as home blood testing. If you are testing for glycosuria you can choose a tablet or stick method. All persons with diabetes should know how to test for urinary acetone. This procedure also involves a tablet or stick method. Remember to follow the directions for testing exactly as stated on the label. Choose the correct materials for your lifestyle. Store your materials in a cool, dark place. Finally, record your results whenever you test, and evaluate your tests.

Self-monitoring of blood glucose is rapidly replacing urine testing. Self-monitoring is easy and accurate and involves test sticks and/or reflectance meters. This self-management task allows you to determine the effect of diet, exercise and insulin on your diabetes control. Read on to learn about self-monitoring of blood glucose.

SELF-TESTING OF BLOOD GLUCOSE

A goal of diabetes self-management is to maintain normal blood glucose. In the past, it was difficult to measure blood glucose control because urine testing had inaccuracies and/or laboratory tests were performed infrequently. Today, there are simple, practical and convenient test methods available to use at home to measure blood glucose. In fact, these tests are now portable. The term "home blood glucose monitoring" has been replaced by "self-monitoring" because you can test your blood glucose anywhere at any time.

Self-monitoring can be dor : easily, not only on a daily basis but several times a day. Your blood glucose may vary widely during a twenty-four-hour period. By checking blood glucose frequently during the day, you may observe these variations. In addition, you can evaluate the effects of medication, diet and exercise. "Self-monitoring" will be used in this chapter to describe the procedure of testing your own blood glucose.

The method used to monitor blood glucose is very similar to that used for urine testing. The test sticks have a pad at the end that contains enzymes sensitive to glucose. These are called reagent strips. When the enzyme interacts with glucose, certain color changes can be noted.

Certain strips can be used alone to determine blood glucose; others are used with a meter that interprets the color changes. The meters are called reflectance colorimeters. They convert the depth of color on the reagent strip to a blood glucose number that is then displayed on the front of the machine.

Advantages of Self-Monitoring

There are many advantages to blood glucose monitoring. You become an independent self-manager and no longer have to rely on guessing your blood glucose level from urine tests. Diabetic persons often say that they feel frustrated by seeing negative urine tests and then hearing from their doctor that their blood glucose is elevated. If you monitor your own blood glucose, you have more control of diabetes. Another advantage of self-monitoring is in the realm of pattern control. You can determine disruptions of your pattern and make adjustments as an outpatient. This will prevent you from being hospitalized for regulation of your diabetes control. You can work as a partner with your doctor in determining pattern control while making necessary adjustments in insulin, diet and exercise. The hospital is not the appropriate place to make such changes. (The hospital is an artificial environment where your diabetes management cannot be perfectly adjusted. The timing and preparation of your meals may be different and your physical activity is reduced compared to when you are in the "real world.") Not only will you be able actively to determine blood glucose during any twenty-four-hour period, but you also will be able to monitor your blood glucose in specific instances. For example, you can determine how low your blood glucose is during hypoglycemia. If you have difficulty determining whether you are actually hypoglycemic, self-monitoring can give you an immediate answer. You may also determine blood glucose readings when you have ketonuria or an acute infection. Another advantage to self-monitoring is that you will receive instant feedback. You can see the effect of exercise, insulin and diet on your blood test results.

Many diabetic persons have been hesitant to attempt blood glucose monitoring because a fingerstick must be used to obtain a drop of blood. Yet many people have overcome this hesitancy and have begun self-monitoring on a daily basis. The advantage of control over your own disease outweighs the discomfort of the fingerstick. The first step before using the fingerstick is hand washing. Wash your hands with warm water to increase blood circulation to the hand; hanging your hand at your side will also do this. Use sharp, safe disposable lancets. Lancets such as the Monolets (Sherwood Medical Industries, Inc.) are recommended. These have a point of only ⅛ inch and will not penetrate the skin too deeply.

Use of Automatic Fingerstick Devices

Automatic devices help make the fingerstick procedure easier. The Autolet is a small, simple device which automatically and painlessly performs the fingerstick. It is manufactured by Owen Mumford, Ltd., England. The exclusive United States agent for the Autolet is Ulster Scientific, Inc. Disposable Autolet platforms and lancets are also available. These platforms determine penetration depth and are available in two colors. The orange platform is recommended for adult use in hospitals or clinic settings where long-term monitoring is not expected. It is also recommended when adequate blood circulation is not present. The yellow platform is recommended for children and all adults using self-monitoring on a long-term basis. Unless you have difficulty in obtaining adequate blood for testing, choose the yellow platform.

The Autolet works very simply. A lancet is fitted into the spring-loaded arm. The arm is pulled back against the spring, where it is secured in place by a catch. Your finger is placed against the platform. The fingertip can be seen and reached through a hole in the platform. When the release button is pushed, the lancet automatically pricks the finger. (See Figure 1.) Advantages of the Autolet are that it is virtually painless, produces less trauma to the skin and is not complicated to use. In fact, the whole process occurs so rapidly that often patients do not think it has worked until the drop of blood appears. Another automatic fingerstick device, available from Bio-Dynamics, is the Autoclix. This works on the same principle as the Autolet. Here, the lancet is hidden from your hand as you press down on a platform designed for either light, medium or heavy pressure. Still another automatic device is the Monojector Lancet Device available from the Monoject Company.

You may be nervous when you first attempt to stick your finger for blood testing. Give yourself plenty of time to work with the material so you do not feel rushed. The procedure will take more time in the beginning until you master it. It is recommended that you obtain blood from the sides of the fingertips

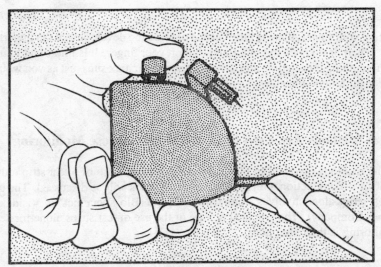

Figure 1. The Autolet is now set to puncture the skin automatically.

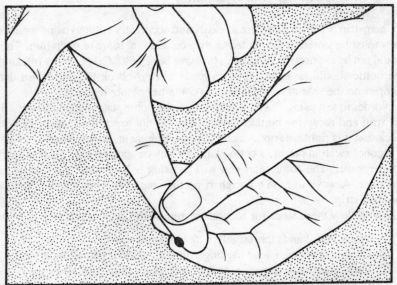

Figure 2. As you push gently on the skin, a drop of blood should appear.
(Illustrations adapted, with permission, from Ulster Scientific, Inc.)

because they are less sensitive than the finger pads. It may also be helpful if you press hard on your fingertip with an opposite finger as you prick it; this partially numbs the area. (See Figure 2.) If you wash your hands regularly before sticking your finger, there is little chance of infection developing at the fingertip sites. There is no need to put a Band-Aid on your finger. It is important to use a different finger each time and to rotate your fingerstick sites just as you would your insulin injection sites.

What Methods Are Used in Home Blood Glucose Monitoring?

The methods involved in blood testing require the use of a test strip either alone or in conjunction with a meter. Both methods will be discussed. The use of test strips alone involves either Chemstrip bG (Bio-Dynamics) or Visidex II (Ames Company). The practical feature of the use of test strips alone for self-monitoring is their simplicity.

Using Chemstrip bG (Bio-Dynamics)

Chemstrip bG strips can be read easily and accurately without using a meter. They must be stored in the container they came in, at room temperature. They should not be exposed to temperatures above 86° F. (30° C.) or below freezing. The bottle should be kept tightly capped. Always check the expiration date stamped on the side of each Chemstrip container before using it.

In order to test using Chemstrip bG, open the bottle, take out one Chemstrip test strip and recap the bottle immediately. Do not touch the reagent pad but check that it is right side up. Assemble your equipment, which should include: an alcohol swab, a lancet, a cotton ball, a clock or watch with a second hand, a paper towel. The color chart you will be using is located on the side of the container. Always use the color chart on the container from which you took your test strip.

Now follow these steps for accurate testing with Chemstrip bG:

1. Wash your hands thoroughly with soap and water.
2. Choose a finger. Clean the fingertip with alcohol and allow it to dry.
3. Drop your hand to your side for 30 seconds. This will allow the blood to flow to your fingertips.
4. Place your hand, palm side up, on a flat surface. Quickly prick the side of your fingertip using the lancet or an automatic finger puncture device.
5. Squeeze your fingertip several times. Using a gentle motion, repeat until a large drop of blood is suspended from your finger.
6. Place the drop of blood on the reagent side of the strip. Cover both the yellow and white squares but do not smear the blood.

7. Begin timing for exactly 60 seconds. Use a clock or watch with a second hand, keeping your eye on the second hand as the blood drops onto the test strip. If you can't remember the starting time, write it down.
8. At the end of 60 seconds, wipe the blood off the strip with the dry cotton ball.
9. You must now wait another 60 seconds. Then compare the two colors of the strip with the color chart.
10. If the colors of the Chemstrip bG strip match 240 mg./dl., you must wait another 60 seconds before making a final comparison.

Many times the colors on the test strip will not match the chart colors exactly. If the colors fall between the color blocks, it is acceptable to estimate the blood glucose reading. For example, if the blue square (bottom) matched 120 and the green square (top) matched 180, the result would be the average of the two numbers, or 150 mg./dl.

When you are learning to use Chemstrip bG strips, you can interpret the color and record the value directly on the strip. Put the strip back into the container for storage. It will retain its color for approximately two weeks. Bring these strips with you when you visit your doctor or nurse, so that your color interpretation can be double-checked.

Using Visidex II (Ames Company)

Visidex is another blood glucose testing procedure that does not require a meter. Visidex strips must also be stored in their container, away from hot or freezing temperatures. Check the expiration date before using the strips, making sure to use them within six months of first opening the container.

This procedure is similar to the one described above. Assemble your equipment, which should include Visidex reagent strips, a lancet, a clock or watch with a second hand, an alcohol swab, a cotton ball, a paper towel. Follow the previously discussed steps 1–5. Then apply the blood to the entire test area. Keep the strip level while you time for 30 seconds. At the end of 30 seconds, wipe the blood off gently with a cotton ball. Wait 90 seconds (2 minutes total elapsed time from when the blood was first put on the pads) and then compare the reacted green pad to the nearest matching green color block. If the test result is less than 110 mg./dl., ignore any slight orange color that may develop on the higher-range pad. If the green pad is darker than the 110 mg./dl. color block, then compare the higher-range pad (orange) to the nearest matching orange color block. If the color falls between color blocks, estimate results. For example, if the color is between 140 and 180 mg./dl., you could estimate your blood glucose at 160 mg./dl. You may notice that another number (mmol./l.) is listed below each color square on the Visidex II chart. "Millimoles per liter" refers to the number of glucose molecules in the blood; 5 mmol./l. is equivalent to 90 mg./dl. There are 18 mg. in 1 mmol., so $5 \times 18 = 90$. Both mg. and mmol. are used on the Visidex II chart.

There are meters used to determine blood glucose and these will now be reviewed.

Use of the Glucoscan Personal Blood Glucose Monitor (Lifescan, Inc.)

This monitor is a portable, pocket-sized meter. It is battery-operated with a built-in timer. Its visual signals remind you of each step in the test procedure. It is used with Glucoscan test strips. The Penlet Automatic Finger Prick Pen is used to make controlled skin punctures. The monitor also comes with a Glucoscan control set, which consists of two control solutions (100 mg./dl. and 250 mg./dl.) which are used to practice the test procedure. The procedure involves pricking your finger with the Penlet and placing a drop of blood on the test strip. The meter signals when 60 seconds have elapsed. You must then blot the blood from the test strip and place it into the meter. The Glucoscan meter then reads and displays your blood glucose level in milligrams per deciliter (mg./dl.).

Use of the Glucometer (Ames Company)

The Glucometer is a small, lightweight, portable instrument for blood testing. It is battery-operated and has a built-in timer and buzzer to assist you in accurately performing the test. It is more compact than the previous model offered by the Ames Company, the Dextrometer. Another advantage of the Glucometer is its easy calibration. Calibration tells the microcomputer in the Glucometer what depth of color on a Dextrostix strip correlates with a particular glucose solution. In order to calibrate for blood glucose readings, the test strips have to be inserted into the meter with artificial solutions on them. The Glucometer has the ability to retain calibration, even when the machine is turned off.

The Glucometer is used with calibration chips, Dextro-check calibrators, Dextro-check control solution (100 mg./dl.) and Dextrostix strips. The strips are similar to the test strips previously described except that those must be washed off with water. The Ames Company supplies a plastic squeeze bottle which should be used to wash off Dextrostix strips. The blood should be gently washed off the Dextrostix as you hold the untreated area of the strip against a cup or inside a sink in order to steady it. The test pad should be all one color if the washing is done properly. Dextrostix should be stored away from humidity and the bottle cap should be closed immediately after a strip has been removed from the bottle.

Use of the Accu-chek (Bio-Dynamics)

Another portable meter available for diabetic individuals is called Accu-chek. This is a small, battery-operated meter for use with Chemstrip bG. It too has a built-in timer and beeper with a digital display. This machine has two convenient features. It provides automatic calibration and does not require washing the strips. It is used with Chemstrips bG 50, which are provided with individual calibration strips.

We strongly recommend the use of blood glucose meters for individuals with Type I diabetes. If you choose any of the blood glucose monitors for blood testing, you must receive careful supervision and "hands on" instruction before self-monitoring. Exact record keeping of blood testing results is just as important as was emphasized in urine testing. If you are self-monitoring four to six times a day, your records will be essential to your diabetes self-management. Remember that performing these tests and keeping records go together. You are obtaining data and interpreting it. Confer with your doctor as to an appropriate range of blood glucose values for you. This range is usually between 80 and 120 mg./dl. fasting. Your doctor may give you more specific examples of blood values to be observed during a twenty-four-hour period.

A question that is often asked is whether blood glucose monitoring replaces visits to your doctor. Self-monitoring works in conjunction with, not in place of, your doctor's guidance. Although self-monitoring of blood glucose will certainly supplement your visits to a laboratory, your doctor will often ask you to have a panel of laboratory tests done, particularly a hemoglobin A_{1C}, so that he may assess your diabetes control. Self-monitoring may bring you into even closer contact with your doctor because you will have more information to share.

Special Benefits of Self-Monitoring

When should you monitor your blood glucose? There are certain cases where blood glucose monitoring is particularly necessary. If you have insulin-dependent diabetes, you should routinely test your blood glucose. Self-monitoring has become essential in the care of the pregnant diabetic woman. The renal threshold is lowered in pregnancy as a result of the increased blood flow to the kidneys. Because of this, urine tests are not appropriate to evaluate control in pregnant diabetic women. The successful outcome of the pregnancy is related to good blood glucose control of the mother throughout the pregnancy. This can be achieved through the use of self-monitoring. Kidney disease affects the renal threshold and may result in inaccurate urine test results or insufficient urine for testing. Diabetic persons with kidney disease may profit from blood glucose monitoring. If a person is color-blind and cannot interpret color values of urine or blood tests, the use of blood-testing meters is essential.

Some people do not wish to monitor their blood on a daily basis, but will monitor blood glucose for specific conditions, such as hypoglycemia. Often diabetic persons will eat in response to what they think is hypoglycemia, when instead they are experiencing anxiety or are hungry. Blood glucose monitoring can document the presence or absence of hypoglycemia. Many people calculate how much of a simple sugar they need to improve their blood glucose if they have experienced hypoglycemia. The use of self-monitoring is helpful for persons on a diet. As obese diabetic individuals begin to lose weight, blood glucose control improves. As they lose weight, they can test their blood glucose and see the improvement in diabetic control. This provides positive feedback. Read the following, which highlights the benefits of blood glucose testing.

WHAT WILL HOME BLOOD GLUCOSE MONITORING TELL YOU?

The obese person who is dieting	Is your blood glucose dropping along with pounds?
The person who is eating constantly to treat "hypoglycemia"	Is your blood glucose really low or is something else triggering your appetite?
The person taking insulin or pills for diabetes	How is your blood glucose control? When is the insulin peaking?
The person experiencing hypoglycemia	How much carbohydrate do you need to raise your blood glucose back to normal?

Costs Involved in Self-Monitoring

There is no doubt that the cost of self-monitoring equipment is high. The costs of the equipment, particularly meters, may be covered by private medical insurance, or Medicare, if prescribed by a doctor. You must ask your doctor to write a letter describing how self-monitoring equipment is necessary for control of your diabetes. Shop around and look for sales, particularly in November, National Diabetes Month, when you may have access to supplies that you can store.

It is important that you appreciate the cost benefits of self-monitoring. Diabetes-related expenses, such as hospitalizations, doctors' fees, tests, surgery or work disability, may be reduced by having your blood glucose controlled through self-monitoring. It has become an important aspect of diabetes self-management. Its continued use will aid in your blood glucose control. Begin to use blood glucose monitoring as you become a self-manager of your diabetes.

There are many advantages to self-monitoring of blood glucose. You become an independent self-manager. It becomes easier to see disruptions in your pattern and allows you to make the proper adjustments. Self-monitoring can document the occurrence of hypoglycemia or hyperglycemia, especially during illness. It is an essential task during pregnancy and for those with kidney disease. The benefits of improved control and independence make self-monitoring very worthwhile.

4

Weight Control

Are the following statements true or false?

1. Once you become overweight it is virtually impossible to lose excess pounds.

2. After the age of forty, obesity is an inevitable problem.

If you answer those questions as true, you have much to learn about obesity and how it can be avoided. This chapter will review what obesity is, the determinants of food intake, how people go about losing weight through safe or hazardous methods, as well as the best way to lose weight and keep it off.

WHAT IS OBESITY?

Most experts suggest that 30 percent of Americans are obese. If you are obese, you are 20–30 percent above your ideal body weight. Obesity, or excess accumulation of body fat, is determined in many ways, aside from the fact that you can simply look in the mirror and recognize the accumulation of fat on your body. You can also have your skin folds measured. A special type of caliper is used which measures the thickness of the skin fold at different body sites. The sites include the triceps muscle area (located on the back of your arm between your elbow and shoulder), the shoulder blade and the front of the thigh. The caliper estimates the amount of fat under the skin.

Overweight is quite different from obesity. Overweight is weight in excess

**Table 6 Desirable Weights Age 25 or Over
From Metropolitan Life Insurance**

	WOMEN				MEN		
Height	Small	Medium	Large	Height	Small	Medium	Large
4'10"	102-111	109-121	118-131	5' 2"	128-134	131-141	138-150
4'11"	103-113	111-123	120-134	5' 3"	130-136	133-143	140-153
5' 0"	104-115	113-126	122-137	5' 4"	132-138	135-145	142-156
5' 1"	106-118	115-129	125-140	5' 5"	134-140	137-148	144-160
5' 2"	108-121	118-132	128-143	5' 6"	136-142	139-151	146-164
5' 3"	111-124	121-135	131-147	5' 7"	138-145	142-154	149-168
5' 4"	114-127	124-138	134-151	5' 8"	140-148	145-157	152-172
5' 5"	117-130	127-141	137-155	5' 9"	142-151	148-160	155-176
5' 6"	120-133	130-144	140-159	5'10"	144-154	151-163	158-180
5' 7"	123-136	133-147	143-163	5'11"	146-157	154-166	161-184
5' 8"	126-139	136-150	146-167	6' 0"	149-160	157-170	164-188
5' 9"	129-142	139-153	149-170	6' 1"	152-164	160-174	168-192
5'10"	132-145	142-156	152-173	6' 2"	155-168	164-178	172-197
5'11"	135-148	145-159	155-176	6' 3"	158-172	167-182	176-202
6' 0"	138-151	148-162	158-179	6' 4"	162-176	171-187	181-207

of a normal range, which is determined by standard height and weight tables. Metropolitan Life Insurance Company (MLI) tables are used most often. New height-weight tables were published in February 1983. The new tables try to show the best weight associated with the lowest death rate. This means that those very underweight may be as unhealthy as those very overweight. Therefore many of the recommended weights have increased for some heights. For example, according to the new table, short women can weigh 10 pounds more than they did on the previous tables. However, most experts still agree that your weight should be on the lean side. The higher weights do not give you freedom to eat and gain weight as you please. In fact, the higher weights simply mean you may have fewer pounds to lose.

Table 6 above lists desirable weights for men and women from MLI. You may also want to obtain a more exact desirable weight rather than use the weight range. You can do this by determining the midpoint between weight ranges. For example, if your weight range is 150–165, the midpoint would be 157.5 pounds.

WHO ARE THE OBESE?

Your age, sex and physical activity are all variables in the development of obesity. Adolescence is a period of life when overweight frequently develops. In this case, excess calories may be coming from more junk food as well as a decrease in physical activity. Middle age can be a prime time for the development of obesity, as a result of too many calories and/or too little exercise. After this time, not as many people are obese. Obesity is more often seen in women than in men. This may be related to socioeconomic class.

THE DEVELOPMENT OF OBESITY

Obesity develops due to an imbalance between calories ingested and calories utilized. Several theories have been put forward to explain the development of obesity. A fat (or adipose) cell is made up of adipose tissue and water, in different proportions. These proportions change throughout life. The fat cell theory states that overweight during infancy is due to the development of a large number of fat cells. Once the fat cell number increases, it remains the same throughout life. So, if an infant is overfed, the number of fat cells increase. If weight gain first occurs in adulthood, on the other hand, it is due to an increase in the size, rather than the number, of fat cells. In other words, the proportion of fat to water inside the fat cell will change and the fat cell will consist primarily of fat. If the adult then tries to lose weight, the fat cells may decrease in size, but the number of fat cells will always remain the same. So during infantile obesity a large number of cells develop. Later in life the size of the cells may increase as weight gain progresses.

There have been some genetic explanations for the development of obesity. Obesity can be transmitted in particular strains of mice. There are also some hereditary diseases that are characterized by excess fat, which can be transmitted from parent to child. Studies with twins and adopted children have attempted to show that the development of obesity may be genetic rather than environmental. The weight of adopted children was compared with that of their foster and natural parents. When the adopted children were compared with the foster parents, there was no correlation with body weight. However, the weight of the child and that of the natural father and mother were very similar. In this case, weight seems to be more related to genetic makeup. Twins raised in the same environment have small differences in body weight. However, twins raised separately tend to show vast differences in weight. In this case, it appears that the environment is a more significant factor than heredity.

DETERMINANTS OF FOOD INTAKE

Intake of food is regulated by a part of the brain called the hypothalamus. Signals from the brain as well as other parts of the body work together to produce sensations of hunger, appetite and satiety (fullness). Hunger, or the need for food, is basic to man. Hunger may cause you to experience many negative or unpleasant sensations. When you go for one or two days without food you may almost feel that you would fight to be able to eat anything. Your appetite is intertwined with the taste, sight and smell of food. Satiety is the sensation that causes you to stop eating because your hunger and appetite have been satisfied.

If you want to lose weight, you should begin by appreciating the many factors that affect your food intake. There is an interaction between biological, experiential and environmental determinants (or factors) that control your food ingestion and selection.

BIOLOGICAL AND EXPERIENTIAL DETERMINANTS

The biological determinants of food intake are complex and usually interact with the other determinants. Your physiological desire for certain tastes, such as sweet, salty or bitter tastes, will determine the type of food you choose. Your own feeling of fullness or hunger caused by experiencing stomach contractions will also determine your ingestion of food.

The experiential determinants (previous experiences with food) include the psychological, cultural and family factors involved in food intake. Can you remember your early learning experiences with food? During childhood you learned about foods through family and social interactions. Someone in the home usually has the role of the "gatekeeper," or the person responsible for bringing food into the home and serving it. Many of your food likes and dislikes may be related to past life experiences. For example, cake may be a favorite food because of its association with pleasant family gatherings. On the other hand, you may intensely dislike liver because you were forced to eat it as a child and told "it was good for you." Food may be used as a reward or punishment. You may have received an extra helping of dessert for being a "good child" or deprived of dinner if you were naughty. You can see that parents play very significant roles in influencing the food habits and weight of children.

Your socioeconomic status will also be an important food intake determinant. Those who grew up in the Depression may recall periods of extreme poverty as well as food deprivation. Commonly consumed foods at that time often included potato sandwiches or beans and rice. Today, while the Depression is behind us, many are still in economic straits. Those who have risen into a higher socioeconomic level are fortunate enough to choose more expensive types of foods. Those persons might find it difficult to eat foods associated with the Depression because that was such an unhappy and trying period of time.

ENVIRONMENTAL DETERMINANTS

Factors in your immediate environment are significant in developing strong associations between food intake and the environment. A variety of lifestyle changes can influence your food intake. Changes in your life, such as marriage, divorce, the starting or stopping of a job, will be significant factors influencing your food intake.

Social situations influence food intake. These include barbecues, coffee breaks, and dinner parties, all of which involve eating and socializing. When reviewing this factor, think of the sabotage or support systems that play a role in your ingestion of food. Do your friends always bring cake to your home? Or do they try to show support by helping you avoid temptations? Also think about your outside interests. Does your life revolve around food or do you have other hobbies or goals that make for an interesting life? Here again, your socioeconomic status may determine your intake of food. For example, is your job conducive to overeating? Can you keep food at your desk and can you eat it at any time? Do you have an expense account and frequently dine out?

Don't for a minute forget the media! Today, there are so many advertisements about food on television, on the radio and in the newspapers. It is difficult to walk down any large city street without seeing one, two or three different types of restaurants per block. Almost every page of a newspaper will have an advertisement about food. Television and radio have several commercials every hour. Also, we live in a fast-food culture, with many of us eating on the run. Many convenience foods are being consumed both at home and away.

Other factors, such as the time of day, the place where you eat, as well as whether or not you are standing up or sitting down, will determine your food intake. Very often you get accustomed to eating when the clock says it is lunchtime rather than when your body tells you you're hungry. You may get into the habit of eating or snacking at other times during the day when you are not hungry. The place where you eat can become a significant factor for food intake. This may be your office, desk, kitchen, living room, bedroom or even your automobile. The physical position you are in may cause excessive food intake. For example, have you ever found yourself standing in front of a refrigerator, just grabbing every edible item in sight? Or do you like to lie in bed and eat?

The people with whom you socialize as well as the atmosphere in which food is being served will play a role in food intake. Take, for example, the family who sits around the dinner table with bowls of food on the table. In this situation, dinner may be the time when family members converse and discuss the happenings of the day. It is also a time when you continue to eat while you talk. Eating occurs without thinking and without getting in touch with internal cues that determine the feelings of fullness.

DETERMINANTS OF FOOD INTAKE

Biological

Taste
Genetic predisposition
Nervous system
Stomach contractions

Experiential
(psychological, cultural and family factors)

Attitude toward weight
Learning history
Food likes and dislikes
Amounts of food
Attitude toward food and its use
Age, sex, mental status
Economic status
Social status
Family/social interactions

Immediate Environment

Perceived hunger
Tolerance of hunger
Time of day
Place
Availability of food
Food advertising
Exposure to food cues
Palatability
Perceived fullness
Social aspects of situations
Physical position

Adapted with permission from Leonard S. Levitz, Ph.D., and Henry A. Jordan, M.D., *Behavioral Techniques for Dietary Management,* Institute for Behavioral Education, King of Prussia, PA.

WHY LOSE WEIGHT?

As you review your life, you can probably think of many factors which have caused you to overeat. So what if you became overweight? What are the implications of obesity? Why is it the nation's number-one health problem? Excessive body weight is associated with a higher death rate (mortality) according to the 1979 Build and Blood Pressure Study. In addition, weighing somewhat less than average was associated with a longer life. The causes of higher death rates associated with obesity are diabetes mellitus, cardiovascular disease, gallbladder disease and hypertension. Obese individuals frequently suffer from arthritis and toxemia of pregnancy. They are also higher surgical risks.

OBESITY AND DIABETES

There are approximately 6 million persons in the United States with diabetes. Of these, about 80 percent are obese. The obese person with diabetes has insulin resistance resulting in hyperglycemia.

Insulin is released from the pancreas but (due to the obesity) it does not allow the glucose in the blood to enter the cells. This results in an elevated blood glucose and an increase in insulin secretion. Thus, the obese person has an increased amount of blood insulin, or hyperinsulinemia. Weight reduction causes a drop in insulin levels and an increase in the number of insulin cell receptors. In fact, for some individuals, losing only ten pounds may be enough to increase the number of insulin receptors, reducing blood insulin levels and lowering blood glucose levels.

The distribution of fat on your body may also be an important factor in the association between obesity and diabetes. The classification of obesity based on body fat distribution may be a way to determine the susceptibility of obese women to diabetes. Women with upper-body obesity (obesity of the neck, shoulders and abdomen) have glucose intolerance more often and have higher blood insulin levels and larger fat cells than women with lower-body obesity (obesity of the buttocks and thighs).

ENERGY BALANCE

Obesity develops when an imbalance occurs between calories ingested and calories expended. Very simply put, calories eaten must not exceed calories used, or else the excess calories will be stored as fat, as seen in Figure 3. Energy is the capacity for your body to do work. Your source of energy is food. The energy for your body is comparable to the gasoline used in a car. You simply must have it in order for your body to function. Food provides calories. A calorie is a measure of energy. It is the amount of heat needed to raise the temperature of one gram of water one degree from 15° to 16° C.

FIGURE 3

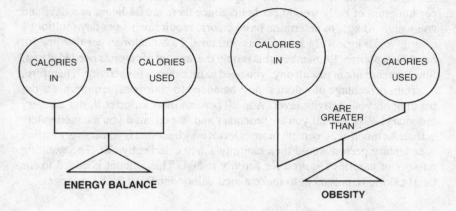

Two aspects of energy balance require calories. These include the basal metabolism and the level of physical activity. Basal metabolism is the amount of oxygen consumed in a resting state, or the amount of energy needed at rest for the body to perform vital functions. Some examples of vital functions are breathing and circulation of the blood. The basal metabolism will vary according to several factors. It is slightly higher in men than in women; it is higher in infancy and then decreases each year afterward. Basal metabolism increases during growth spurts, such as puberty, and in pregnancy.

However, since your body does not perform only vital processes, you need extra calories for physical activity. These activities may include food shopping, cleaning the house, driving the car or going to work. Extra calories needed for activity must be added to your basal metabolic requirements. Energy or calories are obtained by eating according to food preferences, food composition and environmental events. You can determine the amount of calories you need daily. This can be done by calculating the calories needed for basal metabolism and adding the additional calories you need for activity.

You may find it interesting to calculate your individual caloric needs for your present weight. Often patients are surprised at the number of calories eaten just for weight maintenance.

CALCULATION OF INDIVIDUAL CALORIC NEEDS

The first step in estimating the number of calories you need per day to maintain your weight is to take your weight in pounds and change it to kilograms. You do this by dividing your weight by 2.2. For example, if you weigh 154 pounds, divide by 2.2 to get 70 kilograms. The second step involves calculating your needs for basal metabolism. An average basal metabolic rate (BMR) is 1 calorie per kilogram of body weight per hour. Since there are 24 hours in a day, and you weigh 70 kg., to determine basal caloric requirements per day multiply 1 calorie × 70 kg. × 24 hours; thus you need 1,680 calories per day just for basal metabolism. Remember, this is only the amount of calories needed at rest. Since you are not at rest all day, you need extra calories for activity. Therefore, a certain percentage of calories must be added to your basal requirements depending on your activity level. Add 20 percent more calories if you are very sedentary, 30 percent if you are sedentary and 40 percent if you are moderately active. As much as 50 percent more calories may be added if you are very active. A sedentary person would then multiply 1,680 calories by .30. The resulting number of calories required for activity is 504. This amount is added to the basal caloric requirement to make a total caloric intake of 2,184 calories.

CALCULATING INDIVIDUAL CALORIC NEEDS

1. Divide your weight in pounds by 2.2

    154 ÷ 2.2 = 70 kg.

2. Multiply your weight in kilograms by 24

    70 × 24 = 1,680 calories for basal metabolism

3. Determine the percentage of extra calories you need for activity

    20% = very sedentary
    30% = sedentary
    40% = moderately active
    50% = very active

4. Multiply your basal metabolism by the percentage

    1,680 × .30 = 504

5. Add the calories for activity to your basal requirements

    1,680 + 504 = 2,184 calories per day

   The calculations are approximations based on average values of caloric needs. Some people of the same weight differ in calorie needs for basal requirements. Also, your estimate of your activity level is subjective. Therefore, your calculations should be considered estimates of your daily need.
   Let's look at a woman who is 5 feet 1 inch tall and weighs 115 pounds. Her

daily basal calorie requirement is 1,248 calories (2.2 divided into 115 = 52 kg.; 52 × 24 = 1,248). If she is sedentary her calories for activity will total 374 (1,248 × .30 = 374). Her total daily caloric need to maintain her weight is 1,622 calories (1,248 + 374 = 1,622).

Well, what happens if you want to gain or lose weight? Remember the concept of energy balance. One pound of fat is equal to 3,500 calories. Therefore, to lose one pound per week, you can simply decrease your total caloric intake by 500 calories per day and you will reduce your intake by 3,500 calories per week. To lose two pounds per week, you decrease the total intake of calories by 1,000 per day. The reverse would hold true if you wanted to gain weight. Simply add 500 calories per day to gain one pound per week or add 1,000 calories per day to gain two pounds per week.

The individual eating 2,184 calories to maintain weight would have to eat approximately 1,684 calories per day to lose one pound per week, and 1,184 calories per day to lose two pounds per week. The woman who is overweight at 115 pounds would have to reduce her intake to 1,122 calories to lose just one pound per week. Your rate of weight loss should not exceed two to three pounds per week if your weight-loss method is to be safe as well as effective.

WEIGHT-LOSS STRATEGIES

Weight-loss strategies must be tailored to individual needs. Your approach to weight loss depends on the amount of weight you want to lose, your age and your previous successful experiences or failures with weight-loss techniques. Weight-loss programs for those who are 20–30 percent overweight differ significantly from those for persons who are morbidly obese, or 100 percent above their ideal body weight. For most patients, weight loss should occur with a balanced diet of at least 1,000 calories per day. Regardless of the diet you follow, weight loss is simply the result of caloric restriction. If you eat more calories than you need, the scale will continue to go up. Restricting your intake of calories while following a healthy diet can only lead to weight loss. For weight maintenance (keeping weight off) to be successful, nutrition education and behavior modification should be components of the program.

For the morbidly obese, intensive medical or surgical intervention may be required. For these people, the high risks of diets of fewer than 1,000 calories per day may be justified. Group support systems are helpful since these people rarely do well on their own. All persons who must lose more than a few pounds need a long-term program utilizing a team approach. The team may consist of a doctor, nutritionist, nurse and psychologist. Nutrition education is needed to learn the caloric and nutrient composition of food. These programs must involve a commitment of at least one to two years. In the obese, very rapid weight loss can be hazardous, especially if you have other medical problems. In this case, quick weight loss should be undertaken only after other weight-reducing techniques have failed. Then, frequent visits to a trained physician who will monitor you with physical examinations and blood tests are essential.

FAD DIETS AND DRUGS

Obese individuals frequently use a variety of fad diets for weight control. The diets usually promise painless, fast weight loss. The word "diet" tends to connote something temporary; it seems that you could go "on and off diets" forever. In addition, fad diets tend to be rigid and monotonous. The claims of quick weight loss virtually ignore anything to do with maintenance of weight loss.

High-Protein, Low-Carbohydrate Diets

Almost every year a high-protein, low-carbohydrate diet hits the newsstand and is promulgated by TV shows. These include the Stillman and Atkins diets. People mistakenly believe the "rationale" that the elimination of one food group, primarily carbohydrates, will promote weight loss. Another "rationale" is that protein takes longer to digest; therefore digestion burns more calories, resulting in weight loss. The dietary components include as much protein as you can eat. Large intakes of protein usually result in large intakes of fat. Therefore, you may be eating high-calorie foods. Portion sizes of food on these diets are usually not advised. Thus, you could conceivably eat a sixteen-ounce steak at each meal. In addition, without dietary carbohydrates, ketones become the source of fuel for the body. The presence of ketones usually results in a loss of appetite. The objection to this type of diet is that weight loss may not occur, because you eat more calories than needed. If you do lose weight, you may not keep it off. The diets are very high in fat, sometimes resulting in high blood cholesterol levels. There are no data on long-term weight reduction and there is no maintenance program, so this diet produces only temporary weight loss. This diet is not recommended if you have diabetes.

The Scarsdale Diet is another example of a high-protein, low-carbohydrate diet. It is supposedly designed to cause weight loss by eating the "proper combination of foods'' and by burning body fat through ketosis. The diet advocates a quick weight loss of twenty pounds in two weeks. It allows for protein bread, lean and fatty meats and some fruits and vegetables. All other food items, including alcohol and simple carbohydrates, are eliminated. It is recommended that you use your best judgment when determining portions of food. In other words, no advice is given and it is often stated that you may eat as much as desired of protein foods. This diet is only for short-term weight loss. What happens after two weeks is up to you. The author states that the diet is not intended for anyone with medical problems or those with insulin-dependent diabetes. We agree.

The Beverly Hills Diet

This diet is high in carbohydrates but low in protein. Supposedly, weight loss occurs from a plan of combining enzymes obtained from specific foods. There is no scientific evidence that this really occurs. During the first week of the diet, you must eat only fruit. In the following weeks, foods permitted include fruit, nuts and occasionally protein in the form of meat. One particular day calls for up to eight ounces of dried apricots. This amounts to over 500 calories and over 120 grams of carbohydrates. The diet is extremely high in simple carbohydrates and may cause elevations in blood glucose levels. It is rigid, allowing no choices. The author states that the diet is not for use by diabetic persons. In addition, some persons have experienced diarrhea, with resulting loss of fluids and minerals such as sodium and potassium. Finally, the protein content of the diet is much too low to promote good health.

Appetite Suppressants

Appetite suppressant pills are also used for weight reduction. The rationale is to decrease weight by reducing your appetite. Dietary components include some high-protein foods as well as water. The objections to this type of dieting is that weight gain usually follows cessation of the pills. The pills do not change your eating behavior, and weight loss is not permanent. A number of side effects result from commonly used appetite suppressants. They may be habit-forming and overstimulate the nervous system. Blood pressure levels may rise. They also cause a dry mouth and insomnia. The medical profession has tried to police "diet doctors" who prescribe these dangerous drugs inappropriately. The over-the-counter appetite suppressants are also dangerous and should not be used.

Starch Blockers

The starch blockers are another recent weight-loss drug. These diet pills are made from an extract of kidney or northern beans. Other beans may also be used, all of which supposedly stop the action of an enzyme in the small intestine that digests starch. There are about 100 manufacturers of the pills who claim the product allows you to eat large amounts of starch without a weight gain. The pills are taken before meals and may prevent digestion of up to 700 starch calories. Manufacturers also make it clear that this does not mean you can eat unlimited quantities of food, or that the pills prevent absorption of calories from sugar, fat or protein. Some people taking the pills reported to the FDA that they experienced side effects of nausea, vomiting, diarrhea and stomach pains. If the FDA receives convincing scientific evidence that the pills work, they may be permitted for sale as a drug either by prescription or over the counter. However, as of July 1982, the FDA has not received sufficient data to show that the pills are safe or effective, and has banned their sale until further tests are performed.

Liquid Protein Diets

The liquid protein diet hit the market a few years ago. The goal for this diet was to decrease weight with fewer calories by substituting a packaged "food" for high-calorie meals. The dietary components consisted of a few tablespoons of liquid formula made from collagen. Collagen is a protein that is of poor biological value. This means it does not contain all eight essential amino acids. The objection to this diet was that weight loss was temporary. In addition, some people died, possibly due to an imbalance of fluids and minerals such as sodium and potassium.

INCORPORATED WEIGHT-LOSS PROGRAMS

National Weight-Loss Centers

Different types of weight-loss and diet centers have developed across the country. The individual programs may vary. However, they generally are profit-motivated and promise rapid weight loss. The programs usually allow you to pay a weekly fee or one set fee. Individual counseling as well as group behavior modification may be included. A variety of trained and untrained personnel are employed at the centers. Weight loss usually occurs because the diets are quite low in calories. Some allow you to eat what you want on the weekend. Another diet requires you to purchase all your food from the company. These diets are not recommended for diabetic individuals because they may be too low in calories. While initial weight loss may be rapid, it probably would not be maintained. The diets may be dangerous because of lack of medical supervision.

Pritikin Longevity Centers

Pritikin centers offer patients a nutrition program designed to be effective against many diseases (especially the vascular diseases) that now require drug therapies or expensive surgery. The diet provides for 10 percent of the total calories from fat, 10 percent from animal protein and 80 percent from complex carbohydrates. It is low in fat, low in cholesterol and high in fiber from whole grains, vegetables and fruit. Simple carbohydrates (except fruit), caffeine, beef and eggs are excluded. Exercise is also an integral component of the centers.

This diet program may be quite difficult for many Americans to follow since it requires a reduction of fat intake from the customary 40 percent to 10 percent of total calories. The eating plan is designed to last your lifetime, rather than being a temporary diet. The diet may be inadequate in iron as well as calcium. Also, any claims that clogged arteries have been "unclogged" are unproven. The diet may have some benefits for those with diabetes in light of the newer research supporting a higher intake of complex carbohydrates and fiber. However, remember that any claims stating that persons with diabetes can eliminate their insulin injections are related only to the non-insulin-dependent person who presumably has lost weight through the program.

Weight Watchers

Weight Watchers has undergone many changes since it was first developed. The diet is higher in complex carbohydrates today than in the past. The diet allows for a specific amount of complex carbohydrates per day (rather than per week). In addition, it places a limit on animal protein per day. For example, females should not exceed nine ounces of protein daily. Weight Watchers also has a behavior modification program, in which program modules are frequently used. Here a different aspect of behavior modification is reviewed weekly. Each module or weekly session builds on the next module, providing continuing education. The program encourages food monitoring and also has a built-in weight-maintenance program. Those with diabetes may take advantage of the behavior modification aspect of Weight Watchers. However, you may need individual guidance from a nutritionist to help you coordinate your diabetic meal plan with the Weight Watchers meal plan.

Strategies for Weight Reduction

Now that you are aware of some of the facts about obesity and some of the hazardous techniques for losing weight, you may be wondering if there is a healthy way to lose weight. The answer to this question is "yes"! There are a variety of ways to do so. A good reducing diet should meet the following standards: The diet should satisfy all nutritional needs. It should be in accordance with your lifestyle and food preferences. The diet should protect you from between-meal hunger and should be easy to follow outside the home. Finally, the most important characteristic of a good reducing technique is that you can follow it over a long time to retain your new eating habits and maintain weight loss.

Behavioral Strategies for Weight Control

Traditional weight-loss methods can be used for successful treatment. However, calorie-reducing diets can be quite frustrating for the person who has a lot of weight to lose. If you are such a person, perhaps you have searched for an alternative method. It is known that many obese people who lose weight will not remain in therapy. Of those who do remain in therapy, most will not lose much weight. Usually, weight lost is regained. Many psychologists and nutritionists have turned to behavior change as an important component in permanent weight reduction.

Behavior therapy for weight control or behavior modification involves changing specific characteristics of your environment to increase or decrease eating behaviors, or learning a new response or behavior to a familiar cue. You see, the obese person is more sensitive to external food-related cues. In other words, the obese eat more because of external or environmental factors rather than internal factors. For example, when you walk past a bakery, the sight or smell of food (external factors) may increase your desire to eat. Therefore, you must change the environmental factor. So you may actually try a different route in order to avoid walking past the bakery.

Psychologists use these behavioral theories in programs for weight control. A significant number of persons lose weight through behavior modification methods. Weight is lost gradually and many have maintained weight loss for at least a year. These results are very encouraging and have led many nutritionists to urge their patients to embark on a behavior change program.

TABLE 7 EATING PATTERN

	Where Eaten	Activity	Hunger	With Whom or Alone	Mood While Eating	Food	Amount	Calories
6 a.m.								
10 a.m.								
12 a.m.								
4 p.m.								
8 p.m.								
12 p.m.								

H -HOME	0-NO HUNGER	A-ANXIOUS E-ANGRY
W-WORK	1	B-BORED F-HAPPY
C-CAFE OR	2	C-TIRED G-NONDESCRIPT
RESTAURANT	3	D-DEPRESSED
R- RECREATION	4	
	5-STARVING	

The starting point for behavior change is self-monitoring of your food intake. This can be done by using a self-monitoring food record (see Table 7). The food record is kept on a daily basis for a minimum of ten weeks or the duration of a program. The food record is a form that details various aspects of your eating behavior. It includes environmental factors (such as the time when you start and stop eating), where you are when you eat (your home or your office), whether you are standing or sitting, your mood (happy, bored, tired, depressed), whom you are socializing with when you eat, the number of meals and snacks eaten per day as well as your activity (such as watching TV) while eating. The purpose of the food record is to make you more aware of your food intake. The food record can interrupt your normal routine of eating because you must write everything down right after you consume it.

The food record is a tool to help you identify the ABCs of eating. The ABCs stand for the antecedents, behaviors and consequences of food intake. Anything that occurs prior to eating is a cue or antecedent to eating. This can be the time of day, the person you are with or where you are. The behavior of eating is the rate and frequency of your eating; that is, how fast and how many times per day you ingest food. The consequences of food intake have to do with your long- and short-term goals for weight loss. For example, a short-term consequence of eating an ice-cream sundae is that you may not lose weight. A long-term consequence may be that you will not fit into a smaller size for another month. Consequences of food intake also include your feelings about eating. Another benefit of the food record is that it can be reinforcing if used over time. For example, after completing the form for one week, many ABCs will be identified. If you continue to use the food record and complete it, by the tenth week you will be aware of many changes in your eating pattern. You can see for yourself the changes from the first to the tenth week.

After the ABCs have been identified, it is important to understand how you can initiate behavior change. Behavior change takes time, and that is why six months to a year should be allowed for the completion of such a program. You can expect to lose approximately two to three pounds per week. Changes must be made slowly, on a daily basis and practiced over time. An example of a slow change would be practicing to sit down each time you eat rather than standing up, if standing up was identified as a particular problem causing overeating.

The food record will also show you the times of day or the situations you are in when you eat a lot of food, or a lot of high-calorie food. Then, very slowly, perhaps on a weekly basis, one antecedent at a time should be changed. For example, you may preplan meals. You may begin to eat at specific times. You may begin to eat in a designated eating place, such as one specific room in your home. You may decide that when you eat you will avoid other activities. You may resolve to minimize your contact with the sight of food. Whatever it is, one antecedent should be chosen per week and practiced daily. The next week another antecedent is chosen and practiced along with the first, and so on.

Goal setting is an important aspect of behavior change. Goals should be stated in specific behavioral terms. They should be realistic for your lifestyle and should be short-term. An example of a specific goal is: "When I watch TV next week, I will snack only four evenings out of seven." Notice, the behavior deals with snacking, the time period is next week and four out of seven nights is more realistic than avoiding snacks every night. By developing behavior modification skills you can learn to change your thoughts, activities and eating behavior patterns. You can gain information on how to make appropriate food choices and take responsibility for what happens to your weight.

There are many specific strategies available for changing your eating behaviors. One way is called environmental engineering. Using this technique, you remove food from all the rooms of your house except the kitchen. This means that your fruit, nut and candy bowls are taken from the living room or den and kept in the kitchen. In this way you are not tempted to eat, by the sight of food in other rooms. Environmental engineering also deals with "cleaning up" the kitchen. Leftovers should be kept in opaque containers in the refrigerator. Problematic snack foods should be kept in the tallest cabinets out of your reach. Some people have gone so far as to take the light out of the refrigerator to make it difficult to see inside.

Another strategy is called the competing response. This involves engaging in an activity or hobby you especially enjoy whenever you feel an urge to eat. This may occur when you are bored or tired. Competing activities such as needlepoint, puzzles, walking, talking to a friend, using a bicycle or any other activity can compete with the act of eating. It is important that this be something you enjoy, so that it is a satisfying substitute for food.

The use of positive self-talk is extremely important during any weight-loss endeavor. Talk to yourself and congratulate yourself when you are able to make a behavior change. If you're able to sit down for every meal and snack, rather than stand up in front of the refrigerator, you deserve a pat on the back. If you're able to avoid snacking while you're watching TV for a few days, tell yourself you did a good job. If you're able to say "no" to the hostess who is continually encouraging you to eat, congratulate yourself for that too.

If you decide to use behavior change as your method of weight reduction, begin by explaining this technique to your family. You'll be engaged in a variety of activities that may be quite different from previous techniques you used to lose weight. You may be preplanning and recording what you eat, you may be slowing down your food intake, you may delay snacks, you may not be eating many things that your family and friends are eating. Therefore, you must let them know that this technique is different. It focuses more on changing the way you eat than on calorie counting or food deprivation.

In addition, the use of family and friends as support systems must be included in a weight-loss method of this kind. You need people to observe and compliment your behavior changes. You need those same people to ignore your mistakes. Try to avoid people who bring food to your house as a token of appreciation of friendship. When the pounds start coming off, you need people to tell you you're doing a good job and look great.

Finally, try to understand the concept of self-control as opposed to will power. Often people think of will power as power you received at birth and if you didn't happen to get it then you are out of luck. Therefore that is why you are obese and totally out of control when it comes to food. Will power is not a magical power, mysteriously granted to a chosen few. A more positive approach to your overeating and previous lack of adherence to specific meal plans is the concept of self-control. Self-control means you are in total control of everything you do and eat. You are the one who will choose to use or ignore your ability to exert self-control. It is within your control to refuse or accept dessert from an insistent hostess. If you want to snack while standing in front of the refrigerator, rather than sitting down, that is your lack of self-control. If you usually snack in the den while you're watching TV and you are able to avoid this four out of seven nights, that is pretty good. It was your self-control that helped, not your will power. It doesn't take "will power." Behavior is learned and is in your control. Finally, be realistic in your goal setting for weight reduction. If you were overweight for a long time, it is unrealistic to think that the weight will come off rapidly. It is also unhealthy to try a reducing technique that will cause rapid weight reduction, unless you are morbidly obese. Two to three pounds per week is very good and can be achieved through the use of behavior change.

As you can see, behavior modification is a complete program for permanent weight loss. If you only have ten pounds to lose, some additional tips may be useful.

You can follow a calorie-reducing diet which may range from 1,000 to 2,000 calories. The caloric restriction depends on your ideal body weight for your height as well as your specific goal for weight reduction. You will probably have to count calories daily, and you may find these diets are rigid. Calories do count and there are some ways you can decrease your caloric intake without even counting them.

Food Preparation

Food preparation techniques can be changed to avoid excess calories. All your food should be broiled, baked, boiled or poached. Try to avoid frying. Each ounce of meat, fish or poultry that is breaded and fried will absorb approximately one teaspoon of oil. Therefore, if you fry a 3-ounce chicken cutlet, which is about 165 calories, you will ingest an extra 120 calories from the oil (3 teaspoons of oil for 3 ounces of chicken). Instead of margarine, oil or gravy, use diet margarine or mayonnaise, low-calorie spray fats and low-calorie gravies.

Food Shopping

You can change your shopping habits by purchasing lower-calorie foods and avoiding convenience or junk foods. Shopping from a list gives you an idea of essential items you need in your home. Adhering to the list helps you to avoid buying foods that are not needed. Shopping from a list is also an economy technique. If you shop when you are hungry, the sight of food, especially in supermarkets, can be a cue to their purchase. So make sure you have eaten before food shopping.

Portion Control

Decrease the amount of food you eat by controlling portion size. This can be achieved by using measuring cups, measuring spoons and a food scale. This activity does not have to be done every day. However, use of these items periodically for a couple of weeks will help you become familiar with portion sizes of various foods. Keep measuring utensils within easy reach for use after food is cooked. Weigh steaks, chicken and other meats on a scale to determine the correct number of ounces. A measuring cup can be used for cereal as well as macaroni. Finally, use measuring spoons for fats and oils. For example, when preparing a peanut butter sandwich how many times have you just plunged a knife into the jar and scooped out some peanut butter? You can use a measuring spoon to really get a good idea of what one tablespoon of peanut butter looks like. Then, in the future, when you plunge the knife into the jar, you can have confidence that you know the correct portion size to take out.

Physical Activity

Another way to lose weight is to increase your activity level. Your activity must be increased enough to use excess calories. This topic will be discussed in Chapter 9.

Treatment for Morbid Obesity

The morbidly obese person is at least twice his ideal body weight. These patients often regain weight lost. Only 10–20 percent maintain weight loss after a few years. Special medical and surgical techniques have been used in those morbidly obese who have failed to lose weight with diet, hypnosis, behavior modification, drugs or group therapy. Treatment programs should include the team approach and very low-calorie diets. Medical or surgical treatment becomes more hazardous if the patient is 50 years or older. Very low-calorie diets may be employed because patients must lose so much weight. Surgical techniques include jaw wiring, intestinal bypass, gastric bypass and gastroplasty. Weight loss has occurred with all types of surgery. All have significant risks and need frequent monitoring by a physician.

The protein-sparing modified fast has been used with many obese patients. The rationale for this diet is to suppress the appetite and promote rapid weight loss. It is thought that eating a low-calorie, high-quality-protein diet will do two things. First, it will allow for rapid weight loss. Second, it will prevent the body from breaking down its own protein stores such as body organs and muscles. The latter has not been scientifically proven. This diet is experimental and is for the obese diabetic who has attempted and failed at previous weight-loss methods. While on this diet, the patient develops ketosis, so the appetite is reduced. As the body begins to produce ketones, weight loss ensues. The dietary components include high-quality protein such as meat, fish, poultry or egg white. In addition, vitamin and mineral supplements are included plus six to eight glasses of water per day. An obese patient with diabetes remains on this diet for a maximum of three to four months and only with very close medical supervision. Behavior modification techniques must be incorporated into the weight-loss program to facilitate learning about eating habits. The metabolic success of the diet is excellent. Blood glucose, blood pressure and blood lipid levels are reduced along with the weight loss. Weight loss is in the range of two to seven pounds per week. Often insulin or oral hypoglycemic agents as well as antihypertensive medications may be discontinued. The objections to this diet are that it is rigid and very calorie-restricting. In addition, overeating, especially carbohydate binges, while on this or any other starvation diet may cause severe fluid retention and even heart failure. Remember, close supervision with a doctor is essential if you follow this diet.

Jaw Wiring

Jaw wiring has also been used in treating the morbidly obese. The procedure used is standard for broken jaws. It is called maxillo-mandibular fixation or immobilizing the jaw with wires. After fixation, calories are limited to 800 per day, usually provided in a liquid or very soft form. To be considered a candidate for this procedure, you must undergo a dental exam since the teeth and gums may deteriorate with fixation. Oral hygiene practices must be monitored and poor dental conditions must be corrected prior to the procedure. Patients can lose thirteen to twenty pounds in the first month. This will level off to two to ten pounds by the end of six months. At the end of eight months, some researchers have reported an average weight loss of 64 pounds. Jaw wiring seems to produce considerable weight loss with few side effects. Unfortunately, the consequences of unwiring are often rapid and progressive weight gain.

Intestinal bypass involves connecting one part of the small intestine to another, while bypassing a third segment. Some studies report weight loss of 65–125 pounds one year after surgery. Gastric bypass involves the creation of a small upper stomach which is then connected to a part of the small intestine. Patients have lost 30 percent of their initial weight in one year, with a range of 55 to 120 pounds. Gastroplasty involves "stapling" or suturing part of the stomach to form a small pouch. Some problems associated with intestinal and gastric bypass procedures follow.

PROBLEMS ASSOCIATED WITH BYPASS PROCEDURES

Intestinal Bypass	Gastric Bypass
Malabsorption and diarrhea	Gallstones
Fatty liver and cirrhosis	Ulcer
Dermatitis	Temporary hair loss
Reduced vitamins and minerals: vitamins A, D, K and folic acid; iron, zinc, magnesium and calcium	Reduced vitamin A levels
	Dumping syndrome
	Nausea and vomiting after meals
Kidney stones	
Gallstones	
Anemia and malnutrition	

After surgery, food intake may or may not be reduced. Weight loss occurs due to decreased food absorption caused by the surgery. The bypass causes a disease state of malabsorption. Results from some studies show that the body can adapt to the surgical procedure and weight gain may recur. Other studies show that only a small amount (20 pounds) is gained back, most patients maintain weight loss after the first six months.

Diabetes, hypertension and cardiorespiratory function may be improved by the weight loss. Patients report an increased enjoyment of life and a feeling of well-being. All surgical candidates must be carefully assessed prior to the surgery because of the high morbidity and mortality rates associated with the treatment. Patients must be monitored by their medical doctors and surgeons. Nutritionists and psychologists may also participate in the care of the morbidly obese.

Researchers have reported a five-year follow-up on patients who underwent intestinal bypass. Five years after the surgery, more patients had experienced low blood levels of several vitamins and minerals. In addition, more patients suffered from gallstones, kidney stones or liver disease. Gastroplasty is now considered the preferred surgical technique, as intestinal surgery is no longer justified. However, long-term results must be carefully documented to determine the advantages of this procedure.

Hypnosis

For the morbidly obese person, hypnosis may be another alternative. Hypnosis is an altered state of consciousness. The procedure makes use of your own natural ability to reach a state of intense concentration or awareness. Hypnosis works by enhancing your already existing commitment to stop something—in this case, overeating. Today, hypnosis is being used to help people break bad habits of overeating. Using hypnosis, participants can be deliberately induced into a trancelike state. The trance is used to make useful suggestions. If you seek the help of a hypnotist, make sure you check his medical credentials and experience in hypnosis. The hypnotist should be a psychologist, a psychiatrist or another trained physician.

In this chapter you have read the whys, wheres and hows of weight reduction. Try to develop strategies for your specific food problems. For example, if you eat at irregular times, plan to eat three meals per day or try to eat only at specific times. If you eat many high-calorie foods, try to eat low-calorie snacks, use low-calorie recipes and avoid tasting food while cooking. Try to use measuring utensils, serve meals hotel style, avoid second helpings, use smaller dishes and have someone else clear the table. If you encounter many behavioral food problems, develop a hobby to replace problem eating. You can decide to eat in only one place and avoid other activities while eating. Avoid purchasing problematic foods, and sit down and enjoy your meal. If you are interested in weight reduction, the use of behavior change may be worthy of consideration. Remember, for the person with diabetes, losing excess pounds is necessary to normalize blood glucose levels.

5

Oral Hypoglycemic Agents

Pills to lower blood glucose have been available to diabetic persons for more than thirty years. These drugs are classified as sulfonylureas. They are chemically related to "sulfa" drugs, but they do not fight off infections. Since their function is to lower blood glucose and they are taken by mouth, they are called oral hypoglycemics or oral antidiabetic drugs. Presently, the sulfonylureas are the only drugs available in the United States to lower blood glucose. In the past, another class of oral agents, the biguanides, was available. The main biguanide used in the United States was phenformin (DBI or Meltrol). This was used from 1957 to 1977, when its sale was banned in the United States because of its side effects.

THE ACTION OF ORAL HYPOGLYCEMICS

The sulfonylureas are not an oral form of insulin. Initially, they increase the release of insulin from the beta cells of the pancreas. Long-term treatment with the sulfonylureas increases insulin receptor sites. Because the first action of the oral hypoglycemics is to stimulate the release of insulin, these drugs should be used only in patients who have adequate beta cell function (non-insulin-dependent diabetic persons). A person with Type I, insulin-dependent diabetes is unable to produce insulin and so needs insulin injections. In addition, if the pancreas of a Type II diabetic person has a very limited capacity to produce insulin, sulfonylureas will be ineffective. Therefore they often do not work in the lean Type II diabetic person.

For the non-insulin-dependent diabetic person, blood glucose control is always tried through diet and exercise alone. Oral hypoglycemics are prescribed only when additional help is needed; they are not prescribed to replace diet and exercise. Unfortunately, some people have become used to taking pills and may not place enough emphasis on diet. Oral hypoglycemics are less effective if a patient is overweight. Weight reduction remains important when using this medication.

IMPORTANCE OF DIETARY CONTROL

There is no substitute for dietary control. Oral sulfonylureas will only work in conjunction with weight control. Oral agents do not take the place of insulin that is still working in your body. Most overweight non-insulin-dependent diabetic people have high blood levels of insulin due to obesity. The oral agents do not cause weight reduction; only reduced calories or increased exercise will accomplish this. All too often, we see patients continuing to overeat while their blood glucose remains uncontrolled with sulfonylureas. Weight gain occurs, causing more resistance to the effect of insulin. Eventually, the pancreas cannot overcome the insulin resistance and blood glucose levels rise. The oral agents are then considered ineffective. In actuality, weight control was ineffective. Pills alone will never allow you to have control over your disease if you ignore important dietary principles.

TYPES OF SULFONYLUREAS

Four commonly prescribed sulfonylureas will now be described. Their characteristics are summarized in the following table. They differ in their metabolism and excretion. Drug metabolism refers to how a drug is broken down and changed to an inactive form before it is excreted. Excretion refers to how the drug leaves the body, which usually is in the urine.

ORAL HYPOGLYCEMIC AGENTS

Tolbutamide (generic name) (pronounced: tole-BYOO-ta-mide)
Orinase (trade name) (Upjohn Company)
Shape: round
Dose: 250 mg.; color: white
Dose: 500 mg.; color: white
Usual daily dose: 0.5–3 g., usually in a divided dose
Duration of action: 6–8 hours

Tolazamide (generic name) (pronounced: to-LA-za-mide)
Tolinase (trade name) (Upjohn Company)
Shape: round
Dose: 100 mg.; color: white
Dose: 250 mg.; color: white
Dose: 500 mg.; color: white
Usual daily dose: 0.25–1.5 g. in 1 or 2 doses daily with meals
Duration of action: 12–18 hours

Acetohexamide (generic name) (pronounced: a-SEAT-oh-HEX-a-mide)
Dymelor (trade name) (Eli Lilly and Company)
Shape: capsule
Dose: 250 mg.; color: white
Dose: 500 mg.; color: yellow
Usual daily dose: 0.25–1.5 g. in 1 or 2 doses daily before meals
Duration of action: 12–18 hours

Chlorpropamide (generic name) (pronounced: klor-PRO-pa-mide)
Diabinese (trade name) (Pfizer Laboratories)
Shape: D-shaped
Dose: 100 mg.; color: blue
Dose: 250 mg.; color: blue
Usual daily dose: 0.1–0.5 g. in one daily dose with breakfast
Duration of action: 24–36 hours

Tolbutamide (Orinase) is the shortest-acting of the four listed hypoglycemics. This drug is broken down rapidly. Almost all of the drug is excreted in the urine within twenty-four hours. It is usually given in divided doses with a maximum daily dose of 2–3 grams. Tolazamide (Tolinase), has an intermediate action. Eighty-five percent of the drug is excreted in the urine within twenty-four hours. It is given in single or divided doses with a maximum daily dose of 1.5 grams. Acetohexamide (Dymelor) is also quickly broken down, with 60 percent of the drug excreted in the urine within twenty-four hours. This drug is metabolized in the liver. It is given in single or divided doses with a maximum daily dose of 1.5 grams. Chlorpropamide (Diabinese) is the longest-acting of the four drugs. Less than 1 percent is broken down in the liver and 60 percent of the drug is excreted in the urine within twenty-four hours. It is given in a single dose with a maximum daily dose of 0.5 gram.

SECOND-GENERATION ORAL HYPOGLYCEMICS

Sulfonylureas that are more potent in lowering the blood glucose have recently been developed. Since they are newer drugs, they have been called second-generation sulfonylureas. They are presently in use outside the United States. They may be approved for use in the United States in the near future. These drugs act similarly to the four sulfonylureas previously described but may have certain advantages. They are effective in much smaller doses, stimulating the release of a maximal amount of insulin. They have a longer duration of action, fewer side effects and decreased drug interactions.

Two drugs to be marketed are Glyburide and Glipizide. Look for Glyburide to be marketed by Hoechst-Roussel Pharmaceuticals as Diabeta and by the Upjohn Company as Micronase. This drug will be available in 1.25, 2.5, 5 and 10 mg. tablets with the effective dose being between 1.25 and 10 mg. daily. Glipizide will be marketed by Pfizer as Glucotrol. This will be available in 5 and 10 mg. tablets with the effective dose being between 5 and 40 mg. daily.

PREVENTION OF HYPOGLYCEMIA

Your doctor will carefully assess your total health picture before prescribing these drugs. Since sulfonylureas are broken down by the liver (except for Diabinese) and excreted by the kidneys, you must have adequate liver and kidney function. If the liver does not break down the drugs, their level will build in the blood, causing toxicity (damage to other organs). Because these drugs lower blood glucose, prolonged and severe hypoglycemia can occur if kidney and liver function is not adequate.

If you take an oral hypoglycemic, hypoglycemia may also occur if you skip meals or take too many pills by mistake. Weight loss should be your primary goal if you are overweight. Yet if you are taking a sulfonylurea, you should eat regularly scheduled meals. If symptoms of low blood glucose occur, eat or drink something containing sugar immediately. Instruct someone with you to take you to a doctor or a hospital if you think you are going to pass out. Even if your symptoms are easily corrected, notify your doctor of hypoglycemia. The effect of these medications may last for days, with hypoglycemia reappearing after its first occurrence.

SIDE EFFECTS OF ORAL HYPOGLYCEMICS

Side effects of the oral hypoglycemics are usually minimal. At times, nausea, vomiting, diarrhea and allergic reactions have been reported. While taking oral hypoglycemics, be cautious about your exposure to sunlight, especially if you have a history of sun sensitivity. The disulfiram reaction, also known as the Antabuse effect, may occur with the use of chlorpropamide (Diabinese). Antabuse is a drug used in the treatment of alcoholics. When people taking Antabuse drink alcohol, a severe reaction occurs. This same reaction occurs if you take oral hypoglycemics and drink alcohol. You may suffer a sudden flushing of the face and skin, nausea, vomiting, dizziness, sweating and a pounding headache. Check with your doctor regarding his recommendations concerning drinking alcohol when taking oral hypoglycemics. Water retention is a side effect of chlorpropamide. If you take Diabinese, be alert to swelling or puffiness of the face, hands or ankles as well as fatigue, shortness of breath or muscle cramps. Notify your doctor if such symptoms occur.

DRUG INTERACTION

Any medication that you take may react with other medications. Often people with diabetes have other medical conditions that require the use of drugs. Usually these drugs do not interfere with the action of the oral hypoglycemic drugs, but certain interactions should be discussed.

A possible interaction may occur between the sulfa antibiotics and the sulfonylureas; both have a similar sulfa base. Although the oral hypoglycemics do not work as antibiotics, the combination of drugs, particularly with tolbutamide (Orinase), may cause hypoglycemia. As previously mentioned, an Antabuse effect is seen in combination with alcohol and sulfonylureas, particularly Diabinese. Here, the action of the oral agent is affected by the use of another drug, alcohol.

Propranolol (Inderal) is often prescribed for hypertension, angina and other conditions. This drug blocks insulin release from the beta cells that is stimulated by the sulfonylureas. It also may mask signs of hypoglycemia, so it must be used cautiously in diabetic persons. Thiazide diuretics are types of "water pills" that may be prescribed for treatment of hypertension or edema. These, together with oral hypoglycemics, may block insulin release, causing hyperglycemia. Potassium stores may be lost as a result of the diuretic's action. This also raises blood glucose. Therefore, if you take a thiazide diuretic and an oral hypoglycemic, potassium replacement is necessary.

Diabetic persons who have arthritis or gout must monitor their medication. Aspirin and sulfonylureas may work together to lower blood glucose. Your dose of the oral hypoglycemic may have to be decreased to prevent hypoglycemia. Glucocorticoid steroids (cortisone and its derivatives) may be used for asthma or arthritis. Glucocorticoids cause hyperglycemia by increasing gluconeogenesis. Allopurinol (Zyloprim), a medication used in the treatment of gout, may cause a tendency toward hypoglycemia, particularly if you are taking Diabinese. See the following list for a review of drug interactions with oral hypoglycemic agents.

DRUG INTERACTIONS WITH ORAL HYPOGLYCEMICS

These drugs may increase the action of oral hypoglycemics:

   Alcohol
   Aspirin
   Sulfa antibiotics
   MAO inhibitors (medicine for depression)
   Phenylbutazone (anti-inflammatory drug)

These drugs may decrease the action of oral hypoglycemics:

   Steroids
   Furosemide (diuretic)
   Oral contraceptives
   Thiazide diuretics
   Propranolol (Inderal)

In today's world, where you may see many doctors for varied complaints, it is important to tell them you have diabetes and the medications you take. Knowing the names and dosages of your medication will help to prevent drug interactions. Before you take any new drug, ask your doctor and pharmacist about specific associated drug interactions and side effects.

THE UGDP STUDY

The importance of diet was emphasized in the University Group Diabetes Program Study. This study compared different treatments of non-insulin-dependent diabetes. The investigation concluded that a combination treatment of diet and oral agents was no more effective than diet alone for the non-insulin-dependent diabetic person. Other results of this study were controversial and should be examined.

Between 1961 and 1969, 823 participants in the UGDP Study received four different treatments for their non-insulin-dependent diabetes. The UGDP Study failed to demonstrate a benefit of any of the treatments. Excessive deaths from cardiovascular disease were found among those patients taking tolbutamide. These results caused a major controversy. On the basis of these findings, many doctors chose not to use oral hypoglycemics. Other doctors critically analyzed the study and felt that its conclusions were not valid. The disagreement over the UGDP Study has not been totally settled. Whether oral hypoglycemics should be used has now become a decision to be made by the doctor in conjunction with the patient. Doctors prescribe this medication after considering your health needs, your success with diet and your general health. If used properly, oral hypoglycemics can be effective in lowering blood glucose. Nonetheless, sulfonylureas are chemical substances which are not normally present in the body. All drugs are expected to have side effects. No one will disagree that weight loss is preferable to the use of drugs. There is no risk to your health in being of normal weight!

WHO SHOULD OR SHOULD NOT TAKE ORAL SULFONYLUREAS?

While there is still controversy concerning whether sulfonylureas should ever be used, the following is what we consider reasonable advice.

1. Sulfonylureas should *not* be used in persons with Type I diabetes.
2. Sulfonylureas should *not* be used as a substitute for weight reduction in the obese Type II diabetic person.
3. Sulfonylureas should *not* be used in persons with Type II diabetes who are rapidly losing weight because of hyperglycemia (use insulin).
4. Sulfonylureas should *not* be used (or used cautiously) in patients with heart failure, liver or kidney disease.
5. Sulfonylureas should *not* be continued if they are unsuccessful in controlling blood glucose.
6. Sulfonylureas should *not* be used in children or pregnant women.
7. Sulfonylureas *may* be used in the Type II diabetic person who has lost weight and remains hyperglycemic.
8. Sulfonylureas *may* be used in the obese Type II diabetic to control hyperglycemia while he is losing weight.
9. Sulfonylureas *should* be used in the Type II diabetic person with symptoms of hyperglycemia who cannot or will not take insulin.

PRIMARY VS. SECONDARY FAILURE

There are cases where oral hypoglycemics do not work (primary failure or secondary failure). In primary failure, the oral agent never adequately controlled blood glucose from the beginning of therapy. Primary failure occurs within a period of one month. About one-third of all patients who appear to be candidates for the use of oral hypoglycemics fail to respond. Thin Type II diabetic persons will often not respond to their use. Primary failure may also be due to not taking the drug or overeating.

Secondary failure occurs after the drug has been working for some time. This may also occur in one-third of all patients taking oral hypoglycemics. The UGDP Study found that the natural course of Type II diabetes is for the blood glucose to increase with time. This is probably because, as years pass, the pancreas is able to produce less insulin. Eventually, the oral hypoglycemic may not adequately control blood glucose and a switch to insulin becomes necessary. Some patients, though, have been taking oral agents for over twenty years with good control. See Table 8 for the standards of blood glucose control the American Diabetes Association (ADA) has set up regarding treatment with oral hypoglycemics.

TABLE 8
STANDARDS OF CONTROL WITH ORAL AGENTS

Relation to Food	Degree of Control		
	GOOD	FAIR	POOR
	Whole blood glucose in mg./dl.		
Fasting	110	130	All Other Readings
1 hour after food	150	180	
2 hours after food	130	150	
3 hours after food	110	130	

("Standards of Control with Oral Agents", ADA, *Present Status of Oral Agents*, used with permission.)

GUIDELINES FOR TAKING ORAL HYPOGLYCEMICS

In order to obtain the best effect from oral hypoglycemics, it is essential that you follow these guidelines:

1. Follow your diet closely. This medication will not work if you neglect your diet.
2. Know the full name of your medication, its correct spelling, pronunciation, dosage and the times you are to take medication. Know expected effects of the drugs and its side effects.
3. Take this medication only as your doctor directs. Taking more of the medication thinking that it will improve your condition is dangerous. Taking less of a medication than the doctor has prescribed is also harmful. Take your medication at the same time each day.

4. If you forget to take one dose of your medication, take it as soon as possible after remembering. If it is almost time for your next dose of medication, do not take the missed dose at all and *do not* double the next dose. Return to your normal schedule.
5. If you have difficulty remembering to take your medication, you may wish to sort out a week's supply into separate containers with labels.
6. Do not take any other medication unless your doctor has prescribed or approved it. Many people abuse over-the-counter drugs such as medication for colds and appetite-control pills.
7. Continue home testing while taking oral antidiabetic medication. You will be able to judge whether your diabetes is controlled, as well as to observe any early problems with diabetes self-management.
8. Wear or carry identification stating that you are taking this medication for diabetes.
9. Tell other doctors as well as your dentist that you take oral hypoglycemics.
10. Finally, do not hesitate to ask any questions about the medication you are receiving. It may be helpful for you to write down questions and bring them to the attention of your doctor or pharmacist.

In conclusion, oral hypoglycemic agents can be used to lower your blood glucose if you do not have Type I diabetes. However, they are not oral insulin. They work by increasing the release of insulin from the beta cells and by increasing insulin receptors. Sulfonylureas must be used with diet and exercise. Dietary control is a major component of treatment. There are many different types of oral agents with different durations of action. If you take this medication, take precautions to avoid hypoglycemia and be aware of possible side effects as well as interactions with other drugs you may be taking.

6

Pharmacology of Insulin

In 1921, F. G. Banting and C. H. Best, working together in Ontario, Canada, started an important project. They took islet tissues from animals and injected an extract into diabetic dogs. They found that they could lower the dogs' blood glucose levels. After its discovery, the name "isletin" was given to insulin because of its origin in the islet cells. Later, the term "insulin" was used. The insulin you use may be taken from the pancreas of a cow or pig. Pork insulin most closely resembles human insulin, differing in only one amino acid.

"Endogenous" insulin is that which is secreted naturally from the pancreas. "Exogenous" insulin is that which is injected into the body. Insulin cannot be swallowed because it would be destroyed by the stomach juices.

All too often, you may think of the action of insulin only in association with the food you eat. Insulin's role in moving glucose into the cell (thereby helping blood glucose remain normal) is very important. However, insulin does much more than affect glucose metabolism. Insulin has been described in Chapter 1. Now the many roles of insulin will be reviewed.

Insulin has other roles in metabolism, unrelated to food. Important roles of insulin are detailed here. If you think of insulin in general terms as acting only to lower blood glucose, you may forget the other important roles of insulin. Because of this, you may not fully respect the role of insulin. This can lead to a dangerous situation often seen during illness. If you think that insulin works only to lower blood glucose and you become ill, you may not take your insulin. You may think that you don't need insulin because you will not be eating, not realizing that if you omit insulin your blood glucose will continue to rise even if you eat nothing. Keep in mind all of the many roles of insulin. Insulin does not affect blood glucose alone. Its effect is seen on fats, proteins and carbohydrates. Remember, insulin works not only to use glucose properly but also to keep glucose in a normal range.

ROLES OF INSULIN

Effect on Carbohydrates
1. Allows glucose to enter the cell.
2. Stores glucose as *glycogen* in the liver.
3. Inhibits the breakdown of *glycogen* (*glycogenolysis*).
4. Inhibits the new production of glucose (*gluconeogenesis*).

Effect on Fats
1. Allows glucose to enter the fat cell.
2. Stimulates lipogenesis (*fat formation*).
3. Stores fatty substances from dietary fat.
4. Prevents stored fat from being released into the bloodstream (*lipolysis*).

Effect on Proteins
1. Allows glucose to enter the muscle.
2. Stores glucose as *glycogen* in the muscle.
3. Prevents the breakdown of protein and release of amino acids back into the bloodstream.

PHARMACOLOGICAL ACTIONS OF INSULIN

Pharmacology is the study of drugs. Injected insulin is a drug that differs in several ways from the insulin normally secreted by the pancreas. Moreover, the insulin has been chemically changed to achieve a variety of pharmacological actions. Three important pharmacological aspects of different types of insulins are the onset, peak and duration of action. You will not be able to self-manage diabetes properly without a knowledge of these aspects. Onset of action refers to the time period when the specific type of insulin begins to work. Peak of action refers to the time when insulin is working at its strongest. Duration of action refers to the time period that a particular insulin's action will last. All of these are usually expressed in terms of hours.

INDIVIDUAL HUMAN RESPONSE TO INSULIN

The action of insulin may differ among individuals. Insulin's action may be affected by a variety of factors, such as diet, exercise, infection or illness. The injection site, the depth of the injection and other medications may also influence its action. The duration of the action of insulin may be changed by the development of antibodies. Exogenous insulin is a foreign substance, so the body will react to it by producing antibodies. These antibodies bind with the insulin and may vary the timing of onset, peak and duration from individual to individual. For example, Regular insulin has an average onset within thirty minutes to one hour, with a peak activity within two to four hours. In certain people, the onset of action may be lengthened to two hours and the peak activity not seen until a later time.

TYPES OF INSULIN

Insulins are divided into three major categories according to their duration of effect. These are: short-acting, intermediate-acting and long-acting insulins. Regular insulin is a short-acting insulin. It was the first insulin developed and the only one available for fifteen years. It is composed of zinc insulin crystals in a clear solution.

Modifications have been made in insulin since 1921, in order to make its use more flexible. Fifteen years after Regular insulin became available, PZI insulin was developed to avoid multiple injections of Regular insulin. PZI stands for protamine zinc insulin. PZI insulin, a long-acting insulin, was made by adding a protein, protamine. The insulin becomes bound to the protein and its action is extended because it is absorbed more slowly from the site of injection. A buffer, phosphate, was also added. There are disadvantages to using a long-acting insulin. The peak of PZI insulin often comes during the middle of the night, causing hypoglycemia when you are asleep. An intermediate-acting insulin was developed to prevent this.

NPH stands for neutral protamine Hagedorn. A mixture of PZI, Regular insulin and a phosphate buffer was found to produce an intermediate-acting insulin. NPH is a cloudy insulin. Because of the ratio of the protamine in NPH insulin, NPH insulin can be mixed with Regular insulin. Each insulin retains its own properties even though it is mixed with the other.

Other types of insulin to be aware of are part of the Lente family of insulins. Lente insulins are made up of zinc crystals. Zinc delays the absorption of insulin. By increasing the size of the zinc crystals of Lente insulin, the time of action of the insulin lengthens. Semilente insulin is similar to Regular insulin in its action. It is of short duration and contains an acetate buffer. Smaller-size zinc crystals cause its rapid action. Ultralente insulin is the large crystal form of zinc insulin. It is long-acting. Lente insulin is a mixture of 70 percent Ultralente and 30 percent Semilente insulin. It has almost the same characteristics as NPH insulin. Remember that these are average characteristics and that the actions of insulins may vary greatly among individuals. On an average, short-acting insulins have an onset of ½ to 1 hour, a peak of 2 to 4 hours and a duration of 5 to 7 hours. Intermediate-acting insulins have an onset of 1 to 3 hours, a peak of 6 to 12 hours and a duration of 24 to 28 hours. Long-acting insulins have an onset of 4 to 6 hours, a peak of 14 to 24 hours, and a duration of over 36 hours.

STRENGTH OF INSULIN

The dosage of most medications is measured in weight as milligrams or grams. Insulin, however, is measured in units. A unit is an international standard that is the same for every insulin. One unit measures specific blood-glucose-lowering activity or strength. The strengths of insulin are expressed as a U followed by a number. This number represents how many insulin units are dissolved in one cubic centimeter or milliliter. U-100 insulin means that there are 100 units of insulin in 1 cc. One cubic centimeter (cc.) is equivalent to one milliliter (ml.) or 1/30th of an ounce. In 1971, the American Diabetes Association and the Food and Drug Administration agreed that only one concentration of insulin should be available. U-100 insulin was introduced in the United States early in 1973. In the past, insulin strengths varied from U-40 to U-80. U-80 insulin (80 units of insulin in 1 cc.) is no longer available. Today, U-100 insulin is the most widely available and most often used strength of insulin.

U-100 insulin has certain advantages. It makes calculations simple. It is more highly concentrated and purified. Less volume needs to be injected. For example, using U-100 insulin, 100 units equals one milliliter. With U-40 insulin, 40 units equals one milliliter. In the past, if you took 40 units daily and used U-40 insulin, you would need to take an entire milliliter as a dose. Using U-100 insulin and taking 40 units daily involves taking less than 0.5 milliliter (cc.) of insulin, less than 0.5 cubic centimeter of a syringe of insulin. Remember, a unit size remains the same because one unit of U-40 insulin performs the same as one unit of U-100. The strength does not vary, only the amount given. The dosage of insulin prescribed for you is determined as the amount necessary to maintain good control. The requirement of 40 units instead of 30 units does not mean that diabetes is "worse" in individuals who require 40 units.

PURITY OF INSULIN

Since the discovery of insulin, much effort has been exerted to improve the concentration, duration of action and purity of insulins. When insulin is extracted from the pancreas of a cow or pig, other substances such as proinsulin, glucagon and somatostatin are also present. These are considered contaminants. The FDA regards the proinsulin content as an indicator of insulin purity. All insulins sold in the United States have a proinsulin content under 25 p.p.m. Under ordinary circumstances, there is no proven advantage in using "purified" insulins (less than 10 p.p.m.).

U.S. Pharmacopeia (USP) refers to the standard that all pharmaceutical products must match in order to meet the FDA requirements. Modern techniques have greatly improved the purity of insulins. In 1972, Eli Lilly and Company introduced a more refined product called single peak insulin. Single peak insulin referred to electrochemical studies that showed that insulin is composed of mostly one substance. From 1980 to the present time, Lilly insulins have undergone further purification. Lilly's Iletin I insulins have a proinsulin content of less than 20 p.p.m.; Lilly's Iletin II insulins have a proinsulin content of less than 10 p.p.m.

Two purified insulins are new to the United States, although they have been available in Europe since the mid-seventies. Novo insulin is highly purified, having less than 1 p.p.m. of proinsulin. Novo Laboratories has recently associated with Squibb to form Squibb-Novo, Inc. This company now conducts marketing activities for a full range of insulins produced by Novo and sold in the United States by Squibb. The Squibb "new" insulins have a proinsulin content of less than 25 p.p.m. These insulins are available as Regular (pork), Isophane (NPH) (beef), Lente (beef), Semilente (beef), Ultralente (beef) and Protamine Zinc (beef). Novo's insulins are now manufactured as Actrapid (Regular, pork), Monotard (Lente, pork), Lentard (Lente, beef/pork), Semitard (Semilente, pork) and Ultratard (Ultralente, beef).

Nordisk's insulins are purified pork insulins with a proinsulin content of less than 10 p.p.m. Nordisk's insulins are manufactured as Velosulin (rapid-acting), Insulatard, NPH (intermediate-acting) and Mixtard (intermediate-acting, premixed).

Pork insulin is most similar to human insulin. The best type of insulin and purity content for you must be decided in consultation with your doctor. There are certain situations where the use of purified pork insulin is indicated. For example, patients who are on temporary insulin therapy during times of stress or pregnancy may develop insulin antibodies due to the use of insulin therapy. For this reason, patients who will be using insulin for a short period of time only should be using purified pork insulin since they may need insulin again in the future. Other examples will be given later in the chapter.

HUMAN INSULIN

The field of recombinant DNA (deoxyribonucleic acid) technology has allowed a genetic message for the production of human insulin to be placed into bacteria. DNA is the cellular material containing genetic messages which tell cells how to act. This message enters the bacteria and instructs them to produce human insulin. As the bacteria grow, the insulin message is duplicated. We know that bacteria can grow rapidly, so mass production of human insulin is possible. Chemically, the insulin produced by these altered bacteria is identical to human insulin. Treatment with human insulin is now being used in the United States. Its importance is twofold. Human insulin produced through recombinant DNA may cause fewer immunological problems than other insulins derived from animal sources. Human insulin will also increase the potential supply of insulin throughout the world so you will not have to depend on an animal supply. Eli Lilly and Company has introduced Humulin (human insulin of recombinant DNA origin) in the United States. Squibb-Novo has recently produced human insulin as well. This insulin preparation is not made by recombinant DNA technology. Instead, pork insulin is changed chemically (through an enzymatic conversion of amino acids) into human insulin.

INSULIN TREATMENT REGIMES

At the present time many different kinds of insulin treatment programs are being used. For years scientists worked at obtaining an insulin that would last all day. Prior to this, once Regular insulin was introduced, people were injecting insulin as often as four to six times a day. The NPH type of insulin was considered of benefit because it necessitated only one daily injection. Then Regular insulin therapy fell out of favor. Now, in order to achieve blood glucose control, a variety of insulin regimes are being used. Doctors and patients are realizing that one injection a day will not adequately control diabetes in most Type I patients. Think of the human body without diabetes, with 10 million beta cells detecting the blood glucose level, and instantly secreting insulin when necessary. Then contrast this to the daily administration of a single dose of exogenous insulin. You can easily see the imperfection of a single-dose system.

Insulin is normally constantly present in the circulation, but in different amounts. In the fasting state, a basal or low level of insulin is needed to control metabolism. This small amount of insulin is required in the absence of eating to prevent hyperglycemia and ketosis. Additional insulin is needed each time food is eaten, in order to use the food (and thereby keep blood glucose from large fluctuations). When Type I diabetes first occurs, one injection of intermediate-acting insulin may be adequate when the pancreas still produces some insulin. The single injection is adequate to supplement the basal insulin deficiency. However, in time, as the amount of insulin secreted by the pancreas decreases, a single injection may not be sufficient. All you can get from a single injection of intermediate-acting insulin is the basal insulin requirement with an afternoon peak. Although the FBS (fasting blood sugar) may be normal, blood glucose will rise after meals because the extra insulin needed to metabolize food is neither secreted nor injected. Thus, there are two goals of insulin treatment (just as there are two purposes of normal insulin secretion): (a) to provide adequate basal insulin to control metabolism when not eating and (b) to provide supplementary spurts of insulin before eating so that food may be used appropriately. The former may be achieved with intermediate- or long-acting insulin; the latter is achieved with supplementary injections of Regular insulin. Often patients ask, "Can't I just take Regular insulin before my meals?" Regular insulin may adequately lower blood glucose for a short period during mealtime but will not control gluconeogenesis when you are not eating. An intermediate- or long-acting insulin is necessary for this. Simply, the basal insulin supply prevents elevated blood glucose in the fasting state by controlling gluconeogenesis and glycogenolysis. You need additional insulin to prevent elevated blood glucose after eating. This may be achieved by taking intermediate- or long-acting insulin once a day with Regular insulin before meals, by taking two injections of mixed insulins or by using an insulin infusion system.

Some doctors recommend a long-acting insulin with multiple injections of Regular insulin before meals. Others may recommend using two separate injections to control blood glucose. When you take a morning dose of NPH or Lente insulin, you may have a high fasting blood glucose. This is because the insulin is not working as effectively as needed during the early hours prior to breakfast. The addition of an evening injection of NPH or Lente may be the answer.

The thought of taking a second injection may be difficult to accept. You may feel that a second injection means your diabetes has worsened. This is a major misconception. If you are trying to set a goal of generally improving your diabetes control, increasing your insulin to two injections a day (split dose) may achieve this. If your doctor suggests two injections a day, proper planning will enable you to fit this into your lifestyle. So try not to look at this idea as one that is filled with problems and fear. Rather, begin to think of it in a more positive way, as a means to improved blood glucose control.

Another insulin treatment is that of "mixed doses," which involves mixing a short-acting and intermediate-acting insulin together. One type of insulin in the morning may not be enough to control your blood glucose after breakfast. You may have to add Regular insulin in order to obtain better control. If you are taking two intermediate-acting insulin injections (one in the A.M. and the other in the P.M.) but are still experiencing hyperglycemia after breakfast or dinner, this therapy may not be adequate in preventing a rise in blood glucose after meals. Instead you may need an insulin treatment regime called a "split and mixed dose.'' You would then take two injections a day of both an intermediate-acting and a short-acting insulin. An example of this would be taking 25 units of NPH insulin and 5 units of Regular insulin in the morning and 15 units of NPH insulin and 5 units of Regular insulin in the evening. Most people with insulin-dependent diabetes can be managed on this insulin treatment regime. A final treatment would be the use of an insulin infusion system and this will now be described.

INSULIN INFUSION SYSTEMS

Normal pancreatic beta cells produce the correct amount of insulin in response to blood glucose levels. The pancreas works in response to the feedback it receives from blood glucose concentration. In an effort to provide this type of feedback system, alternative methods of insulin delivery have been devised. This has led to the development of the insulin pump, also known as CSII (continuous subcutaneous insulin infusion). A CSII device consists of a small pump that you can wear. Insulin is constantly infused, through the pump, to meet your basal (daily) insulin needs. Boluses of insulin (a certain amount of insulin delivered at once) can be given at mealtimes to prevent hyperglycemia after meals. All portable insulin pumps differ slightly in design, but most have the same general characteristics. The pumps use a portable syringe that may be connected to a microcomputer to regulate insulin flow. The syringe is attached to a long catheter (12–40 inches) which is connected to a needle (27 gauge, ⅝ inch). The needle is inserted subcutaneously and taped in place. The site of insertion of the needle must be changed about every two days.

The pumps used today are compact and convenient to wear. They are small, usually measuring 5¼ × 3¼ × 1 inches, and lightweight, 10–13 ounces. The pump is worn twenty-four hours a day but can be removed for showering, sexual intercourse or any type of vigorous exercise. Regular insulin, alone or diluted, can be used in insulin pumps, depending on the model.

These pumps are referred to as ''open loop'' systems because they do not have a feedback system. The insulin is given continuously without a built-in report of blood glucose range. Instead, the diabetic patient must provide the answers to ''close the loop'' by careful self-monitoring of blood glucose. A closed-loop insulin pump would automatically determine blood glucose levels and properly adjust the insulin delivery rate. Although closed-loop devices are available in research settings, they are not yet being used for ambulatory patients.

You may be wondering, if the pumps offer good control as well as ease of use, why don't all patients use them? The use of a pump demands that you be responsible, capable and highly motivated. Much education is necessary for the proper care and functioning of the pump. The program of diet, exercise and emphasis on self-monitoring that accompanies the insulin pump must be rigidly followed. Assessment of whether you are psychologically ready for the pump must be made before you decide about its use. The presence of an insulin pump is an outward, noticeable sign of diabetes that is not appealing to everyone with diabetes. Interpersonal relationships with spouses, family and co-workers will be affected. Yet the benefits of improved control outweigh some of these adjustments. It is important that you discuss these things with your doctor prior to starting insulin pump therapy.

Ask your doctor about the kind of education available to you if you start to use CSII. You need comprehensive diabetes education prior to the start of therapy. Some doctors feel that hospitalization with five to seven days of education is necessary at the start. Adequate follow-up and twenty-four-hour emergency resource help is essential. Patients must also closely adhere to diet therapy when using the pump. Self-monitoring and adequate dietary adherence are necessary to the successful use of the pump.

Certain patients are considered prime candidates for insulin pump therapy. Women who are pregnant and diabetic persons who have unstable (poorly controlled) diabetes fall into this category. If your doctor does not feel that your diabetes warrants CSII treatment, ask him about the use of modified insulin and multiple doses of Regular insulin. Treatment with this intensive conventional therapy has given successful results similar to those achieved with pump therapy. The major advantage of the insulin pump, aside from the improved control, is the lifestyle flexibility the pump can offer. If you take an injection of an intermediate-acting insulin in the morning, you are committed to eating at a certain fixed time to avoid hypoglycemia. Because the bolus injection of insulin is given prior to meals with CSII treatment, hypoglycemia should not occur if meals are slightly delayed. Many patients like this freedom of lifestyle that the pump affords.

A major concern of insulin pump therapy is the prevention of hypoglycemia. Some patients have inadequate responses of contrainsulin hormones to hypoglycemia. Therefore, when they become hypoglycemic from insulin, they may not readily recover. Recently tests have been proposed to identify those patients who are at special risk for the development of hypoglycemia with CSII or intensive conventional insulin therapy. Doctors take great care in selecting patients for intensive blood glucose control using the pump. Because of the continuous supply of insulin, it is essential to avoid hypoglycemia. Dietary consistency as well as intensive self-monitoring will help to achieve this. Doctors often ask patients to monitor their 3 A.M. blood glucose to verify that they are not hypoglycemic during the night and to prevent their fasting glucose from being too low. This testing is often done in the first stages of insulin pump therapy, until control is established. Hypoglycemia is also prevented by filling the insulin syringe with only one day's dose at a time.

Although many diabetic patients may be interested in pump therapy, not everyone is a candidate for its use. If a person has not participated in diabetes self-management activities in the past, he would not be considered for the pump. Motivation and a good understanding of what is expected from you is crucial to pump therapy. You will have to read about the subject and attend classes on diabetes education. You will need to take meticulous care of insulin sites and change the sites according to your doctor's or nurse's directions. You will have to learn how to work the pump better than anyone else. You will find that, when using a pump, you must assume responsibility for your diabetes self-management, with the health-care team acting as advisers.

Many diabetic patients have misconceptions about the insulin pump. They think that they will now have total freedom from injections. This is not true. With the pumps available today, the catheter must still be inserted at regular intervals. People also think that they may now be able to eat anything that they wish. This, too, is false. If you do eat simple sugars while on the pump, you may still be able to control your blood glucose. Yet these simple sugars will nevertheless cause damage. You will eventually gain weight. Diet and weight maintenance remain important. Finally, some diabetic patients think that the pump is for everyone, a cure for diabetes. The pump is only for insulin-dependent patients, particularly those who are not well controlled on conventional therapy. It is an addition to therapy that includes diet, blood monitoring and exercise.

Insulin pumps are expensive but reimbursement is available. The success in obtaining reimbursement has varied from state to state. A letter from your doctor stating the necessity of the pump and a copy of the doctor's prescription for the pump are necessary to obtain reimbursement. Often, direct communication by the doctor with the insurance carrier is helpful.

A few of the insulin pumps in use today will now be described. Their manufacturers' addresses may be found in the "Community Resources" section at the end of this book.

One pump used for insulin delivery is the Flint Laboratories Auto-Syringe Model AS-6C-U-100. This pump has been reduced in size from its original model and now weighs under 10 ounces and measures 3.3 × 6.3 × 1 inches. It delivers a basal rate and bolus rate. The bolus rate is delivered when the patient pushes a button and holds it until the desired dosage is delivered. The digital display indicates the number of insulin units delivered. After the bolus rate is given, and if the patient forgets to switch back to the basal rate, the pump will automatically switch back to the basal mode. This machine also has an alarm system. It is priced at about $1,200. The pump uses U-100 insulin and does not need dilution.

Cardiac Pacemaker, Inc.'s Model 9100 portable insulin pump became available in August 1981. This device has a microcomputer which provides a controlled subcutaneous insulin infusion. The pump weighs 3 ounces and it can be easily programmed to deliver a basal dose, bolus doses and a supplemental dose (programmed for delayed delivery). It has several special features such as a "hold" to stop insulin delivery without erasing the programming, a lockout to prevent accidental reprogramming and an alarm system. The pump uses any commercially available Regular insulin without dilution. It is supplied with three rechargeable battery packs, a recharger, disposable syringes, infusion sets and a diary for recording blood glucoses. It is priced at $1,995, which includes supplies for approximately two years.

Other insulin pumps available in 1983 include the Delta Medical Industries pump; the Markwell Medical Institute, Inc., Pen Pump Infuser; the Medix Corporation Medix 209-100 pump; the Orange Medical Instruments, Inc., Beta I Infusion pump; the Pacesetter Systems, Inc., Micromed pump; and the Windsor Medical Inc. Mark I Ambulatory Infusion Device (AID). Continued research is helping to make insulin pumps more lightweight, efficient and usable.

The "closed loop" devices are now being studied. These are more sophisticated devices that have a feedback system to control the delivery of insulin. The insulin delivery rate is automatically adjusted on the basis of the internal monitoring of blood glucose. The key to this device is the miniaturization of the glucose sensor. The glucose sensor acts like your pancreas, sensing blood glucose and releasing the appropriate amount of insulin. A form of this "artificial beta cell" has been made by the Life Science Instrument Division of Miles Laboratories, Elkhart, Indiana. It is known as the Biostator and is used only in investigative studies. Implantable open-loop infusion pumps have been developed and are being tested at the present time. These insulin infusion devices are small enough to implant (like a pacemaker) yet large enough to hold a sufficient reservoir of insulin, allowing freedom from catheter lines.

You now have much information about what insulin does, how kinds of insulin differ and how they are often prescribed. The next chapter will discuss some practical aspects of insulin administration.

7

The Use of Insulin

This chapter will discuss more practical aspects of insulin. You will learn specific information about taking care of insulin supplies as well as the actual technique of insulin injection.

BUYING AND STORING OF INSULIN

When you buy insulin, check the box and bottle for the proper name of the insulin. Check that the proper strength of the insulin is listed as well as the expiration date. Plan ahead for an emergency. Always store at least one extra bottle of insulin to use if something happens to your present bottle. Rotate your supplies, using your oldest supplies of insulin first. The pharmacy will exchange unopened bottles that are past the expiration date.

Storage of insulin should pose no problem. Insulin you are not using can be stored in the refrigerator. Avoid freezing insulin (this will cause it to become less potent). Avoid high temperatures (above 72° F.). Insulin in current use should not be refrigerated. Fewer skin problems at the injection site will result if you store it at room temperature. All insulins retain their strength at room temperature for many months.

Check your insulin bottle carefully. Regular insulin should be clear. Discard any bottle of Regular insulin that is cloudy. Discard any bottle of insulin that is discolored. When you are examining your insulin bottle you will see that there is a number on it that says 10 cc. This tells you that there are 10 cubic centimeters of insulin in the bottle. U-100 insulin means that there are 100 units in each cc. of insulin. If there are a total of 10 cc. in the bottle, the bottle contains 1,000 units (10 cc. × 100 units = 1,000 units). If you divide the 1,000 units by your daily dosage of insulin, you will find how many days one bottle of insulin will last. For example, if you are taking 10 units of insulin daily and using a bottle of U-100 insulin, divide 1,000 units by 10 units. You now know that you will be using this insulin for a little over three months, or 100 days.

You will need to purchase needles and syringes in order to administer your insulin. Needles for insulin can vary in size but are approximately one-half inch long. The needle gauge size indicates the thickness of the needle and is usually 28. The lower the needle gauge, the thicker the needle. For example, an 18-gauge needle is very wide; a 28-gauge needle is very thin. Needles should be thin and sharp to decrease discomfort at the injection site.

Syringes hold the insulin and are usually labeled in numbers of up to 100 units, or 1 cc. New syringes have been developed for patients who are taking less than 50 units. These syringes hold 0.5 cc. and are called Lo-dose (Becton Dickinson) or Mini Syringes (Monoject). These may help you to administer the insulin more easily since they are divided into 1-unit measurements. Both Becton Dickinson and Monoject, which are the primary syringe makers for insulin, produce 0.5 cc. and 1 cc. syringes. Both companies are trying to produce the finest insulin syringe and needle that will produce the least discomfort.

Some people are unable to inject themselves because they fear discomfort. Automatic injectors are available for those who are unable to inject themselves. An automatic injector may be used in special circumstances. A syringe is filled with insulin and then placed in the injector. When the injector is set against the skin the needle is triggered to go through the skin. The patient must then push the plunger down to inject the insulin. One type of instrument like this is the Injectomatic, available from the Monoject Company.

The injection itself may pose a psychological problem for many people. Syringes have long been associated with pain, discomfort, hospitals or illness. The first major problem encountered by many diabetic persons is the necessity of having to take insulin. Insulin administration is only a technique that once mastered can become a routine part of your life. Other factors of diabetes self-management are far more important than mastering the insulin injection alone. Yet if the idea of insulin self-administration is the most frightening one to you, this becomes the first important problem to solve. It helps if you speak to others about their feelings regarding insulin administration. Recognize that insulin self-administration is a difficult task. Speak about any fears or anxieties that you have to health professionals or other members of your own support group. Oftentimes, the fear of the insulin administration is worse than the act itself. We see an example of this in the use of oranges in a hospital setting. Often when someone is newly diagnosed, he is told to practice insulin administration on an orange. If days go by and the person is left practicing on the orange and not giving himself the injection directly, his fear of the pain, discomfort and difficulty in injecting intensifies. For this reason, we recommend that a person be instructed immediately, if willing, in self-injection. The worst injection is the first one. Before you learn more about other areas of diabetes self-management, you should feel comfortable with giving yourself your own insulin in a safe and accurate manner.

INSULIN ADMINISTRATION

Insulin administration begins by gathering your equipment. You can decide whether to use a glass or plastic syringe. Today, because of the convenience of disposable plastic syringes, few people in the United States use glass syringes. If you use a glass syringe, it may be reused, but it must be kept clean. Glass syringes can be purchased with disposable needles. After use, the glass syringe must be taken apart and boiled for at least five minutes. Then replace the syringe, without touching the inside of the plunger, and store it in alcohol. Prior to using the syringe again, make sure that the alcohol has dried off inside the syringe. You can do this by repeatedly drawing air in and out of the syringe. Disposable syringes are made of plastic and should never be boiled. Purchase extra syringes just as you would extra insulin.

Your equipment should be spotlessly clean, as should the skin area where you inject the insulin. Skin can never be sterilized. "Sterilization" refers to the total absence of bacteria. Some bacteria always remain on the skin, but cleaning the area well will reduce any chances of infection. Infections at the site of the injection are rare and are usually caused by poor hygiene practices. Insulin in the bottle is sterile and must remain so. The needle, too, must be sterile because it enters the bottle and your skin. Avoid contamination of the insulin syringe needle, the plunger and the inside of the barrel of the syringe since they will come in contact with the sterile insulin.

How do you select a site for insulin injection? The site selection and rotation must be individualized. You will develop your own system based on the number of injections you take each day. Insulin is injected into the subcutaneous tissue. This tissue lies between the fat layer just under the skin and the muscle layer below. The following areas are preferred for insulin injections because they lie away from joints, nerves and large blood vessels: the front and side areas of the thighs, the upper outer aspect of the arms, the upper outer aspect of the buttocks, and the abdomen (see Figures 4 and 5). Avoid the area of the navel and waistline, where friction from a belt could cause irritation. Avoid injecting into areas that you will be exercising. Insulin may be absorbed more rapidly from them. Choose one of these areas and inject into it for 5–7 days, making

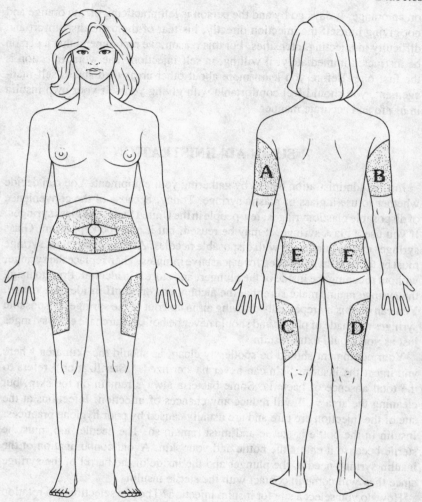

Figures 4 and 5. Insulin injection sites. The gray areas show where insulin may be safely injected. (Adapted with permission from Site Selection and Rotation, *Becton Dickinson and Company.)*

sure that each injection is 1½ inches apart. Keep a record of each injection, marking the date on the calendar shown in Figure 6. Keep a record of your insulin site rotations. This will remind you of where you last gave your injection. This is particularly important when you are taking two injections on a daily

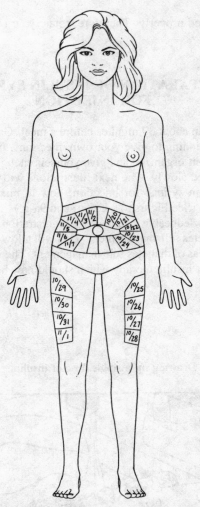

Figure 6. Calendar of sites for injection. You may draw your own body calendar of where and when you have injected your insulin.

basis. Insulin site rotation is done to prevent skin problems at the area of injection. Examine insulin sites carefully for any signs of redness, bruising and inflammation. If you constantly give an insulin injection in only one area, the area may harden into a lump, known as hypertrophy. If this develops, insulin will not be absorbed properly. Therefore, rotate your sites according to your record.

PREPARATION OF INSULIN SYRINGE
FOR INJECTION

Take your insulin about 30 minutes before a meal. Gather your equipment. If you are just beginning to give your own injections, find a private area, try to relax, get yourself organized and give yourself enough time so that you are not rushed. Proceed slowly. The next illustrations will help describe how to prepare your insulin syringe for injection, how to mix insulins and how to administer insulin. (See Figures 7a-h, 8a-j and 9a-g.)

Careful and knowledgeable insulin self-administration will put you in control of this part of diabetes self-management. This will allow you to concentrate on other important areas of diabetes self-management. There are three other areas of complications of insulin therapy which should now be addressed.

Drawing up a single dose of insulin.

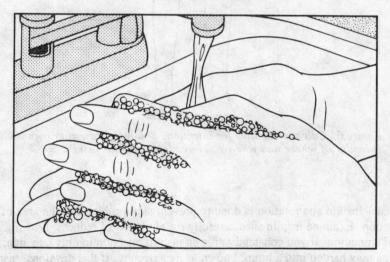

Figure 7a. Before beginning, wash your hands vigorously with hot water and a mild soap.

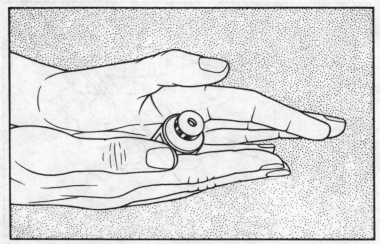

Figure 7b. Rotate the bottle of insulin in the palms of your hands to gently mix the insulin. Do not shake the bottle.

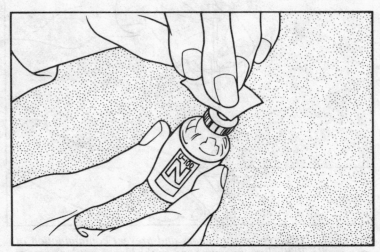

Figure 7c. Wipe the tip of the insulin bottle with a cotton ball soaked in alcohol or an alcohol swab. Place the insulin bottle on a flat surface.

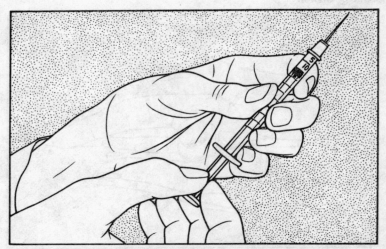

Figure 7d. Remove the needle cover and pull the plunger back to the unit that marks your dose, in this case, 10 units. You have now filled the syringe with air.

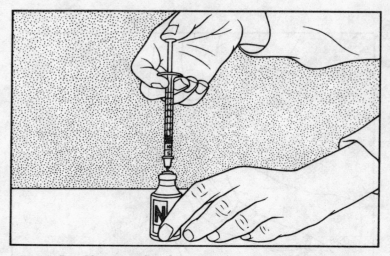

Figure 7e. Observe safety factors and prevent contamination of the needle. While keeping your hand on the insulin bottle to steady it, push the needle into the rubber bottle cap. Push the plunger so that air is pushed inside the bottle.

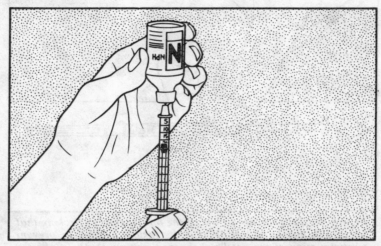

Figure 7f. Now invert your bottle of insulin, holding it in the palm of your hand, and pull the plunger about five units past your dosage mark. Make sure that you are drawing insulin back into the syringe.

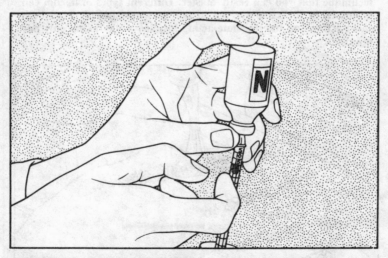

Figure 7g. Check the syringe for air bubbles. Remember that the danger from air bubbles is that they displace insulin in the syringe. You will get less insulin than your prescribed dose. Remove air bubbles by flicking the syringe softly with your finger. Then push the plunger back to your dosage mark.

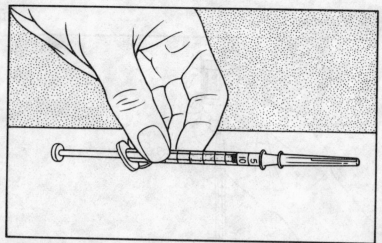

Figure 7h. Take the needle out of the bottle, slowly checking that no insulin has been lost. Recap the insulin syringe to prevent contamination of the needle. You are now prepared to give your insulin injection. At times, you may take a mixture of two different kinds of insulin. You would then mix the insulins, as directed by your doctor or nurse, in one syringe. Figure 8 illustrates how this is done.

Mixing insulins may seem complicated but is, in fact, another technique that you can easily master. Different types of insulin can be mixed in the same syringe so that you may benefit from both short-acting and intermediate-acting insulins while taking only one injection.

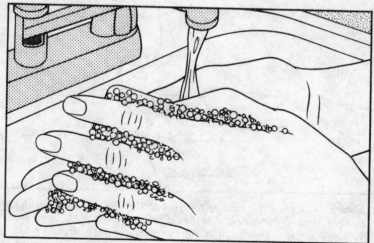

Figure 8a. Wash your hands and organize your equipment as previously described.

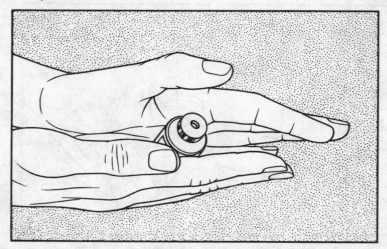

Figure 8b. Mix each bottle of insulin by rotating it slowly in your palms.

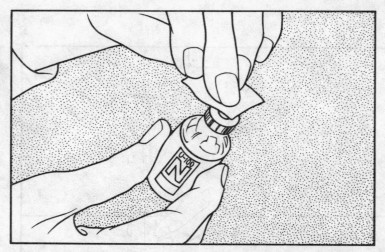

Figure 8c. Clean the top of each insulin bottle with alcohol.

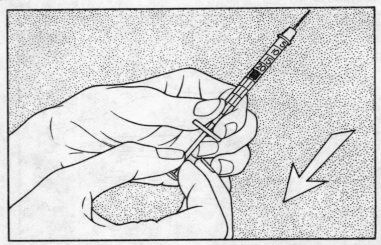

Figure 8d. In this example, you will be drawing up 20 units of NPH insulin and 10 units of Regular insulin. Determine the total amount of the mixed dose by adding the doses of Regular and modified insulin together. First draw 20 units of air into the syringe by pulling the plunger back to 20 units.

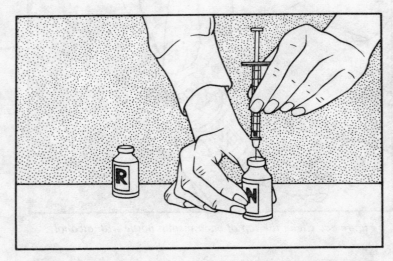

Figure 8e. Insert the needle into the bottle of NPH insulin. Push the air into the bottle. Pull the needle out of the stopper without drawing up any insulin. Be careful not to contaminate the sterile needle. You have just put air pressure into the bottle for later use.

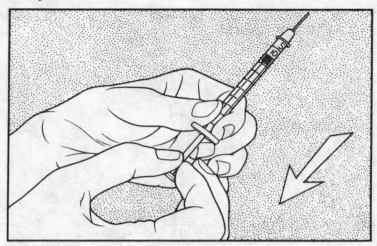

Figure 8f. Now draw 10 units of air into the syringe by pulling the plunger back to 10 units.

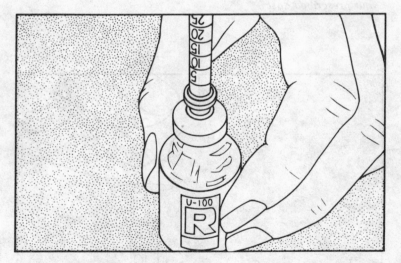

Figure 8g. Inject the air into the Regular insulin by pushing on the plunger. Leave the syringe in the bottle this time.

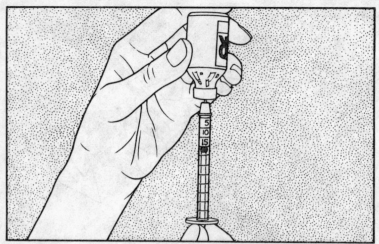

Figure 8h. Turn the bottle of clear insulin upside down with the syringe in it. Keep the needle under the level of insulin in the bottle and cradle the insulin and the syringe in the palm of your hand. Pull back on the syringe to an amount about 5 units past your prescribed dose.

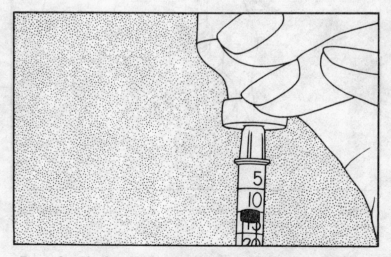

Figure 8i. Check again for air bubbles. Push the plunger back to your prescribed dose and withdraw the correct amount of Regular insulin.

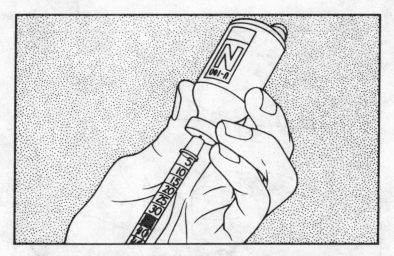

Figure 8j. Reinsert the needle into the bottle of NPH insulin and immediately withdraw the amount required to make up the total dose of the mixed insulin. In this case, the total would be 30 units.

Always follow the same routine in drawing up the clear insulin first and the cloudy insulin second. In this way you will prevent contamination of the Regular insulin bottle. (It may be necessary to use Regular insulin later on during an emergency.) Make this part of your daily routine to prevent errors in the future. You are now prepared to give your insulin injection.

Administration of insulin

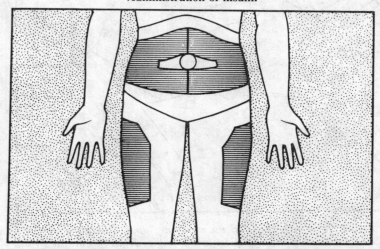

Figure 9a. Choose your insulin site after checking your record to see where your next injection should be given.

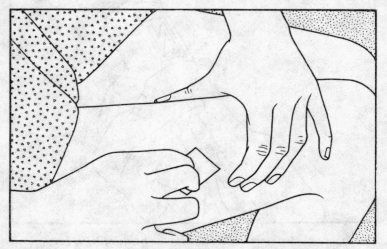

Figure 9b. In a circular motion, clean a small area around the injection site with alcohol.

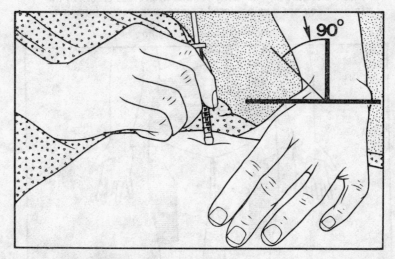

Figure 9c. Pinch the skin up with one hand. Point the needle straight toward the skin. Use a 90° angle. Hold the needle in a dartlike fashion and firmly and steadily inject.

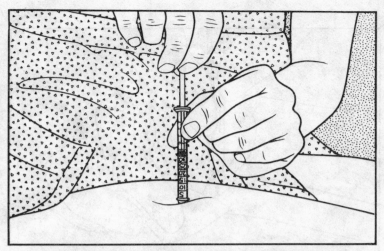

Figure 9d. Many people will check to see if blood comes into the barrel of the syringe. This is done by pulling up slightly on the syringe. If blood appears, remove the needle and begin again. Only very small blood vessels are present in the area where you are injecting, and the return of blood is not likely to be harmful. The best practice in diabetes self-management, though, is to begin again.

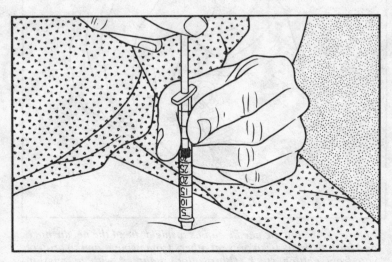

Figure 9e. If no blood appears, inject the insulin by pressing the plunger down at an even, steady rate. This should take three to six seconds, depending on the dosage.

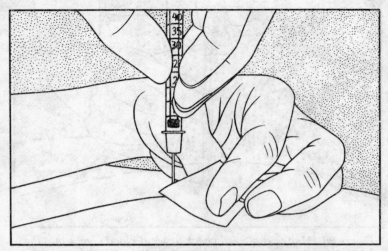

Figure 9f. Remove the needle. Wipe the skin once more, but do not rub the area.

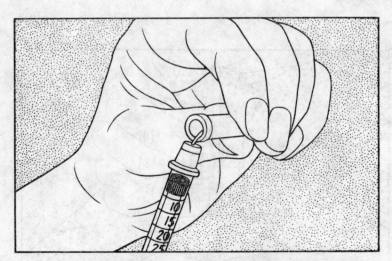

Figure 9g. Using the needle cap as a shield, bend the needle back and forth to break it, to prevent others from using it and to protect you from getting stuck. (Illustrations adapted with permission from Getting Started, *Becton Dickinson and Company.)*

INSULIN RESISTANCE

Immunological insulin resistance is said to occur when a person's insulin requirements rise dramatically. Insulin resistance has been defined as the need for more than 100–200 units of insulin per day for a period longer than two days, in the absence of infection. This is an unusually large amount of insulin. The condition of immunological insulin resistance is caused by antibodies. These are produced when the body recognizes beef or pork insulin as a foreign substance. In this condition, there are high levels of antibodies that neutralize insulin's action. Because these antibodies neutralize the effect of insulin, the insulin dosage is increased to high levels to control blood glucose. An insulin known as U-500, with 500 units of insulin in 1 cc., is available for use during insulin resistance. Other methods of dealing with immunological resistance include the use of purified pork insulin or human insulin as well as cortisone. Six weeks to three months after beginning insulin therapy, all patients develop antibodies that bind insulin to a certain extent. Binding of insulin prevents it from working effectively. The binding that occurs may involve less than 10 units, but when insulin resistance develops, binding is 6 to 1,000 times that amount. This may occur less commonly with the current use of more purified insulins.

Non-immunological resistance may occur in conjunction with obesity, infection or certain endocrine and liver diseases. Large numbers of fat cells present in an obese patient are not receptive to the action of insulin. In other words, insulin is not working properly. When weight reduction occurs, insulin's effect improves. Many times we have seen obese Type II patients taking insulin and overeating. Their insulin dosage is increased to keep their blood glucose normal and they gain more weight and become more resistant to insulin. Such patients may be taking hundreds of units of insulin per day. We admit them to the hospital, place them on a very low-calorie diet and stop their insulin. Their blood glucose usually drops, sometimes dramatically, even without insulin.

INSULIN ALLERGY

Another complication of insulin therapy is insulin allergy. You have already learned about antibodies that neutralize insulin. Other antibodies can cause the release of substances associated with allergies. Insulin allergy may occur both locally and systemically (pertaining to the whole body rather than parts). Various causes of insulin allergy include impurities in the insulin and/or the species source (pigs or cows).

Local insulin allergies are seen as skin reactions, such as redness at the site of the injection. This allergy is often seen when insulin therapy is begun. Firm, red areas at the site of the insulin injection may develop 24–48 hours after the injection and may require 7–10 days to subside. At times, redness or itching may develop in parts of the body away from the injection site. Local insulin allergy is treated by first examining your insulin administration technique. See if you are giving your insulin accurately. Poor technique may cause local irritation. Antihistamines may be used for treatment. If the insulin allergy persists, you may be switched to purified pork insulin, desensitized or switched to human insulin.

Systemic insulin allergies result in skin eruptions but may also include respiratory problems or gastrointestinal symptoms. Hypersensitivity to insulin has been found to occur more frequently in people who have had previous short-term treatment with insulin. Reintroduction of insulin is thought to stimulate the production of insulin antibodies. If a person needs insulin and is allergic to it, he may need desensitization. Pork insulin is used as a desensitizing insulin. Desensitization is the process by which gradual exposure to a foreign substance causes tolerance to the substance. Desensitization to pork insulin is performed in a hospital setting. During the process, dilute insulin injections are given over a period of eight to ten hours for three to four days. During desensitization, patients are protected from allergic reactions and hypoglycemia.

LIPODYSTROPHY

Another complication of insulin therapy is lipodystrophy. Lipodystrophy is a disturbance in the fat pattern of those taking insulin. Insulin hypertrophy occurs when adipose tissue accumulates where the insulin has been administered. Patients with hypertrophy may have a history of constant use of one injection site. A buildup of painless scar tissue occurs. Because the injection site is painless, most individuals continue to use it. Insulin tends to be absorbed less completely from hypertrophied sites; as a result, blood glucose levels rise. This condition may mimic insulin resistance. You can treat hypertrophy by not injecting into the hypertrophied areas. Purified pork insulin may be necessary, and the rotation of injection sites is part of the *prevention* as well as the *treatment* of hypertrophy. If a site rotation pattern is followed, hypertrophy will usually be avoided.

Another form of lipodystrophy is insulin atrophy, a loss of fat at the injection site. This is seen most commonly in children and adolescent girls. It may occur within the first few months of insulin therapy. The cause has not been definitely established. Now that human insulin is available, this may become part of the treatment plan. Present treatment involves injecting purified pork insulin directly into the affected areas and around their perimeter. Treatment lasts three to four months until the atrophy clears. This treatment is thought to work because insulin stores fat. After the affected sites begin to fill in, they must be rotated so that hypertrophy is avoided. Leaving insulin at room temperature may also help avoid lipoatrophy. Lipoatrophy may become less common now through the use of the more purified U-100 insulins.

Hypoglycemia, too, must be considered a complication of insulin therapy. All people taking insulin must learn to avoid, recognize and treat hypoglycemia. Chapter 10 deals exclusively with hypoglycemia.

Insulin has many functions other than moving glucose into the cell. It is involved in the metabolism of proteins and fats. Exogenous insulin is obtained from animals, but recently human insulin has been developed. There are many kinds of insulin, each having different onset, peak and duration of action. You must know when your insulin works as well as your correct dosage. Insulin administration is only one task in diabetes self-management. Though it may seem frightening at first, remember that it is only a task. Try to get over the fear of self-injecting by communicating with others, so you can feel comfortable injecting and can learn more about other areas of self-management.

8

Meal Planning Using the Exchange System

Food is an important part of our culture, and is essential in fulfilling certain physiological and psychological needs. This chapter will be devoted to the meal plan or Exchange System for the insulin-dependent person as well as the non-insulin-dependent person who takes insulin to control hyperglycemia. If you are overweight and not taking medication for diabetes, it is not essential that you use this meal plan. However, increasing your knowledge of the meal plan can help you learn more about nutrition and the nutrient composition of foods.

The nutrition goals of persons with diabetes are the same as the goals for the general population. A diabetic meal plan is a nutritious diet that promotes health; it does not differ in calories or nutrients from what non-diabetic individuals should eat. However, for those who require exogenous insulin, your intellect must replace the pancreas. You must balance food and exercise with the exogenous insulin that was injected at the beginning of the day. This may be a frustrating process initially, for two reasons. It requires learning a great deal about nutrition and it demands careful thought throughout the day about eating. Every time you think about diet, insulin or exercise you are reminded that you have diabetes. However, for those who adjust to diabetes and effectively plan their meals, the reward is good control. Moreover, with practice, meal planning becomes a habit and requires very little effort.

If you take insulin, use the Exchange System as a means to achieve blood glucose control. An important concept to remember is that *anticipation* of meals and special occasions plus *consistency* of meals can lead to improved control. Anticipation means that you preplan for meals, you are familiar with the Exchange System and you know how to work with the system. Consistency means that you are prepared to eat at about the same time each day, with the same amounts and types of nutrients in each meal. These important concepts are inherent in achieving blood glucose control. Insulin-dependent persons cannot be well controlled unless they achieve dietary consistency.

NUTRITION GOALS AND OBJECTIVES

There are two major nutrition goals corresponding to the two types of diabetes. The goal for the insulin-dependent person is to focus primarily on achieving consistency in the meal plan. The goal for the obese non-insulin-dependent patient is weight loss. A 1979 position paper by the American Diabetes Association cites four objectives useful in achieving these goals. The first is to improve your overall health by maintaining optimum nutrition. This objective can be achieved by eating a wide variety of foods and obtaining all essential nutrients. The second objective is to try to maintain your ideal body weight. If you are overweight, your meal plan must be restricted in calories yet be nutritionally adequate. If you are underweight, your meal plan must provide adequate calories to achieve a desirable weight. The next objective is to maintain blood glucose levels as near normal as possible. One way to do this is through the use of the Exchange System, calorie control and consistency in the meal plan. The fourth and final objective is to prevent or delay future complications. This is achieved by meeting the three previous objectives.

NUTRITION STRATEGIES

While the goals are the same for all persons with diabetes, the strategies are quite different. If you take insulin, you must also have the same daily intake of calories and nutrients. Consistency in the timing of meals is required. You should be eating all your meals and snacks at about the same time each day. Approximately the same amount of calories as well as grams of carbohydrate, protein and fat should be consumed in each meal. This must be done for the following reasons. With diabetes your pancreas does not secrete sufficient insulin in response to eating. One to three injections of insulin may be needed in an attempt to keep the blood glucose normal. This obviously cannot match the second-to-second response of a normal pancreas. Therefore, the timing and composition of meals must be the same if one to three injections of insulin are used. Moreover, injected insulin works most effectively at peak times. Food must be available to prevent hypoglycemia at those times. Your meal plan must be individualized and tailored to your specific needs. In addition, you may need extra food if you engage in unusual exercise. Your goal must be blood glucose control.

If you have Type II diabetes and are obese, your total intake of calories should be decreased. Consistency is not as important for you. You do not have to eat exactly on schedule nor must you eat specific proportions of carbohydrate, protein and fat. However, very careful attention must be paid to your intake of total calories. You will not need extra food for unusual exercise. You will use stored body fat as the main fuel during exercise. If you are not taking insulin to control hyperglycemic symptoms, you will not need extra calories to prevent hypoglycemia, and it is not mandatory that you follow the exchanges. The following strategies are for both groups of persons with diabetes.

Diet Strategy	Persons Not Taking Insulin	Persons Taking Insulin*
1. Decrease calories	yes (if obese)	calories to maintain ideal weight
2. Increase number of meals and/or snacks per day	no	yes
3. Achieve consistency of calories, carbohydrates, protein and fats at each meal	not necessary	very important
4. Achieve consistency in the timing of meals	not necessary	very important
5. Consume extra food for unusual exercise	not necessary	very important
6. Use food to treat or prevent hypoglycemia	not necessary	very important

WHAT WAS THE "DIABETIC" DIET LIKE BEFORE?

Historically, the meal plan for persons with diabetes has undergone many revisions according to the changing philosophy of physicians. The diet for diabetes dates back to prehistoric times. In 1500 B.C. the Ebers Papyrus provided the world with its oldest recipe for polyuria. It consisted of fresh grits, wheat grains, green lead earth and water.

---

* Includes Type I and Type II individuals who take insulin for control of hyperglycemia.

Hindu doctors prescribed weight reduction for the obese person with diabetes. However, in 1797 the first systematic attempt to remove carbohydrates from the meal plan of persons with diabetes was undertaken. Dr. John Rollo, Surgeon General of the British Royal Artillery, treated an army captain with diabetes. The patient was confined to a room and fed a limited diet of milk plus lime water with bread and butter for breakfast. Lunch was blood pudding made of blood and suet. Dinner was game or fat and rancid old meats, such as pork, eaten in moderation. On this diet, the patient improved and was able to return to service. Later, the diet was expanded to include cabbage, lettuce, boiled onions and radishes. So began the first era of carbohydrate restriction, its rationale including partial starvation.

In the mid-1800s, Dr. Apollinaire Bouchardat gave patients with diabetes gluten bread and fresh vegetables and allowed them a moderate alcohol intake. He was the first to use fast days to control glycosuria. Fast days were times when the patient would eat little or no food. In the later nineteenth century, Arnoldo Cantini of Italy advised dietary restriction through carbohydrate deprivation. Patients were allowed one pound of cooked meat per day and were locked in their rooms to assure dietary adherence. Fast days were also included at least once per week. As you can see, diets prior to the insulin era were horrible. Dietary adherence was quite difficult. Thankfully, research has led to more scientific and rational philosophies.

In the late 1800s, Bernhard Naunyn first observed the differences between the insulin-dependent and the obese person with diabetes. He recommended an adjustment of carbohydrate intake according to each patient's tolerance and caloric needs. Carbohydrate was limited to an amount that did not cause glycosuria.

Finally, the philosophy of dietary treatment for diabetes devised by Dr. Frederick M. Allen prevailed from 1914 until insulin was discovered in 1922. Dr. Allen recognized that diabetes was a problem of total fuel metabolism, not just carbohydrate metabolism. Patients fasted for one to ten days initially, until glycosuria disappeared. During this time, they were allowed to eat only bran muffins and fluids; then green vegetables, fruit, meat and fats were added. Patients were asked to fast every seventh day and the caloric intake was slowly increased. If the patient was free from glycosuria, he was discharged and put on a diet of restricted calories and bulk foods. Fast days were recommended every one to two weeks. This treatment did improve the life expectancy of patients with diabetes. This was accomplished by starvation and carbohydrate restriction.

Once insulin was discovered, diet therapy changed so much that patients no longer had to starve themselves. In 1950, the Exchange List for Meal Planning was developed. It provided a wide variety of foods. It was easy to use because patients did not have to calculate calories or grams of carbohydrates, proteins and fats. They were able to exchange or change foods within each food group but not between different food groups. In 1950, meal plans were designed to provide approximately 40 percent of the total calories from fat, 40 percent from carbohydrate and 20 percent from protein. This meant that if you were on a 1,500-calorie diet, 600 calories would come from fat, 600 from carbohydrate and 300 from protein. However, many patients found dietary adherence to the Exchange System quite difficult. Often the diet was not individualized and did not fit into the patient's cultural or economic lifestyle. The meal plan may have been different from the eating pattern of the patient's family and friends. The patient may not have understood the basic mechanism of the Exchange System or he may have misunderstood the general goals.

WHAT IS THE DIET OF TODAY?

In 1976, the American Dietetic Association and the American Diabetes Association developed a new Exchange List for Meal Planning. This was done in cooperation with the National Institute of Arthritis, Metabolism and Digestive Diseases, the National Heart, Lung and Blood Institute, the National Institutes of Health, the Public Health Service and the U.S. Department of Health, Education and Welfare. Meal plans developed after 1976 are designed to provide approximately 50–60 percent of the total calories from carbohydrate, 12–20 percent from protein and the remaining calories from fat. This means that if you are placed on a 1,500-calorie diet, you would receive approximately 825 calories from carbohydrate, 225 from protein and 450 from fat.

The amount of carbohydrate in the present diet has increased while fat has decreased. The amount of protein is a little less or the same. The fat composition of the diet was changed because diabetes contributes to cardiovascular disease. Dietary intervention may prevent this. Blood cholesterol can be reduced by lowering the intake of saturated fat. Some controversy continues over the reduction of dietary cholesterol and the inclusion of polyunsaturated fat. However, the American Diabetes Association notes that saturated fat should be decreased and partially replaced by polyunsaturated fat. In addition, the diet should contain only a moderate amount of cholesterol. Therefore, the current diet for diabetes reflects the new changes in fat content needed to maintain normal lipid values, in attempting to prevent atherosclerosis.

CARBOHYDRATES ARE O.K.

As the fat content of the diet was reduced, the carbohydrate content was increased. In the present meal plan, complex carbohydrates are no longer disproportionately limited. Complex carbohydrates and simple carbohydrates have different effects on blood glucose levels. Ingestion of simple carbohydrates causes high blood glucose peaks. These elevations in blood glucose are avoided in non-diabetic individuals by the rapid release of an appropriate amount of insulin. In the diabetic, endogenous insulin is not available to prevent erratic blood glucose peaks. Therefore, simple carbohydrates must be avoided. Digestion of complex carbohydrates does not affect glucose tolerance in the same way as simple carbohydrates, for many reasons.

Eating more carbohydrates without increasing the total calories does not increase insulin requirements in the insulin-dependent person. Hyperglycemia is more related to total calories than to levels of dietary carbohydrate. In overweight persons, more carbohydrate does not aggravate glucose tolerance. In fact "calorie control" is more important than "carbohydrate control." Carbohydrates are not fattening, since they provide only 4 calories per gram, whereas fats provide 9 calories per gram. Since the early nineteenth century the intake of complex carbohydrates by the general public has decreased in the United States. However, obesity, diabetes and atherosclerosis have increased. Generally, people in societies that obtain most of their calories from complex carbohydrates are lean, and those that consume diets low in starch are fat.

There was concern that diets high in complex carbohydrates might increase blood triglyceride levels. However, this occurs only in the presence of excess calories, not as a result of the high starch content of the diet. In addition, it does not make sense physiologically to restrict carbohydrates, for your liver has an internal mechanism that allows it to make glucose on its own. Thus, if there is insufficient insulin present, your blood glucose will rise due to gluconeogenesis. Finally, diets high in complex carbohydrates may allow insulin to work more effectively. It is hoped that these explanations will give you extra motivation to begin to enjoy complex carbohydrates daily.

Currently there is new interest in two aspects of carbohydrate use in the diet. Recently researchers added glucose, sucrose, fructose, potato starch and wheat starch to meals for persons with diabetes. No significant difference was found in blood glucose elevation. The research suggests that sucrose may be added to the diet as long as weight reduction is not required and if it is consumed with a meal. Although the research was well publicized, the American Diabetes Association has not changed their present recommendations regarding sucrose. Therefore it is advisable to refrain from its use until much more research is performed.

The second new aspect concerns the effect of starches on blood glucose. Research results are showing that differences exist between the blood glucose response to different foods containing starch. This information suggests that perhaps future dietary recommendations may advise specific foods rather than a choice of foods from food groups.

Remember that research into both these areas is new and constantly growing. More research is continually being done in hopes of developing specific guidelines for you.

ADVANTAGES OF THE EXCHANGE SYSTEM

The 1976 recommendations should not be thought of as rigid requirements. Rather, it is more important that the percentage of calories from each nutrient be adjusted for your individual needs and your specific lifestyle. Day-to-day consistency and distribution of nutrients, however, is still a major goal. Remember, it is virtually impossible to achieve any type of blood glucose control without consistency.

The Exchange System is designed to allow you to eat a variety of foods. The system divides food into six groups. The groups are: milk, vegetables, fruits, breads, meats and fats. Within each food group, an exchange is approximately equal in calories and amount of carbohydrate, protein or fat. Almost any food you can think of can be found on one of the lists. The exceptions to this are foods such as candy, cakes, cookies, pies, jams, jellies, honey and other sugary foods.

Use of the Exchange System does not mean that special foods or special food preparation is needed. You can enjoy meals with your family because the family meals include foods you can eat. The present Exchange System also identifies foods low in saturated fat and high in polyunsaturated fats for preferred food choices. The Exchange System was developed to assist in meal planning, not to be a guide to "all you ever needed to know about the diabetic diet."

Your meal plan must be individualized to meet your specific nutritional and lifestyle needs. Actively participate with a nutritionist in developing your meal plan. Individualization of your meal plan may be based on many factors, such as your weight, social life, medical condition and medications, activity level, daily routine and current eating practices.

You will be the only one who can identify problems once you have implemented your plan. Therefore, your participation in its development cannot be overestimated. Remember that the meal plan is a lifelong commitment. You may need continued follow-up with a nutritionist to assess the suitability of your plan. Each change in your lifestyle may necessitate a change in your meal plan. Changes in your meal plan may be required by physical conditions such as an increased need for nutrients, weight change, change of physical activity, frequent hypoglycemia and social factors such as holidays. Confidence in understanding your meal plan should be attained. Take responsibility in formulating your own meal plan with the help of a nutritionist.

HOW TO START

When you begin learning about the Exchange System try to have some individual counseling with an experienced nutritionist. He or she will help calculate the appropriate amounts of nutrients for you. Use this meal plan for a few weeks to see how it fits into your lifestyle. Before you begin to follow the meal plan read it through in its entirety, along with the Exchange Lists. In this way, you will know which foods are included in each food group. Working with the Exchange System can be simple if you become expert in determining the correct portion sizes of foods. You can use a food scale, a measuring cup and measuring spoons to determine portion sizes.

THE MILK GROUP

The Exchange List starts with the milk group. In this group a serving contains approximately 12 grams of carbohydrate, 8 grams of protein and 80 calories. The best choices in the milk group are those that are fat-free, such as skim milk. A review of portion sizes will help you determine what an 8-ounce or 4-ounce serving resembles. Whole milk, milk containing 2 percent butterfat (2 percent milk), milk containing 1 percent butterfat (1 percent milk) and skim milk each contain the same amount of carbohydrate. The carbohydrate in milk is the simple sugar lactose. However, the advantage of using skim milk is that you will be avoiding calories from fat. If you find it is difficult to switch from whole milk to skim milk, try a gradual approach by going from whole milk to 2 percent milk to 1 percent milk and finally to skim milk. Yogurt is also included in the milk group and is an excellent source of calcium. The low-fat yogurt is an interesting addition to meals and a zesty ingredient in cooking. If you choose low-fat fortified milk products, you will have to omit one additional fat exchange from your total plan. If you choose whole-milk items you will have to omit two fat exchanges.

THE VEGETABLE GROUP

Each half-cup serving from the vegetable group contains approximately 25 calories, 5 grams of carbohydrate and 2 grams of protein. Vegetable choice II, as seen in the middle column, provides the same amount of nutrients in one cup, so you can actually double your serving size with these vegetables. You can eat as much of the free vegetables as you desire. A free vegetable is one that provides a relatively insignificant amount of calories. Notice that starchy vegetables are not included in this list. You can use seasonings such as herbs and spices to enhance the flavor of vegetables without adding extra calories from fat. Frozen or canned vegetables are acceptable as long as no sugar or fat is added.

THE FRUIT GROUP

The fruit exchange contains approximately 40 calories per serving. Each fruit in the appropriate portion size contains approximately 10 grams of carbohydrate. Remember, the sugars in fruits are the simple carbohydrates sucrose, fructose and glucose. Become familiar with the serving size of all fruits. When fruit is included in a meal you can choose any one from the list. Breakfast might include half a banana one day, 2 tablespoons of raisins another day and 4 ounces of orange juice a third day. Purchasing canned fruits packed in water or fruit juice, without added sugar, is also acceptable.

THE BREAD GROUP

Each serving from the bread group contains approximately 70 calories, 15 grams of carbohydrate and 2 grams of protein. Become proficient in determining portion sizes accurately in order to eat the correct amount from the bread group. (The use of a measuring cup, initially, will also help you determine portion sizes.) Starchy vegetables are in this group. Some convenience foods (foods that are partially or completely prepared prior to sale) are also included on the list. These convenience foods contain added fat. Therefore, some fat exchanges must be omitted in order to prevent an intake of excess calories from fat. Choosing a variety of foods from the bread group can help make meals more interesting. A variety of high-fiber food choices, such as breads, cereals and grains, are included in the bread group. The division of the day's bread exchanges might look like this: Breakfast might include two bread choices such as half a bagel and 1 cup of puffed-wheat cereal. Lunch might include two bread choices such as two slices of whole-wheat toast. Two bread choices for dinner might be a half cup of lima beans and a half cup of brown rice. An evening snack might include one bread choice which would be equivalent to 3 cups of popcorn. So you can see the wide variety of foods to include in just one day.

THE MEAT GROUP

The meat group is divided into three categories, based on the amount of fat in each group. The groups are: lean meats, medium-fat meats and high-fat meats. One meat exchange equals 1 ounce (cooked weight) of meat, fish, poultry or cheese.

The lean meats contain approximately 55 calories per ounce. Each ounce provides 7 grams of protein and 3 grams of fat. The lean meat group is the best to choose because these meats are low in fat. Try small portions of red meat trimmed of visible fat, chicken without the skin, turkey, fresh or frozen fish, low-fat cheese and meatless meals made with beans.

The medium-fat meats provide 7 grams of protein, 5 grams of fat and approximately 75 calories per ounce. Medium-fat meats contain more saturated fat than lean meats. You may want to eat them only once in a while (once every one to two weeks). Medium-fat meats include those that are high in cholesterol, such as liver, kidney and sweetbreads. They also include cheeses (such as part-skim milk, mozzarella and ricotta), eggs, peanut butter and a variety of meats that contain more saturated fat than those in the lean meat group.

The third meat group consists of the high-fat meats. These meats contain 7 grams of protein, 8 grams of fat and approximately 100 calories per ounce. Foods in this group include cold cuts, such as salami, liverwurst, bologna, corned beef and pastrami. Examples of high-fat cheeses are American, Muenster, Swiss and other specialty-type cheeses. Frankfurters and other specialty meats, such as sausages, are on this list as well as breast of veal and lamb. Many pork products and fatty cuts of beef are also listed. The high-fat meat group provides much more saturated fat than the lean meat group, so you may want to avoid these food choices entirely, or choose them once in a while.

THE FAT GROUP

The last food group in the Exchange System is the fat group. The fat exchanges are divided into three categories: polyunsaturated fats, monounsaturated fats and saturated fats. You may refer to Chapter 17, on cardiovascular disease, to learn more about each fat. Each food in the fat group, regardless of the type of fat, provides about 5 grams of fat and 45 calories per serving. The portion size of foods listed in the fat exchange varies. For example, ten peanuts comprise one fat exchange, but so does one-eighth of an avocado or one teaspoon of oil. Polyunsaturated fats are your best choices. These are the soft tub margarines, vegetable oils and walnuts. The monounsaturated fats include olive oil and peanut oil. Finally, try to avoid the saturated fats that increase your serum cholesterol level. Fats that are saturated include lard, butter, cream and other animal fats. Your goal should be the inclusion of polyunsaturated fats in your meal plan while you reduce your intake of saturated fats.

The following has been adapted in part, with permission from the American Dietetic Association.

THE MILK GROUP

One serving from the milk choice contains 12 grams of carbohydrate, 8 grams of protein and 80 calories.

Non-Fat Fortified Milk

skim or non-fat milk	1 cup (8 oz.)
powdered non-fat milk	⅓ cup
canned evaporated skim milk	½ cup
skim-milk buttermilk	1 cup
yogurt made from skim milk (plain, unflavored)	1 cup

These are your best choices, as they contain a trace of fat and the least amount of cholesterol and calories.

Low-Fat Fortified Milk

1% fat fortified milk	1 cup (omit ½ fat exchange for each serving)
2% fat fortified milk	1 cup (omit 1 fat exchange for each serving)
yogurt made from 2% fat fortified milk (plain, unflavored)	1 cup (omit 1 fat exchange for each serving)

Whole Milk (omit 2 fat exchanges for each serving)

whole milk	1 cup
evaporated whole milk	½ cup
whole-milk buttermilk	1 cup
yogurt made from whole milk (plain, unflavored)	1 cup

THE VEGETABLE GROUP

Each serving from the vegetable choice provides 5 grams of carbohydrate, 2 grams of protein and 25 calories. The serving size is ½ or 1 cup unless otherwise stated.

Adapted in part from *Diabetes Guidebook: Diet Section* Edition 3, by John K. Davidson, M.D., Ph.D., and Mary P. Goldsmith, B.S., R.D., Grady Memorial Hospital, Emory University School of Medicine, Atlanta, GA 30303.

Vegetable Choice I (½ cup = 1 serving)	Vegetable Choice II (1 cup = 1 serving)	Free Vegetable Choice
artichoke (½ cup or small)	asparagus	chicory
bamboo shoots	beans, string	Chinese cabbage
beets	beans, wax	endive
beet greens	bean sprouts	escarole
broccoli	cabbage	lettuce
brussels sprouts	cauliflower	Boston
carrots	celery	Iceberg
catsup (1 tbs.)	chards	Butterhead
collard greens	cucumber	spinach (raw)
dandelion greens	green peppers	watercress
eggplant	(1 shell raw or cooked)	
kale	mushrooms	
kohlrabi	okra	
mixed vegetables (⅓ cup)	parsley	
mustard greens	radishes (10)	
onions	rhubarb (without sugar)	
pimientos	summer squash	
rutabaga	turnip greens	
sauerkraut	zucchini	
snow pea pods		
spinach		
tomatoes		
tomato juice		
tomato paste (2 tbs.)		
tomato puree (¼ cup)		
tomato sauce		
turnips		
water chestnuts (4)		

THE FRUIT GROUP

One serving from the fruit choice provides 10 grams of carbohydrate and 40 calories.

apple	1 small (2″ dia.)	banana	½ small
applesauce (unsweetened)	½ cup	berries	
apricots, fresh	2 medium	blackberries	½ cup
apricots, dried	4 halves	blueberries	½ cup
apricots, canned	4 medium halves	raspberries	½ cup
		strawberries	¾ cup

cherries	10 large
dates	2
fresh fruit cup	½ cup
fig, fresh	1
fig, dried	1
grapes	12
grapefruit	½
guava	1 small
lemon	1 whole
mango	½ small
melon	
cantaloupe	¼ small
honeydew	⅛ medium
watermelon	1 cup
nectarine	1 small
papaya	¾ medium
peach	1 medium
pear	1 small
persimmon, native	1 medium
pineapple	½ cup
pineapple slices, canned	1½ slices
plums	2 medium
prunes	2 medium
orange	1 small
raisins	2 tbs.
tangerine	1 medium

Juices

apple cider	⅓ cup
apple juice	⅓ cup
cranberry juice (low-calorie)	¾ cup
grape juice	¼ cup
grapefruit juice	½ cup
orange juice	½ cup
pineapple juice	⅓ cup
prune juice	¼ cup

THE BREAD GROUP

One serving from the bread choice provides 15 grams of carbohydrate, 2 grams of protein and 70 calories.

Bread

white (includes French & Italian)	1 slice
whole wheat	1 slice
pumpernickel	1 slice
rye	1 slice
raisin	1 slice
bagel, small	½
English muffin, small	½
plain roll	1
frankfurter roll	½
hamburger roll	½
bread crumbs (dried)	3 tbs.
tortilla (6″)	1

Cereal

bran flakes	½ cup
other ready-to-eat unsweetened cereal	¾ cup
puffed cereal	1 cup
cereal (cooked)	½ cup
grits (cooked)	½ cup
pasta (cooked)	½ cup
spaghetti, noodles, macaroni (cooked)	½ cup
popcorn (no fat added)	3 cups
rice (white or brown, cooked)	½ cup
flour	2½ tbs.
cornmeal (dry)	2 tbs.
wheat germ	¼ cup
barley (cooked)	½ cup

Crackers		Starchy Vegetables	
arrowroot	3	corn	⅓ cup
graham (2½″ sq.)	2	corn on the cob	1 small ear
matzoh (4″ × 6″)	½	lima beans	½ cup
oyster	20	parsnips	⅔ cup
pretzels (3⅛″ long × ⅛″ dia.)	25	peas, green	½ cup
rye wafers (2″ × 3½″)	3	potato, mashed	½ cup
saltines	6	potato, white	1 small
soda (2½″ sq.)	4	pumpkin	¾ cup
		winter squash, acorn or butternut	½ cup
Dried Beans, Peas, Lentils		yam or sweet potato	¼ cup
beans, peas, lentils (cooked)	½ cup		
baked beans (no pork) (cooked)	¼ cup		

Convenience Food Items

biscuit (2″ dia.) (omit 1 fat exchange)	1
corn bread (2″ × 2″ × 1″) (omit 1 fat exchange)	1
corn muffin (2″ dia.) (omit 1 fat exchange)	1
crackers, round butter-type (omit 1 fat exchange)	5
muffin, plain, small (omit 1 fat exchange)	1
potatoes, french-fried (2″–3½″ long) (omit 1 fat exchange)	8
potato or corn chips (omit 2 fat exchanges)	15
pancake (5″ × ½″) (omit 1 fat exchange)	1
waffle (5″ × ½″) (omit 1 fat exchange)	1

THE MEAT GROUP

A 1-ounce serving (cooked weight) of a *lean meat* provides 7 grams of protein, 3 grams of fat and 55 calories. These items contain the least amount of saturated fat and cholesterol.

Beef

roasts
  arm
  chuck (round bone)
  rump (all cuts)
  round
steaks
  flank
  round (bottom, top)

tenderloin
plate skirt

miscellaneous
  baby beef (very lean)
  chipped beef
  plate ribs
  tripe
  lean stew
  ground round (extra lean)

Lamb

leg
rib
sirloin
loin (roast & chops)
shank
shoulder

Pork

leg (whole rump, center shank)
ham
smoked (center slices)

Veal

leg
loin
rib
shank
shoulder
cutlets

Poultry

(meat without skin)

chicken
turkey
Cornish hen
guinea hen
pheasant

Fish

all types (fresh & frozen)

canned salmon,
   tuna, mackerel,
   crab, lobster (¼ cup)

clams, oysters, scallops, shrimp
   (5 or 1 ounce)

sardines (drained) (3)

Cheese/Other

cottage (dry, 1% & 2%) (¼ cup)
pot
baker's
Lite Line
Weight Watchers
Tasty Loaf (Kraft)
CountDown (Fisher Cheeses)
sapago
St. Otho
Laughing Cow (reduced-calorie)
dried beans, peas (½ cup)
   (omit 1 bread exchange)

A 1-ounce serving (cooked weight) of a *medium-fat meat* provides 7 grams of protein, 5 grams of fat and 75 calories. These items contain more saturated fat and cholesterol than the lean meats and should be considered *once-in-a-while* choices.

Beef

roasts
   eye chuck (blade)
   sirloin
steaks
   T-bone
   shoulder

porterhouse
sirloin
rib eye

miscellaneous
   corned beef (canned)
   round (ground commercial)
   round (15% fat)

Pork	Other
Canadian bacon	egg
loin (all cuts)	cottage cheese (4% fat, creamed)
shoulder	(¼ cup)
arm (picnic)	ricotta, mozzarella
blade	Parmesan (3 tbs.)
Boston butt	peanut butter (2 tbs.)
boiled ham	(omit 2 fat exchanges)
	farmer cheese
	Neufchâtel cheese
	liver
	kidney
	sweetbreads

A 1-ounce serving (cooked weight) of a *high-fat meat* provides 7 grams of protein, 8 grams of fat and 100 calories. These items contain the highest amount of saturated fat and cholesterol and should be considered *avoid* choices. If you choose to eat high-fat meats, you would need to omit 1 fat choice for each ounce of meat.

Beef	Pork
roasts	spare ribs
rib	loin (back ribs)
steaks	country-style ham
rib	deviled ham
club	frankfurters
miscellaneous	picnic
flanken	pigs' feet
hamburger	sausage links
(with more than 20% fat)	cold cuts
corned beef (brisket)	pork butt
pastrami	ground
short ribs	
frankfurters	Veal
salami	breast
Lamb	Poultry
breast	duck (domestic)
	goose
	capon

Fish   *Other*

commercially pre-breaded and   most other cheeses not previously
    pre-fried   mentioned

THE FAT GROUP

One serving from the fat choice provides 5 grams of fat and 45 calories.

The following are your best choices because they contain primarily *polyunsaturated oils*.

oils and soft tub margarines made from safflower, sunflower, corn, cottonseed and soybean oils	1 tsp.
salad dressings made with the above oils	2 tsp.
mayonnaise	1 tsp.
diet mayonnaise	2 tsp.
diet tub margarine	3 tsp.
Poly Perx (liquid coffee lightener)	2 tbs.
walnuts	6 small
commercial salad dressings (except those containing cheese)	2 tsp.

The following contain primarily *monounsaturated fat* and should be considered *once-in-a-while* choices. Try to use them only *once per week*.

peanut oil, olive oil	1 tsp.
avocado (4″ dia.)	⅛
olives	5 small
pecans	2 large
peanuts	
Spanish	20 whole
Virginia	10 whole
almonds	10 whole
nuts, other	6 small

The following contain primarily *saturated fat* and should be considered *avoid* choices. These items tend to elevate serum cholesterol levels. Try to use them only *once per month*.

bacon	1 strip
bacon fat	1 tsp.
butter	1 tsp.
cream, light and sour	2 tbs.

cream, heavy	1 tbs.
cream cheese	1 tbs.
lard	1 tsp.
salt pork	¾" cube
powdered coffee lighteners	1⅓ tsp.
liquid coffee lighteners	2 tbs.
solid shortenings	1 tsp.
margarine, stick type	1 tsp.
half-and-half	2 tbs.

PRACTICE PLANNING MEALS

By now you should have a good idea of the foods in the Exchange System and the role that portion control plays in this system. Take your time reviewing the Exchange System so you are familiar with foods included in it. Remember that virtually any food can be eaten except candy, cakes, cookies, pies, jams, jellies and honey. See if you can figure out what foods might be included in the following 1,500-calorie meal plan.

Your 1,500-calorie meal plan might include the following exchanges. Breakfast is one milk, one fruit, one bread, one fat and one lean meat exchange. A midmorning snack is one bread and one fruit exchange. Lunch includes two lean meats, one bread, one fat, one fruit, and one vegetable exchange. An afternoon snack provides one milk and one bread exchange. Dinner is three lean meats, two fats, two breads, one vegetable and one fruit exchange. Finally, an evening snack includes one medium-fat meat, one bread and one fruit exchange. See the following ideas for appropriate food choices.

EXCHANGES FOR 1,500-CALORIE MEAL PLAN

Food Choices

BREAKFAST

1 milk	1 cup skim milk
1 fruit	2 tbs. raisins
1 bread	1 slice whole-wheat bread
1 fat	1 tsp. margarine
1 lean meat	¼ cup low-fat cottage cheese

MIDMORNING SNACK

1 bread	2 graham crackers
1 fruit	4 oz. orange juice

LUNCH

2 lean meats	2 oz. sliced chicken breast
1 bread	1 small roll
1 fat	1 tsp. mayonnaise
1 fruit	¼ cantaloupe
1 vegetable	4 oz. tomato juice

AFTERNOON SNACK

| 1 milk | ½ cup plain yogurt |
| 1 bread | ¼ cup wheat germ |

DINNER

3 lean meats	3 oz. sliced steak
2 fats	2 tsp. margarine
2 breads	1 large baked potato
1 vegetable	½ cup broccoli
	tossed salad and lemon wedges
1 fruit	¾ cup strawberries

EVENING SNACK

1 medium-fat meat	1 tbs. peanut butter
1 bread	3 rye wafers
1 fruit	½ sliced grapefruit

You may find that you need practice planning meals. The following charts show different foods you could choose from if your meal plan provides for the exchanges listed. You can refer to Table 9 for the number of exchanges for each food group for several different calorie levels. As the calories increase, so do the number of exchanges per group. The "More Useful Information" section in the back of this book lists some cookbooks that may be useful.

TABLE 9   EXAMPLES OF EXCHANGES FOR VARIOUS CALORIE MEAL PLANS

	1200	1500	1800	2100	2400	2700	3000
Milk	2 cups	2 cups	2 cups	3 cups	3 cups	4 cups	4 cups
Vegetables	2 Exchanges	3 Exchanges	4 Exchanges	4 Exchanges	4 Exchanges	4 Exchanges	5 Exchanges
Fruit	3 Exchanges	4 Exchanges	4 Exchanges	5 Exchanges	5 Exchanges	7 Exchanges	8 Exchanges
Bread	5 Exchanges	8 Exchanges	9 Exchanges	10 Exchanges	12 Exchanges	13 Exchanges	15 Exchanges
Meat	5 Exchanges	6 Exchanges	7 Exchanges	9 Exchanges	10 Exchanges	11 Exchanges	12 Exchanges
Fat	5 Exchanges	6 Exchanges	8 Exchanges	8 Exchanges	10 Exchanges	11 Exchanges	12 Exchanges

If your meal plan provides for this:	Your food choices might include this:	Calories	or this:
Breakfast			
1 milk	8 oz. skim milk blenderized with ¾ cup strawberries	80	8 oz. skim milk
1 fruit		40	½ banana
2 breads	1 whole-wheat bagel	140	⅓ cup bran cereal and 1 slice whole-wheat bread
1 fat	1 tbs. diet margarine	45	1 tbs. diet margarine
		305	
Lunch			
3 lean meats	tuna-macaroni salad made with: ¾ cup tuna packed in water and	165	3 oz. lean turkey meat
2 breads	½ cup macaroni	70	
	3 rye wafers	70	2 slices rye bread
1 fat	1 tbs. diet mayonnaise	45	1 tsp. mayonnaise
1 fruit	½ cup grapefruit juice	40	1 small apple
		390	
Afternoon Snack			
1 fruit	1 small nectarine	40	½ cup orange juice
1 bread	25 pretzel sticks	70	6 saltines
		110	
Dinner			
3 lean meats	3 oz. shrimp	165	3 oz. ground round hamburger patty
2 breads	1 cup rice	140	½ hamburger bun and ½ cup peas
2 vegetables	½ cup marinara sauce for shrimp and ½ cup string beans	50	½ cup carrots, sliced tomato
1 fat	salad with 1 tbs. reduced-calorie salad dressing	45	salad with 1 tsp. oil and vinegar
		400	
Evening Snack			
1 fruit	2 tbs. raisins	40	¼ cantaloupe
1 bread	2 graham crackers	70	3 cups unbuttered popcorn
		110	

Total 1,315 calories

If your meal plan calls for this:	Your food choices might include this:	or this:	Calories
Breakfast			
1 lean meat	1 slice low-calorie cheese	¼ cup cottage cheese	55
2 breads	1 pumpernickel bagel with	1 whole-wheat English muffin	140
1 fat	1 tsp. margarine	1 tsp. margarine	45
2 fruits	8 oz. orange juice	2 tbs. raisins and ½ cup grapefruit juice	80
			320
Lunch			
3 lean meats	3 oz. lean roast beef on	3 oz. chicken salad	165
2 breads	1 hard roll	6 rye wafers	140
1 fruit	1 apple	¼ cantaloupe	40
1 vegetable	1 tomato	carrot sticks	25
2 fats	2 tsp. mayonnaise	2 tsp. mayonnaise for chicken salad	90
	1 sour pickle		FREE
			460
Dinner			
4 lean meats	4 oz. lobster tail	4 oz. loin lamb chop	220
2 breads	1 baked potato and 1 small roll	½ cup macaroni and ½ cup lima beans	140
2 vegetables	1 cup broccoli	½ cup carrots and ½ cup spinach	50
2 fats	2 tsp. butter for lobster	2 tsp. margarine	90
1 fruit	¾ cup sliced strawberries	1 small pear	40
			540
Evening Snack			
1 milk	8 oz. skim milk	1 cup Alba hot cocoa	80
1 medium-fat meat	1 tbs. peanut butter	1 oz. mozzarella	75
1 bread	1 slice whole-wheat bread	½ bagel	70
			225

Total 1,545 calories

The diabetic meal plan has undergone many changes. A goal for people with diabetes must include following a nutritious diet to promote health. Through this diet, diabetes and weight control become realities.

At present, Type I and Type II persons with diabetes follow different diet strategies that lead to the same important goals of control. The Type I person can achieve consistency in meal timing and nutrient composition. The Type II person can reduce or maintain his weight. All those with diabetes can use the Exchange System, which has undergone many changes. It is now recommended that you eat more complex carbohydrates and less fat. However, this system is not as important for persons who do not take insulin. You can actively participate in planning your diet so it fits into your lifestyle.

9

Exercise

Diabetes control depends on achieving a balance of diet, medication and exercise. In the past, exercise has not been emphasized as much as the other two cornerstones of diabetes management. Fortunately, with the current interest in physical activity, the role of exercise has received more emphasis. Again, another aspect of diabetes self-management, regular exercise, has become important in many people's lives, with and without diabetes.

In this chapter you will learn about the physiology of exercise and its role in diabetes control. You will also be given guidelines on starting an exercise program.

The resting muscle uses free fatty acids for fuel. When mild exercise begins, the muscle shifts to using glycogen stores as a fuel supply. Glycogen is broken down to glucose and released into the blood. As exercise continues, both glucose and free fatty acids are used for fuel. The amount of each fuel used depends on the intensity and duration of exercise as well as the prior nutritional state.

Exercise increases the flow of blood and oxygen to muscle, skin and subcutaneous tissues. It also increases cardiac output, pulse rate and blood pressure. Exercise promotes weight loss; it does not increase appetite. Endurance and coordination improve through exercise. Exercise increases muscle mass and high-density lipoprotein (HDL) levels while reducing serum triglycerides, very low-density lipoprotein (VLDL) and low-density lipoprotein (LDL) levels (see Chapter 17). Exercise helps to reduce stress, improves the quality of life and strengthens social relationships. Finally, exercise is helpful to the diabetic person in that it aids in developing self-discipline. If you are involved in regular exercise, you have already developed self-discipline. The self-discipline that you have gained through an exercise program can help you to cope more effectively with other demands of diabetes self-management.

EXERCISE AND DIABETES

Exercise lowers blood glucose levels. Glucose is used for fuel during exercise. Exercise enhances the effectiveness of insulin. It increases the number of insulin cell receptors as well as the receptors' affinity for insulin. Cells that become more sensitive to insulin in this way will then use glucose more effectively. Because of this, insulin requirements may be lowered through exercise. While exercise is not a substitute for insulin, it may aid in reducing insulin requirements.

Exercise is most valuable when diabetes is controlled. If your blood glucose is high, exercise can worsen diabetic control. Insulin is needed to use glucose efficiently during exercise. Certain hormones are secreted during exercise which elevate blood glucose. These include epinephrine, norepinephrine, growth hormone, cortisol and glucagon. In the person with uncontrolled diabetes, the absence of sufficient insulin and the presence of these contrainsulin hormones can cause elevation of blood glucose and ketosis. You should not be exercising if your blood glucose is above 250 mg./dl. *Do not begin an active exercise program until your blood glucose is controlled with diet and medication.*

AVOIDING EXERCISE-RELATED PROBLEMS

There is a tendency toward hypoglycemia during exercise. Hypoglycemia may also result from increased blood flow to subcutaneous tissues at the injection sites of patients who take insulin. Insulin that is injected into an exercising limb may be absorbed more rapidly. This fast absorption depends on the intensity of the exercise, the injection site and the type of insulin used. Since more insulin is available for use, the risk of hypoglycemia increases. Therefore, if you take insulin, avoid injecting into an area which you will vigorously exercise. For example, avoid injecting into your right arm if you will be using that arm to play a game of tennis.

The obese non-insulin-dependent diabetic person can exercise without eating extra food. In these individuals, body fat stores can meet energy needs. This will lead to weight loss, a major advantage of exercise. However, if you are insulin-dependent, hypoglycemia is also likely to occur when too little food has been eaten prior to exercise. You will need to preplan a snack to avoid hypoglycemia during exercise. If you take insulin, you must replenish glucose and glycogen stores prior to intense exercise. For a mild activity of short duration, only a simple carbohydrate such as an orange may be necessary. Moderate exercise, such as brisk walking, might require taking one fruit every hour. Exercise such as intense tennis may require 20 grams of carbohydrate per hour. Runners may need food every twenty minutes. Slowly absorbed foods such as crackers are beneficial during strenuous activities of long duration. Rapidly absorbed simple carbohydrates, though, must also be available during exercise. Be alert to the possibility of hypoglycemia occurring after exercise. The blood-glucose-lowering effect of exercise may continue for twenty-four hours after exercise has stopped. Therefore, you need to be consistent in eating meals.

HOW TO START AND WHEN TO STOP

Because exercise changes your blood glucose according to your fuel needs, check with your doctor regarding your control before beginning an exercise program. Exercise could worsen retinopathy, heart disease or hypertension if these conditions were unnoticed and untreated. The doctor is the best person on the health-care team to decide if, in your present physical state, you should begin an exercise program. He or she would determine this by a variety of methods. First, he would assess your diabetes control. He would then look at your weight. If you are obese, he might ask you to lose weight before beginning a strenuous exercise program. This would decrease stress on your cardiovascular system. He would also check your extremities to be sure that peripheral vascular disease and foot problems will not interfere with exercise. The doctor may then test your cardiovascular system by doing an exercise stress test. A stress test or stress EKG is performed while you exercise on a treadmill. You walk on a gradual incline while your heart rate, EKG and blood pressure are monitored. The doctor is able to observe possible heart problems as well as how your heart responds to physical stress. Should certain abnormalities become apparent, he or she may advise you to modify your activity. These abnormalities may include irregular heartbeats, signs of coronary artery disease, angina pectoris (chest pain occurring during exercise) and uncontrolled high blood pressure.

As important as exercise is, it is just as essential to recognize when you should stop exercising. Always stop exercising if you develop an insulin reaction. Nausea, dizziness, shortness of breath, chest pain, muscle pain or swollen ankles should make you stop exercising. Blisters or ulcers on your feet are definite reasons to stop exercising.

OBJECTIVES OF EXERCISE

There are two separate objectives of exercising. For the lean insulin-dependent person, exercise is necessary to improve general health and blood glucose control. It is important to regulate the amount of time you exercise so that you achieve daily consistency in activity, diet and insulin. For the obese non-insulin-dependent person, weight loss may be the primary goal.

TYPES OF EXERCISE

Physical fitness has been defined as a person's ability to complete daily activities without fatigue and yet have enough reserve energy to meet extra demands placed upon the body. Factors that reflect your physical fitness level include strength, flexibility, agility, balance, power and endurance. Aerobic exercises will lead to cardiovascular fitness. Choose an aerobic exercise program. Here, your muscles use oxygen to carry out the exercise. You are training and improving the fitness of the entire cardiovascular system (the heart and blood vessels). Aerobic exercises stimulate the heart and lungs while increasing circulation and improving muscle tone. Aerobic exercises should be started slowly and increased gradually.

Exercises that increase aerobic fitness are continuous, nonstop exercises using large muscle groups over an extended period of time. Muscles contract, relax and move in rhythm. Walking, jogging, running, bicycling, cross-country skiing, swimming and rowing are all exercises which improve aerobic fitness. Exercise should be progressive in nature. When the body adjusts to a particular level of activity, the exercise can safely be increased to a more difficult level. Endurance exercises improve physical fitness. This means that they are done for more than five to ten minutes at a time. Your goal should be to participate in a regular exercise program that lasts for at least thirty minutes, three to four times a week. Make sure your exercise program is comfortable. Fatigue should never be an end point or by-product of proper exercise.

There are other kinds of exercises, such as calisthenics, isometrics and anaerobics. Calisthenics improve strength and flexibility. These include activities such as sit-ups, knee bends and push-ups. They are not particularly beneficial for the cardiovascular system but may be helpful in "warming up." Isometric exercises involve the tightening and releasing of muscles and are used to improve muscle tone. An example of this would be pushing or pulling your hands together or apart with no subsequent motion or movement. These exercises do not improve cardiovascular fitness. Anaerobic exercises are the same type of exercises as aerobic but they are done not only for a shorter period of time but also at a higher intensity. An example of this type would be a fifty-yard dash. Short-term strenuous exercises are not as helpful in improving general cardiovascular fitness.

You do have a variety of exercises from which to choose. Remember, aerobic exercises are beneficial for people with diabetes since they also improve cardiovascular fitness. The other types of exercise, in particular calisthenics, are useful in warming up and stretching your muscles prior to beginning an aerobic exercise program.

PRECAUTIONS

Some precautions are necessary to avoid harm and gain maximum benefit and enjoyment from exercise. Avoid exercising in bare feet. Wear two pairs of cotton socks to prevent blisters. Wear properly cushioned shoes. Although certain athletic shoes are expensive, they are a wise investment to protect your feet. Keep your feet dry and clean with toenails properly filed or clipped. If you exercise with someone, it is important to say that you have diabetes. If unexpected hypoglycemia occurs, you may need help. Always wear identification when you exercise. You should carry a simple carbohydrate and money. An emergency coin can be tucked in the pocket of a warm-up suit. It can be used if you become ill while exercising and need to call someone for help.

TRAINING EFFECTS OF EXERCISE

Many of you who are reading this book for the first time may not actively participate in a regular exercise program. You should begin slowly. At first, you may want to increase the amount of daily walking and other activities of daily living. For instance, you might climb stairs at work rather than wait for the elevator. Others of you may have made physical fitness and training a part of your daily life and diabetes self-management. For those who are interested in fitness, the effects of regular exercise will be reviewed. When you are vigorously exercising, it is important to monitor your body's response. What is occurring in the cardiovascular system? Monitoring can easily be accomplished by taking your pulse. Maximal heart rate varies with age. There is a limit to how fast your heart can beat no matter how long or fast you exercise. For example, a man in his early twenties may be capable of attaining a maximal heart rate of 195 beats per minute. A man in his sixties may be able to attain a maximal heart rate of 160 beats per minute. Maximal heart rates are predicted by graphs as well as by the simple approximation of 220 minus your age. When you exercise you should not attempt to achieve your maximal heart rate, but rather 70 percent of your maximal heart rate. You can best monitor this by taking your pulse. This will help you to assess the cardiovascular fitness benefits of exercise. Exercise will not improve cardiovascular capacity unless 70 percent of the maximal heart rate is achieved. (This may vary depending on medication.) Exercise must be done on a regular basis, three to four days per week, for at least thirty minutes.

You can take your pulse by placing the first three fingers of your left hand on your right hand, at the point where the wrist meets the beginning of your thumb. Press down slowly and feel for a few seconds to detect the rhythmic beating of the pulse. Once it is clearly felt, count the number of pulse waves for ten seconds and multiply by six. This will equal your pulse rate.

RECORD KEEPING

Keep a record of the type of daily exercise you do. Note the duration of the exercise as well as signs and symptoms of hypoglycemia or any cardiovascular symptoms, such as shortness of breath, chest pain or weakness, that may have occurred. Your pulse rate should be recorded when you exercise.

EXERCISE AND CORONARY HEART DISEASE

Exercise may be advantageous in preventing or delaying coronary heart disease. A sedentary lifestyle increases the risk for heart disease. Regular exercise can change that lifestyle. Physical fitness increases the HDL levels. An elevated HDL level is a protective factor against the development of coronary heart disease. In addition, exercise can reduce the VLDL and LDL. Finally, while exercise may not affect total blood cholesterol, it does reduce blood triglyceride and blood pressure levels. It is believed that regular aerobic exercise helps to develop coronary collateral circulation. This refers to the formation of additional blood vessels in an area of poor circulation of the heart. You have an improved chance of surviving a heart attack if collateral circulation is present. If there is an interruption in the blood supply to the heart due to atherosclerosis (that is, a heart attack), and you have developed collateral circulation, you will already have additional blood supply. This may help to limit the size or severity of a heart attack.

Cardiac rehabilitation programs are designed to allow participants who have cardiac conditions to achieve an optimal level of physical fitness. Usually you must obtain medical clearance from your doctor to participate in these programs.

Goals of the program include weight loss, improved muscle strength and tone and improved cardiovascular fitness. For diabetics who have already experienced some cardiovascular difficulties, additional benefits may include a decrease in exercise-induced shortness of breath, a reduction in exertional chest pain, a decreased resting heart rate and lower blood pressure. Many cardiac rehabilitation centers offer supervised exercise programs under the guidance of a coronary-care nurse and doctors familiar with exercise testing and therapy.

EXERCISE AND GENERAL HEALTH

Health includes a feeling of well-being. Exercise provides this, probably through the release of endorphins. Endorphins are opiate-like substances that are released from the brain. They have been found to reduce the pain threshold and produce sedation. They become active when the body experiences stress, such as during exercise. Endorphins produce the feeling of well-being seen in many people who exercise. Runners are familiar with the "high" during running that results from the release of endorphins.

You should not be unrealistic about the role of exercise in weight reduction. Calorie restriction will always remain the primary way to lose weight, with exercise seen as an important aid. For example, if you were to expend 2,400 calories per day and were placed on a 1,200-calorie-per-day weight-reduction plan, you would create a 1,200-calorie-per-day deficit. One pound would be lost in approximately three days (one pound of fat equals 3,500 calories). However, look at how much exercise you would need to achieve the same effect: three hours of tennis or six hours of walking or two hours of running per day. See the following table for other exercise/calorie equivalents. You can immediately see the difficulty here in using exercise alone to reduce weight. Yet exercise is vital in aiding weight loss and should be viewed as an excellent addition to your diabetes self-management program.

CALORIE USAGE

(per hour)

Bicycling (5½ m.p.h.)	270
Bicycling (13 m.p.h.)	670
Hill climbing (slope 1 in 5.7, with 11-pound load)	640
Roller/ice skating	350
Running (6 m.p.h.)	630
Running (10 m.p.h.)	900
Skiing (10 m.p.h.)	600
Snowshoeing (soft snow, 2½ m.p.h.)	830

Squash and handball	610
Swimming (crawl, 45 yds. per minute)	690
Table tennis	360
Tennis	430
Walking (2½ m.p.h.)	220
Walking (3½ m.p.h.)	290
Wood chopping	420

GUIDELINES FOR EXERCISE

Follow these guidelines when engaging in an exercise program:

1. Exercise should be started slowly and increased gradually; never tire or push yourself to unnecessary limits.
2. Exercise on a regular basis, eventually for at least thirty minutes a day, three to four times a week.
3. After any illness or cessation of exercise, even for a short time, start again slowly. Check with your doctor and resume your exercise at a slower pace.
4. Avoid exercising in weather extremes, such as unusual heat, cold or humidity.
5. Showers following exercise should always be tepid, not too hot or cold. Saunas cause added stress to your cardiovascular system and should be avoided.
6. Avoid competition, either with yourself, with others or with the clock. If you enjoy participating in games or sports, such as basketball, tennis, badminton and softball, these may be a welcome addition to a life of physical fitness. However, avoid the overcompetitive edge that may prevent you from realizing the benefits of exercise.
7. Exercise should be primarily of an aerobic nature. Avoid isometric exercises. Use calisthenics to warm up slowly and then start an aerobic form of exercise. Avoid spa machines, which may be dangerous if you have diabetic neuropathy, which may prevent you from feeling irritations. These machines will not help in weight reduction or change fat distribution.
8. Avoid hypoglycemia by eating a light snack prior to exercising and by carrying a simple carbohydrate with you while exercising. This applies only to those who are taking insulin.
9. It is wise to avoid alcohol consumption during exercise. Both alcohol and exercise have a hypoglycemic effect. It will also be helpful to avoid

exercising when your insulin is peaking. Remember not to inject insulin into a site that will be exercised strenuously.

10. Dress comfortably in a lightweight, loose-fitting outfit of at least 50 percent cotton. Never wear rubber suits.

11. If participating in water sports, take care of your feet. Wash and dry them thoroughly in order to avoid possible infection. Be alert to the dangers of athlete's foot when using public locker rooms.

12. If beginning an exercise program, remember that brisk walking is one of the best and safest forms of exercise.

13. Select an exercise program that you can carry out throughout the year. For example, your ability to exercise on a given day should not be influenced by weather conditions.

Physical training to improve your cardiovascular system must be done slowly after checking with your doctor. You must receive guidelines specific for your particular condition. Enjoy exercise as a sport, as a stress-reducing aid and as an aid in improving diabetes control. With proper guidance from your healthcare team, you can enjoy exercise and see its benefits in your self-management program.

10

Hypoglycemia

Hypoglycemia is a low blood glucose level. In this chapter you will learn what causes hypoglycemia as well as how to avoid, recognize and treat it. Hypoglycemia due to insulin administration is also known as an "insulin reaction" or "insulin shock." This must be treated promptly since it is dangerous. Hypoglycemia most often affects insulin-dependent people, but may also occur in individuals taking oral hypoglycemic agents. The causes vary but usually fall within the following categories: too much insulin, too little food or too much exercise.

KINDS OF HYPOGLYCEMIA

There are several illnesses which cause hypoglycemia. These include diseases of the liver and adrenal glands, which may interfere with glucose production. A tumor of the islet cells of the pancreas (insulinoma) produces excessive insulin, causing low blood glucose. This is a rare condition that may be curable. These are only some of the illnesses which may cause hypoglycemia.

A common form of hypoglycemia, functional hypoglycemia, has received much public attention. Symptoms of this condition such as mental confusion and increased perspiration and heart rate usually last for fifteen minutes. Individuals do not lose consciousness and these symptoms may disappear after eating. Some symptoms of hypoglycemia are similar to those experienced during an anxiety attack. They are caused by release of epinephrine from the adrenal glands. As a result, functional hypoglycemia has been greatly overdiagnosed.

This has been compounded by doctor-entrepreneurs who have attributed a variety of symptoms to hypoglycemia. This is so much the case that the term "non-hypoglycemic hypoglycemia" has been used. Functional hypoglycemia should be suspected only when someone has hypoglycemic symptoms occurring one to three hours after eating that are then relieved by additional food. The diagnosis is then confirmed by finding a low blood glucose during a glucose tolerance test or during an attack. However, 15–20 percent of healthy people will have a blood glucose less than 45 mg./dl. during a glucose tolerance test. Therefore, hypoglycemia should not be diagnosed unless the patient's symptoms are reproduced at the time of low blood glucose and are relieved by raising the blood glucose. Functional hypoglycemia is not harmful and can usually be treated by dietary measures. The remainder of this chapter will deal with hypoglycemia caused by supply and demand factors related to insulin.

WHAT OCCURS DURING HYPOGLYCEMIA?

The pancreas has been described as an exquisite glucose sensor. It is able to sense exactly where the blood glucose level is at all times and change that level if it is too high or low. This sensor is necessary for the proper functioning of vital organs such as the brain. The brain, as well as the red blood cells and the kidneys, can use glucose even when insulin is not present. These organs are very sensitive to a lack of glucose. If blood glucose falls, certain physiological changes occur immediately. These changes include the release of glucagon and epinephrine. Some diabetic patients, though, do not release these counterregulatory hormones appropriately in response to hypoglycemia. These patients tend to have frequent and profound insulin reactions.

The early warning signs of hypoglycemia are due to the release of epinephrine. Its effects include an increased pulse and breathing rate, a feeling of hyperactivity, sweating, pallor, trembling, weakness and palpitations. If low blood glucose continues, the central nervous system is then affected. Headaches, yawning and confusion may occur. There is difficulty in remembering familiar things, lack of coordination and incoherent speech. Patients may appear to be drunk. As hypoglycemia progresses, dangerous conditions such as convulsions and unconsciousness may occur. In order to avoid the danger of hypoglycemia you must learn how to prevent, recognize, treat and evaluate it.

PREVENTION OF HYPOGLYCEMIA

An important self-management principle is to prevent hypoglycemia. Hypoglycemia occurs if there is too little demand for insulin or an oversupply of insulin. An imbalance of diet, exercise and insulin may cause this.

Dietary consistency is essential in preventing hypoglycemia. If food is not eaten regularly, insulin will lower blood glucose and hypoglycemia will occur. To prevent this, avoid skipping or delaying meals. Weight reduction also affects hypoglycemia. You will need less insulin to maintain blood glucose control as you lose weight. If you lose several pounds and do not reduce your insulin, hypoglycemia may occur. Talk with your doctor about this. Preventive aspects of hypoglycemia include consistency in the timing and composition of food intake and conferring with your doctor during a weight-loss program.

You will have to prevent hypoglycemia when you exercise. Exercise lowers blood glucose levels. This is beneficial, of course, but you want to avoid hypoglycemia. Review Chapter 9 to understand how to plan your meals prior to exercise. Remember, there is an anticipatory nature to your diabetes self-management. By eating prior to strenuous exercise and carrying a simple carbohydrate with you during the actual exercise, you can avoid hypoglycemia. Knowledge concerning your insulin regime is important. In order to prevent hypoglycemia, review the onset, peak and duration of the insulin you are presently taking. By knowing when your insulin peaks, you will know when you are most vulnerable to the onset of hypoglycemia. Hypoglycemia may also be avoided by consistency in insulin dosage and timing. Insulin is a potent medication and errors in drawing it up must be avoided.

RECOGNITION OF HYPOGLYCEMIA

Consider prevention to be step one in self-management of hypoglycemia; step two is its recognition. Individuals vary in their physical response to hypoglycemia. Some patients have only one or two symptoms, while others have a full-blown classic picture of an insulin reaction. Recognize exactly what symptoms you experience when hypoglycemia develops. Describe them to family members, close friends and health-care providers so they may assist you, if necessary. (See Figure 10.)

What happens to you when you are hypoglycemic? Symptoms include hunger, irritability, lethargy, confusion, palpitations, headache and sweatiness. Trembling, pale skin, weakness, nervousness, loss of memory, incoherent speech, jerky movements and convulsions may also occur. These symptoms have a purpose. The sweatiness and tremors that you feel are your body's inner messages that assistance is needed in raising your blood glucose level. This is similar to your pain reflex which helps you pull your hand away from a hot object to prevent you from being burned. The warning signs of an insulin reaction help you to self-manage hypoglycemia.

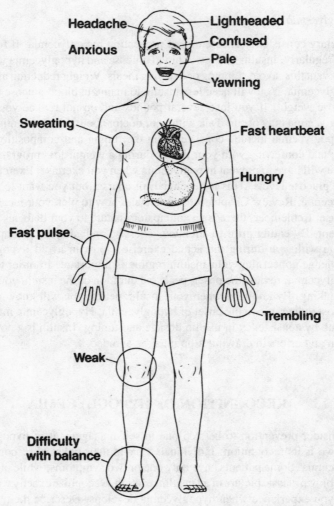

Figure 10. *How would you look and feel if you were having a reaction?*

Symptoms of hypoglycemia may vary depending on the kind of insulin you take. Regular insulin causes a rapid decrease in blood glucose which stimulates the epinephrine-induced symptoms of hypoglycemia. NPH insulin lowers the blood glucose at a slower rate; sometimes only symptoms involving the central nervous system, such as confusion, may become obvious. Certain situations may mask hypoglycemia. Patients with autonomic neuropathy, a diabetic complication affecting the nervous system, may have problems feeling hypoglycemia. Messages through the nervous system are delayed or symptoms involving the sympathetic nervous system are completely absent. Sweating, palpitations and nervousness may not be felt. Those people with decreased circulation to the brain due to atherosclerosis may have problems recognizing symptoms related to the central nervous system. Such people need assistance from others in the treatment of hypoglycemia.

RECOGNIZING HYPOGLYCEMIA AND DRUG INTERACTIONS

Medication may have an effect on hypoglycemia as well. One frequently used medication for hypertension and heart disease is propranolol (Inderal). Propranolol blocks the effect of epinephrine that is produced in the early stages of an insulin reaction. Trembling, sweating and palpitations may not occur. Because of the danger of missing early warning signs of hypoglycemia, a person taking Inderal or other beta blockers may rapidly have a severe insulin reaction. If you take beta blockers, you will need specific education concerning how to avoid hypoglycemia. Self-monitoring of blood glucose becomes especially important.

The oral agents may also cause hypoglycemia. The hypoglycemia caused by the sulfonylureas can be prolonged and dangerous. Hospitalization with intravenous glucose feedings may be needed. Hospitalization has been necessary even for people who are taking short-acting oral hypoglycemics because of the length of time the drugs remain in the body. Some patients experience one hypoglycemic reaction and then hypoglycemia recurs later in a 24- or 48-hour period. For this reason, recognition of hypoglycemia is important for all who have diabetes, whether you take insulin or oral agents.

SITUATIONS MISTAKEN FOR HYPOGLYCEMIA

One of the most common situations mistaken for hypoglycemia is an anxiety reaction. An anxiety reaction may be very similar to a hypoglycemic reaction. Anxiety can be thought of as an uneasiness, dread or apprehension. Your body reacts to anxiety by an increase in the heart rate, palpitations, rapid breathing, frequent yawning, "butterflies in the stomach," pallor, excessive perspiration and headache. During an anxiety reaction, the adrenal glands are stimulated to produce epinephrine, which causes many of these symptoms of hypoglycemia. Hypoglycemia may be differentiated from anxiety by self-monitoring of blood glucose. Measure blood glucose during an attack and you will avoid treating what you may think is hypoglycemia but really is anxiety. Situations resulting in a lack of oxygen to the brain, such as a stroke, may be mistaken for hypoglycemia. Pain, too, may produce some of the symptoms of hypoglycemia, such as tremors, sweating or palpitations. Medical attention has to be sought in these situations.

You have learned how to prevent hypoglycemia and how to recognize a reaction if it occurs. As the third step in self-management of hypoglycemia, you must learn how to treat the reaction.

TREATMENT OF HYPOGLYCEMIA

The counterregulatory hormones will help to stimulate glycogenolysis, the breakdown of the stored form of glucose (glycogen) in the liver. Only 75 grams of glucose are stored in the liver. This helps in raising blood glucose levels, but you must also help by eating extra carbohydrate. This is why it is so important always to carry a simple sugar with you when you take insulin. You can easily pop a Life Saver into your mouth or take a drink of juice, without a fuss, if it is already with you. Ten grams of simple sugar is usually enough to adequately combat hypoglycemia. Simple carbohydrate in liquid form will be digested and absorbed faster than solids. Therefore, orange juice is better than an orange. Nutritious foods such as fruit juice are preferable to non-nutritious sources such as candy. See the following list of foods containing 10 and 15 grams of simple sugar.

SIMPLE SUGARS FOR TREATMENT OF HYPOGLYCEMIA

	10 grams	*15 grams*
Coke	3.5 oz.	5 oz.
7-Up	3.5 oz.	5 oz.
ginger ale	3.5 oz.	5.5 oz.
Life Savers	5	7.5
jelly beans	6	9
sugar cubes	1.5	2.5
honey	2 tsp.	3 tsp.
caramels	5 small	7 small
orange juice	4 oz.	6 oz.
grapefruit juice	4 oz.	6 oz.
grape juice	2 oz.	3 oz.
apple juice	3 oz.	4.5 oz.

Sometimes, 10 grams of a simple carbohydrate is not enough to prevent a recurrence of hypoglycemia. Therefore, you may have to supplement the initial treatment with a complex carbohydrate like bread or a protein-containing food like milk or cheese.

Try not to overtreat an insulin reaction. Both patients and health-care providers working with patients are fearful when an insulin reaction occurs. This may result in overtreating a reaction with perhaps two packets of sugar in a 12-ounce glass of orange juice. This is too much carbohydrate to use to start treating a mild reaction and may lead to hyperglycemia. You can use home blood glucose monitoring to determine how much carbohydrate you need to raise your blood glucose.

Another way to treat an insulin reaction may be to use Instant Glutose or glucose. Each 80-gram bottle of Instant Glutose (Paddock Laboratories) contains 32 grams of glucose in a dye-free gel base. The bottle of glucose solution contains 128 calories and has a lemony flavor. This is quickly absorbed by the body upon ingestion. The usual dose is one-third of the bottle of glucose orally, which can be repeated in ten minutes if necessary. Monojel (Monoject Company) is a lemon/lime-flavored product of a similar nature. It is supplied in individually wrapped packages. This method of treating hypoglycemia may be helpful if you find it tempting to keep candies or other sugars around you.

Dextrasol is another product useful in the treatment of hypoglycemia. Dextrasol tablets are supplied in fourteen pocket-sized packages. Each tablet contains 2.8 grams of glucose which raises blood glucose rapidly. Many patients monitor their blood glucose during a reaction to determine how many tablets are necessary to raise blood glucose. For example, 3 Dextrasol tablets provide approximately 9 grams of simple sugar. This amount may raise blood glucose enough to treat hypoglycemia, but amounts must be calculated for each individual.

Glucose tablets (Becton Dickinson) are available to treat hypoglycemia. Each tablet contains 5 grams of glucose. The usual dose is 3 tablets, providing 15 grams of glucose and 64 calories, but fewer or more may be taken depending on the severity of a reaction. These tablets are chewable, without water. Each foil-sealed package contains two doses and can easily be stored.

THE USE OF GLUCAGON

A discussion of hypoglycemia would not be complete without describing glucagon. Glucagon can be injected, just like insulin, for use during hypoglycemia. It is given by injection if the patient is unconscious or cannot swallow. Ask your family members to read this section.

An important principle of first aid if someone is unconscious is never to force him to eat or drink fluids. Giving food or liquid by mouth to someone who cannot swallow may cause aspiration. Aspiration refers to food that is swallowed that goes into the lungs rather than the stomach and may cause a person to stop breathing. If there is any question that the diabetic person cannot swallow, you must not give him fluid. Instead, position the person by turning his head to the side. If the person is sitting, lean him forward with his head to the side. If he is lying down, roll him on his stomach, placing his head to the side. By placing the head to the side, aspiration will be prevented if vomiting occurs.

After you have positioned the person to avoid aspiration, you may proceed with the administration of glucagon. Glucagon is sold in a package with two vials; one vial contains one unit of powdered glucagon, and the other vial contains the diluting fluid. Glucagon must be reconstituted. This means that the powder and diluting fluid are mixed together in order to use them. Purchase two packages of glucagon and keep them in a cool, dry place. Keep them where you know you can reach them quickly in an emergency. Check the expiration date carefully. Glucagon will be good until that date if it is not mixed. The glucagon is drawn up in the same type of syringe as that used for insulin. (See Figures 7 and 9 in Chapter 7.) Instructions are packaged with the glucagon. A family member or friend who has been trained in giving the glucagon would have to give this injection to the diabetic patient who has lost consciousness. The diabetic person should be observed carefully after being given glucagon. If there is no improved response within fifteen minutes, another injection of glucagon can be given. Call an ambulance so that the patient can be taken to the emergency room for proper evaluation and care.

Even after the diabetic person regains consciousness, you should keep him positioned on his side to avoid problems, for one of glucagon's side effects is vomiting. After the patient awakens, wait a short time and have him eat a complex carbohydrate to avoid a recurrence of hypoglycemia. If the patient is brought to the emergency room, he will usually be given glucose intravenously to help keep his blood glucose elevated. After you have transported the patient to the emergency room and he has received care, remember that you now need to buy more glucagon for future emergencies.

THE NEED FOR IDENTIFICATION

A discussion of the treatment of hypoglycemia would be incomplete without stressing the importance of wearing identification. If you become confused or disoriented during a hypoglycemic reaction, you may not be able to express yourself correctly. People who have experienced hypoglycemic reactions often say they may be aware of what is happening but cannot communicate their feelings and thoughts to others. If you lose consciousness, others around you would not necessarily think of diabetes as a possible cause. Upon admission to the emergency room, there are many causes of unconsciousness to be considered. For this reason, identification stating that you have diabetes should be worn in necklace or bracelet form. A wallet card or key-chain plaque is not sufficient.

If alcohol is taken injudiciously, severe hypoglycemia may occur. This is another reason why the importance of wearing identification cannot be overstressed. If you become unconscious with the odor of alcohol on your breath, someone aiding you in an emergency might think of the alcohol overdose as the first problem, not diabetes. It would only be through your wearing of identification that you could be saved from a misdiagnosis.

The Medic Alert Foundation International is a charitable, nonprofit organization. This organization provides emergency medical identification services. A lifetime membership fee includes a three-part membership plan: a metal identification tag that can be worn as a bracelet or a necklace, a wallet card with additional medical information and an emergency answering service that can be used to obtain more information about your health status. Mediscope (Microdesign Systems) is another identification tag. It is a "telescope" that is worn around the neck. The Mediscope is held up to the eye and looked through. Important information, such as your name and address, condition, current medication, physician's name and address, is listed. Addresses of both these organizations are listed in the directory, "Community Resources," in the back of this book.

Before discussing the final step in self-management of hypoglycemia, evaluation, let us examine two situations related to hypoglycemia. It is often difficult to determine if your symptoms relate to hypoglycemia or hyperglycemia.

IS IT LOW OR IS IT HIGH?

Thorough education is necessary to understand the causes, physical effects and warning signs of both hypoglycemia and hyperglycemia. If you know why the body is reacting in a certain way, and understand the physical symptoms, you will remember how to differentiate between low and high blood glucose. Understanding why symptoms occur is better than memorizing columns of symptoms for either condition. The following list details such symptoms.

DIFFERENCES BETWEEN HYPOGLYCEMIA
AND IMPENDING DIABETIC KETOACIDOSIS

Hypoglycemia

Causes: too much insulin, delayed or omitted meals, unusual amount of exercise
Onset: rapid
Mental status: nervous, anxious
Appearance: pale, moist skin
Symptoms: sweaty, faint, shaking, hungry, weak, pounding heart, irritability
Blood glucose: less than 60 mg./dl.
Urine acetone: negative

Hyperglycemia DKA

Causes: too little insulin, dietary ignorance, infection, fever, stress
Onset: gradual
Mental status: drowsy, sleepy
Appearance: flushed, dry skin
Symptoms: increased thirst and urination, weakness, abdominal pain, generalized aches,
   loss of appetite, nausea and vomiting, heavy labored breathing
Blood glucose: greater than 250 mg./dl.
Urine acetone: large amount

By using blood glucose monitoring at the time of early warning symptoms
of hypoglycemia, you can document whether or not your blood glucose is low
or high. You can also differentiate between low and high blood glucose if you
know that with hypoglycemia you are often shaky and sweating, whereas in
high blood glucose or diabetic coma, you are dehydrated, so that your body is
flushed and dry. Finally, if you are unsure whether glucose is high or low, it
is better to treat for hypoglycemia. If you take 10 grams of a simple carbohydrate
for symptoms that you think are due to hypoglycemia but your glucose is actually
high, those 10 grams of sugar will not drastically increase your blood glucose.
Yet those 10 grams of a simple carbohydrate may immediately bring you out
of hypoglycemia. So when you are uncertain, treat any reaction as hypoglycemic. Of course, we are speaking here of one or two single episodes of uncertainty. You should not continue snacking without properly documenting
hypoglycemia. The best way to differentiate between the two is through self-
testing of blood glucose.

THE SOMOGYI EFFECT

A condition which may be confused with hyperglycemia and which results
from hypoglycemia is known as the Somogyi effect. Hypoglycemia may occur

during the night when symptoms may not awaken you. Counterregulatory hormones are then released. Insulin-dependent patients often overrespond to these hormones. This response, if exaggerated, leads to elevated blood glucose. Even if nighttime hypoglycemia does not occur, patients often experience high blood glucose before breakfast. This is known as the "dawn phenomenon" and is related to low concentrations of insulin in the blood. So if nighttime hypoglycemia results in an overrelease of counterregulatory hormones at the same time that insulin levels are low, you may have an increase in blood glucose. If your insulin dose is increased in an attempt to lower your morning blood glucose, this will only cause more nighttime hypoglycemia. This will result in more secretion of counterregulatory hormones and an increase in morning blood glucose, and will start a vicious cycle.

Some symptoms of the Somogyi effect include headaches occurring in the morning, perspiration during the night, a restless sleep pattern, and recurring nightmares, as well as elevated urine and blood glucose tests (particularly when they follow a series of negative or low results). Another symptom is a low body temperature in the morning. Treatment of the Somogyi effect involves lowering the insulin dose or adjusting the meal plan to prevent nighttime hypoglycemia. Many patients are finding that by using blood glucose monitoring during the middle of the night, they can pinpoint the occurrence of hypoglycemia. Some doctors ask patients to set the alarm clock for 3 or 4 A.M., awaken and do a quick blood test. This can provide extra information to determine if the Somogyi effect is present.

EVALUATION OF HYPOGLYCEMIA

Evaluation is the fourth and final aspect of self-management of hypoglycemia. It is probably the most important. You must ask yourself why hypoglycemia occurred. Review your insulin dosage and the timing of the insulin. Was there an increase in exercise at this time? Did you change your diet or delay a meal? Did you draw up your insulin correctly? Record all hypoglycemic reactions in the comments column of your testing record for review and preparation for the future. Some patients report frequent episodes of hypoglycemia as part of their life with diabetes. You are not supposed to have frequent hypoglycemic episodes as part of having diabetes. Through a proper self-management program you should be able to obtain good blood glucose control without having frequent insulin reactions interfering with your daily life. If you are having frequent insulin reactions and cannot evaluate their cause, bring this to the attention of your doctor or nurse.

There are many symptoms of hypoglycemia. They develop due to the body's reaction to a lack of glucose. Counterregulatory hormones play an important role in helping to raise the blood glucose. But you too must help. Remember to eat your meals on time, preplan your food for extra activity and inject the correct amount of insulin at the proper time. Be aware that hypoglycemia is most likely to occur when your insulin peaks. You can treat hypoglycemia with a simple carbohydrate, often followed by a complex carbohydrate. Other sugar-type pills and solutions are also available. By planning ahead, you can rely on yourself rather than others to treat hypoglycemia. Glucagon can be injected, like insulin, in those who are unconscious. Wear identification stating you have diabetes. Finally, always evaluate why the insulin reaction occurred, to prevent it from happening again.

11

Hyperglycemic
Complications
and "Sick Days"

Two dangerous conditions are associated with marked hyperglycemia. In the non-insulin-dependent person, hyperglycemia can lead to hyperglycemic hyperosmolar non-ketotic coma (the hyperglycemic-dehydration syndrome). In the insulin-dependent person, lack of insulin can lead to diabetic ketoacidosis. In this chapter, you will learn how to avoid these conditions as well as how to evaluate, recognize and treat them. If you are insulin-dependent, illness may increase your chance of developing diabetic ketoacidosis. This chapter will also explain how to handle "sick days."

HYPERGLYCEMIA-DEHYDRATION SYNDROME

Hyperglycemic hyperosmolar non-ketotic coma (HHNC) is also known as the hyperglycemia-dehydration syndrome. It is a dangerous condition that often goes unrecognized. It probably is responsible for 10–20 percent of severe cases of hyperglycemia; 40–70 percent of people who get it may die. This syndrome is characterized by extreme dehydration due to high blood glucose. In order to understand how dehydration occurs, think about how fluids remain in the body. Osmosis has to do with maintaining the same concentration of dissolved particles on either side of a cell membrane. Water passes through cell membranes freely to balance osmolality. If there is elevated glucose in the blood, there is high osmolality in the blood compared with the cells. Water passes from the cells to the blood to maintain osmolality. The water, along with excess glucose, is then excreted in the urine. The excretion of water along with glucose is an "osmotic diuresis." This produces the polyuria of uncontrolled diabetes.

Usually the kidney protects you against a buildup of blood glucose by excreting glucose. If the kidney is damaged it will not be able to excrete glucose efficiently. Blood glucose will increase. Most people who develop HHNC have underlying kidney disease. Another condition that slows the excretion of glucose is the reduced amount of fluid present in the circulation because of the diuresis. As water is lost through diuresis, the volume of blood decreases. Blood flow through the kidney is decreased and glucose cannot be adequately excreted, so blood glucose rises further. As the blood becomes more concentrated, there is a risk of thrombosis (development of a blood clot). The rise in blood glucose, usually above 600 mg./dl., combined with severe dehydration, results in an emergency situation.

The hyperglycemia-dehydration syndrome occurs due to a lack of insulin. Blood glucose rises but ketones do not accumulate in the blood. It is believed that ketosis does not occur because the deficiency in insulin secretion is not as severe as in Type I diabetics.

AVOIDANCE, RECOGNITION AND TREATMENT OF HHNC

How would you avoid developing hyperglycemic hyperosmolar non-ketotic coma (HHNC)? Knowing the causes of its development will help. Usually, the syndrome starts when a non-insulin-dependent person is ill. This condition may arise if you are not producing or taking enough insulin. Stress from burns, heart attacks, kidney failure, infections or strokes may also cause its development. Certain medications, such as thiazide diuretics, glucocorticoids or propranolol, may also predispose certain individuals to HHNC. Following sick-day rules, calling your doctor, adhering to your diet and medication prescription will all help you avoid HHNC.

Many patients experiencing HHNC are mistakenly diagnosed as having a stroke because they may exhibit mental changes. Here you can see the necessity of wearing identification stating that you have diabetes. Sleepiness, seizures and loss of speech are common signs. Polyuria, weakness and polydipsia may often be experienced. Be aware of these symptoms; do not allow them to persist without attention.

Treatment involves replacing lost fluids with intravenous fluids. Regular insulin is used to lower blood glucose. Potassium, which is lost during dehydration, is given. Any underlying problem, such as infection, is treated. In conclusion, if you have non-insulin-dependent diabetes, you must be alert to signs of HHNC. Its occurrence is usually related to illness. Be aware that in times of stress Type II diabetic persons may require insulin. Call your doctor if your glucose becomes elevated. You can take an active role in prevention, by monitoring blood glucose levels. Again, through self-management skills, you will be able to prevent and/or control this dangerous complication of hyperglycemia.

DIABETIC KETOACIDOSIS

Diabetic ketoacidosis (DKA) may best be viewed as an absolute lack of insulin. The lack of insulin is greater than in the hyperglycemia-dehydration syndrome. Sixty-five percent of all hospital admissions of diabetic patients up to the age of 19 are for DKA. It is a significant problem in adults as well, with an admission rate of 6 percent in patients above the age of 25. DKA is an emergency. Uncomplicated DKA has a mortality rate of 1–2 percent (for every 100 episodes of DKA one or two patients will die).

In order to understand diabetic ketoacidosis, you must first learn about acid/base balance. A substance is more or less acid, depending on its concentration of ionized hydrogen. An acid is a compound that has enough hydrogen ions to give some away. A base takes up ionized hydrogen. An acid or base's strength is expressed by the symbol pH (power Hydrogen). A pH of 7 is considered neutral. Solutions with a pH above 7 are alkaline; below 7 they are acidic. The more acid a solution is, the lower is its pH number. The range of pH is 0–14. The pH of living things is very important because all the chemical reactions in the cells are sensitive to pH. Although urine usually has a pH of 5 or 6 and stomach secretions usually have a pH of 1 to 4, the blood pH must remain in a very narrow range. In fact, a blood pH below 7 or above 8 is not compatible with life. The waste products of cells are acidic. Buffers constantly neutralize excess acids (or bases). Buffers are compounds that help to keep the blood pH in a narrow range. Excess acids are also eliminated through the respiratory and urinary systems. The way the buffers in the respiratory and urinary systems act together to keep the blood pH at about 7.4 is an example of homeostasis (acid/base balance).

Remember that insulin works to prevent the breakdown of fats as well as to store glucose properly. In DKA, two main problems arise, hyperglycemia and ketosis. These work together to create the emergency state of DKA. Without sufficient insulin, glucose in the blood is not properly used and is also overproduced by the liver. Hyperglycemia occurs as a result of gluconeogenesis and the decreased use of glucose by the cells. As glucose builds up in the blood, excessive loss of water and electrolytes occurs, with accompanying symptoms of polyuria and polydipsia. Thus, hyperglycemia leads to dehydration.

At the same time that dehydration is occurring, fats are being broken down (lipolysis). Insulin deficiency increases lipolysis, and fats are converted to fatty acids and glycerol. The glycerols can act to further increase blood glucose. The fatty acids will go to the liver and form ketoacids in large quantities. Ketoacids build up in the blood. They are excreted, along with glucose, in the urine. Sodium bicarbonate stores are lost. Bicarbonate acts as a buffer to reduce the blood's acidity. Without bicarbonate, acidosis progresses. The pH drops dangerously. In addition, dehydration worsens ketoacidosis. In this uncontrolled state, protein stores break down to amino acids. The liver converts excess amino acids to glucose and hyperglycemia worsens. As ketoacidosis worsens, all systems slow down and accumulated ketones are broken down slowly. The lungs attempt to remove excess acids but they may become overtaxed. Deep, labored breathing (Kussmaul's respirations) begins and the breath may have a fruity odor of acetone. Ketoacidosis is a stressful state. The adrenal glands cause the liver to increase gluconeogenesis. More glucose becomes available, only worsening the problem. (See Table 10.) The cycle can be reversed only with insulin.

TABLE 10   CYCLE OF DIABETIC KETOACIDOSIS

Insulin Lack

Hyperglycemia
(Blood Glucose Rises)   Glycerol ←— Lipolysis (Breakdown of Fat)

Osmotic Diuresis   Free Fatty Acids

Loss of Electrolytes and Fluids   Free Fatty Acids Burned

Dehydration   Ketones Produced

Ketoacidosis

Although DKA is serious and its emergency nature cannot be overemphasized, it is almost always preventable and treatable. Lactic acidosis is another type of acidosis that occurs in diabetic persons, though only rarely. Since the removal of Phenformin from the market, fewer cases have been seen. We will now look at the causes, recognition and treatment of diabetic ketoacidosis.

CAUSES OF DKA

The primary cause of DKA is severe deficiency of insulin. This may occur in several situations, such as a new diagnosis of diabetes, stress or failure to take insulin. For the insulin-dependent diabetic, an insulin injection is necessary on a daily basis. If you forget to take insulin, lose your supplies or refuse to take the injection, DKA will occur. Another cause of DKA is illness combined with failure to take insulin. Do not make the grave mistake of not taking insulin when you are ill since you may not feel like eating. If you are insulin-dependent and ill, you will need not only your normal dose of insulin but possibly extra insulin. This will be discussed later on in this chapter.

DKA may be due to unsuspected diabetes. An individual may not be aware he has insulin-dependent diabetes and will miss warning symptoms. If insulin requirements change and are not monitored carefully, DKA may develop. Emotional stress, too, has been shown to raise blood glucose in some individuals and predispose them to hyperglycemia and/or DKA. Menstruation may be a possible cause of ketoacidosis. In some young females, diabetes is more difficult to control during menstruation. This may be due to the pain, anorexia or vomiting that some women experience at this time. Menstruation lowers the renal threshold for glucose, and glycosuria is seen more often. For many patients, acetonuria also occurs during this time. Menstruation is a rare cause of DKA but one that must be kept in mind. Tell your doctor if you find you have acetone in your urine at this time. He may want to evaluate and modify your self-management program during the menstrual cycle.

RECOGNITION OF DKA

If symptoms occur that are similar to those you experienced when you were first diagnosed (polyuria, polydipsia, fatigue), be alert to the onset of DKA. Other symptoms include weakness, abdominal pains, generalized aches, a loss of appetite, nausea and vomiting and heavy, labored breathing. All of these, if untreated, can lead to what is known as "diabetic coma." When the term "diabetic coma" is used, you may think only of unconsciousness. However, a confused state is considered a diabetic coma. Commit the following symptoms of DKA to memory. One sign that will alert you to DKA is ketones in the urine. It is important, though, to realize that spilling a small amount of ketones when you are ill or when diabetes is not yet controlled does not mean you are in ketoacidosis. Ketoacidosis is accompanied by many symptoms, especially those related to dehydration.

Increased urination
Increased thirst
Weakness
Nausea, vomiting
Loss of appetite
Generalized aches
Abdominal pain
Labored breathing
Fruity breath odor
Confusion
Unconsciousness
Remember the definite sign present in DKA:
large amounts of urine glucose and ketones.

In addition, DKA develops gradually. You may read articles that describe the slow onset of DKA compared with hypoglycemic reactions. Yes, hypoglycemia may occur within a time period as short as ten minutes. But DKA may develop within only twelve hours in the insulin-dependent diabetic who omits an insulin injection in the morning. The word "gradual" in this case means hours rather than minutes. Do not be fooled into thinking that DKA only develops over days or weeks. It is a life-threatening emergency that may start slowly, but it will not occur if you are properly educated concerning its avoidance, recognition and treatment.

TREATMENT OF DKA

How would you treat DKA? If you see ketones in your urine, and you experience other symptoms of DKA, call your doctor immediately. If you are able to swallow, try to take fluids. Family members should know the signs and symptoms of DKA and should encourage you to drink fluids. Continue to test your urine and keep in contact with your doctor. If your symptoms involve dehydration, vomiting, weakness and labored breathing, call an ambulance and go to the emergency room. You would be diagnosed in the ER as being in diabetic ketoacidosis, based on blood tests. The treatment for DKA is insulin and fluids. Insulin is needed since it is not present in sufficient amounts. Fluids are needed to replace those that you have lost through dehydration. Regular insulin is given during DKA. Its rapid action is needed in this emergency. It is often given in low doses, 5 to 10 units per hour, through a continuous intravenous infusion. Larger doses of insulin are used if your blood glucose does not decrease. Fluids are given intravenously and patients are given liquids to drink, if possible. Proper treatment of DKA can only occur in a hospital setting where there is access to intravenous equipment, emergency medications and the watchful eyes of doctors and nurses.

HOSPITALIZATION FOR DKA

What can you expect if you are hospitalized for DKA? If you are diagnosed as having DKA, you should expect to stay in the hospital for treatment and observation. Remember, DKA has a profound effect on all body systems. Therefore, you will probably be admitted to the intensive-care unit (ICU) for close monitoring. During this time, in addition to treatment of DKA, its cause and methods of prevention of future episodes will be investigated.

In the emergency room, a short history will be taken and a physical exam performed. If you are confused, a family member or friend can give the necessary information. Again, you can see the need for identification stating that you have diabetes. You will be asked to give a urine specimen or, if you are unconscious, you might be catheterized. This involves passage of a sterile tube into your bladder for collection of urine. This procedure is usually avoided, but if you are not awake, it may be necessary in order to judge kidney function. Blood samples will be taken.

If you are admitted to the ICU, you will find yourself in a specialized unit with close medical and nursing observation. The intravenous infusion will continue in order to provide fluids and medication. DKA can result in the loss of important electrolytes such as potassium. When this occurs, disturbances in the rhythm of the heartbeat may occasionally result. You may be placed on a cardiac monitor that will evaluate your heart rhythm. You will also find that you are having frequent laboratory tests. You may have blood drawn from a vein in your arm as well as from an artery, to determine your pH and the level of oxygen and carbon dioxide in your blood. You will have fingerstick blood determinations of glucose frequently, to monitor the fall in your glucose level. As your condition stabilizes, your ICU stay will end. Usually within one to two days following an episode of DKA, you are ready for transfer to a medical floor. At this time, your diabetes self-management will be evaluated. Use this time for an update or start of education in self-management.

EVALUATION AND PREVENTION OF DKA

The final concept essential to your self-management of DKA is to evaluate it and prevent future episodes. Why did ketoacidosis occur? Was the insulin you injected sufficient to meet your requirement? Did you have an infection? Did you have a fever? Were you inconsistent with your diet? Did you experience emotional stress that may have precipitated DKA? Look at all of the following areas and evaluate what occurred in the past in an effort to prevent this from happening in the future. The next part of this chapter provides guides to the prevention of DKA. Through education, DKA can be avoided. Ketosis can be recognized and prevented from progressing.

EVALUATE WHY DKA HAPPENED:

1. Did you take insulin as prescribed?
2. Are you injecting into areas of hypertrophy?
3. Do you have an infection?
4. Did you forget your insulin because you were sick?
5. Are you following a diet?
6. Have you experienced severe emotional stress?

Find the cause of DKA so you can prevent its future occurrence.

In summary, two dangerous situations develop in relation to hyperglycemia. Hyperglycemic hyperosmolar non-ketotic coma is characterized by elevated blood glucose and dehydration but ketones do not appear in the urine. It usually occurs in non-insulin-dependent persons who are ill, under stress or taking certain medications. Diabetic ketoacidosis is characterized by high blood glucose, dehydration and ketonuria. This may occur in someone previously undiagnosed, or if you forget to take your insulin, are ill and do not take your insulin, or are under stress. Treatment for both includes hospitalization, during which you receive intravenous fluids and medication, especially insulin. Your self-management goals should be to learn these conditions, seek help immediately and evaluate why they occurred. Self-management during sick days will now be discussed.

SELF-MANAGEMENT OF SICK DAYS

Preventing illness is a priority for all people, but particularly for people with diabetes. In this chapter, you will learn about the importance of preventing illness as well as managing your diabetes if illness does occur.

Be aware of principles of general health maintenance. This includes continued care by a doctor and health-care team devoted to diabetes. Meeting with your doctor, nurse, dietitian, podiatrist and ophthalmologist helps you stay in good health to prevent illness. Keep your immunizations up to date and be aware of good hygienic practices. These may include the necessity of tetanus injections after a severe cut, general cleanliness measures in preventing cuts from becoming infected and maintaining good skin care. Recognize and treat symptoms of flu and pneumonia under your doctor's guidance.

With diabetes, you cannot be ill for a day or two and decide to ignore self-management while you concentrate on feeling better. You must be alert to the interaction of diabetes with other illnesses. Any illness, no matter how small or large, will affect diabetes control.

IDENTIFICATION OF ILLNESSES AND INFECTIONS

Identify illnesses that may interfere with diabetes control. These include gastrointestinal upsets such as nausea, diarrhea and vomiting. An episode of influenza, a common cold, a sore throat or a twenty-four-hour virus will also have a detrimental effect on diabetes control. Other signs of infection include fever, chills, vaginal discharge or itching and burning or pain when urinating. An acute illness will make blood glucose control difficult. If blood glucose control worsens, the illness, too, may become worse.

Illness, and particularly infection, will lead to hyperglycemia and its associated symptoms. Infection can cause an increase in the rate of metabolism. Gluconeogenesis may be accelerated as part of this, resulting in hyperglycemia. Of course, by checking your blood or urine, you will know whether your glucose level has increased. Self-monitoring is important in the self-management of sick days and will be discussed later.

SELF-MANAGEMENT GOALS DURING ILLNESS

A primary self-management goal for both the non-insulin-dependent and the insulin-dependent person is to increase contact with your doctor when illness occurs. This may prevent the illness from interfering with diabetes or from developing into anything more serious. With guidance, you may be able to handle your sick days at home.

When should you call your doctor? Most doctors want to hear from you if you find unusually elevated blood glucose readings, have urine test results that are greater than 2 percent during illness, with ketones present, or have fever. It is most important to call the doctor if you are not able to keep any food or liquids down. If you are unable to reach your doctor, and have been vomiting, go to the emergency room for help.

When you contact your doctor, be prepared to give him the information he needs to analyze your present situation. This would include all the signs and symptoms of your present illness. Also tell him your temperature and the results of your blood and urine tests for glucose and acetone. Be prepared to tell him what you have been able to eat within the last twenty-four hours, and if you've had any vomiting, diarrhea or nausea.

If you have non-insulin-dependent diabetes, continue to take your oral medications and increase your home testing to every three to four hours when ill. If your urine glucose shows a level of 1 percent or more, or blood tests are above 250 mg./dl., test for acetone and review the symptoms of hyperglycemia and diabetic ketoacidosis. Be aware that non-insulin-dependent diabetic persons may also go into a coma without showing acetone in their urine.

In the insulin-dependent person, insulin adjustment is the second tool of self-management. One of the most serious self-management mistakes is made during sick days. If you awaken with the flu and decide not to take your insulin because you will not be eating, you place yourself in danger. It is true that exercise, diet and insulin must always be balanced. When you are ill, you may not want to eat or exercise, but taking insulin remains extremely important. It is needed because you are always producing glucose, through gluconeogenesis. If a diabetic person does not take insulin and does not eat, his blood glucose will still be high. This happens because glucose is released from body stores when insulin is not present. Infection may raise the rate of metabolism in the body, causing an even greater need for insulin. Without insulin, glucose cannot enter the cell where it is needed. Your fat stores will break down. Ketones will be produced in the liver and DKA can develop. Insulin is necessary to combat ketoacidosis. You must continue to take your insulin while staying in contact with your doctor. The timing of injections as well as the amounts of insulin may be altered. In fact, you may be told to add Regular insulin in small doses, throughout the day, as a supplement to your normal dosage of insulin. Insulin adjustments are made on the basis of the third tool of self-management, self-monitoring.

SELF-MONITORING

Self-monitoring of blood glucose and urine acetone is necessary during sick days. Why is it important to test for acetone when ill? When fats are broken down, their by-products, fatty acids, are released. Fatty acids are used to form ketones, and ketones can be measured easily in the urine as acetone. The presence of large amounts of acetone should alert you to ketosis. Incorporate testing for acetone into your self-management program. If it is present, contact your doctor.

What if you are too ill to perform self-monitoring? Although the philosophy of this book is dedicated to the individual's being a self-manager, there are times when you must rely on help from others. This is one of those occasions. If you are too ill to test, a family member or friend should continue the urine testing for you. What about exercise? It is essential that you rest, keep warm and not attempt to exercise when you are ill. Have a family member stay with you if you are too weak to perform self-management tasks. Call your *doctor* for advice.

DIETARY INTERVENTION DURING ILLNESS

When you have a fever, your body may lose fluids that must be replaced. Keep a record of all food and liquids taken so that you can tell your doctor. Food is important for two reasons. It will give you the nutritional support to aid in your recovery, and it is important in "covering" the insulin you have taken, so that you will not develop hypoglycemia. If you have taken your insulin and find you cannot keep regular meals down, do not force yourself to eat. Attempt to drink 2–4 tablespoons of a sweetened fluid every twenty minutes. Take sips of sugared juices, ginger ale, soups, broths, teas or cola. Vomiting and diarrhea can cause you to lose electrolytes such as sodium and potassium. These must be replaced. If you cannot take any fluids, contact your doctor. The following is a list of food choices during illness.

FOOD CHOICES FOR SICK DAYS

If you are unable to retain fluids, try 2–4 tablespoons every 20 minutes of:

    regular Jell-O
    regular soft drinks
    orange juice
    tea with sugar
    sweetened applesauce
    sherbet
    ice cream
    beef or chicken broth

If you can retain fluids and food but your appetite is poor, try at least one of the following each hour:

    ¼ cup regular Jell-O
    ½ cup regular soft drinks
    ½ cup orange or grapefruit juice

¼ cup grape juice
1 tbs. honey
½ twin-pop Popsicle
1 banana
1 cup beef or chicken broth/soup

To increase your nutritional status when your appetite is still "not too hot," try:

½ cup eggnog
1 cup creamed soup
1 cup plain yogurt
½ cup sweetened custard
½ cup ice cream
½ cup hot cereal
1–2 soft-boiled or poached eggs
½ cup cottage cheese
½ cup fruit juice
½ cup unsweetened applesauce

If you are able to keep foods down but still have a poor appetite, try easily digestible foods. These include creamed soups, mashed potatoes, cooked cereals, plain yogurt, bananas, ice cream, gelatins as well as juices, broths and regular sodas. Milk choices such as custard or eggnog are also appropriate. Attempt to take one cup of food or liquid at least every two hours. Small snacks that are easily digestible can be taken from bread exchanges such as six saltines, one-half cup of cooked cereal or one-half cup of mashed potatoes.

There are certain differences in diabetes self-management when you are well compared with when you are ill. In the area of nutrition, you normally avoid foods and beverages containing sugar. During illness, this rule is reversed. (At this time you replace other foods and fluids with carbohydrates.) Another difference is the use of extra insulin. If hyperglycemia has occurred, you may need *additional* insulin when sick. This may be used as a supplement every four hours, in a dose each time of 20 percent of your normal daily dose. This sick-day rule may become a standard procedure for you after you have fully discussed sick days with your doctor. For example, if you normally take 40 units of NPH insulin in the morning and you are ill, you would take your daily dose of 40 units of NPH insulin. You may then supplement this with Regular insulin, according to your doctor's orders. This supplement might be 8 units of Regular insulin every four hours, depending on the results of home blood glucose and urine acetone tests. If only acetone was present in the urine, and glucose was not elevated, extra insulin would *not* be necessary. In that case, the acidosis may be due to starvation rather than DKA. Blood glucose monitoring is invaluable during this time. Review the following basic sick-day rules.

BASIC SICK-DAY RULES

1. Contact your doctor immediately.
2. Always continue to take your insulin.
3. Measure blood glucose and urine acetone.
4. Stay in bed, rest.
5. Modify your meal plan:
   a. If you have a fever, increase your intake of unsweetened fluids.
   b. Choose sweetened liquids or foods when your appetite is poor and you cannot retain fluids.
   c. Choose liquids or foods that can replace the electrolytes: sodium and potassium.
6. Obtain help from family members and friends.
7. Take supplements of Regular insulin, as directed by your doctor.
8. If you are vomiting, seek help immediately.

RECOVERY FROM ILLNESS

As part of your recovery from illness you need to evaluate your sick-day management. Were you able to increase the frequency of blood and urine testing? Did you take your normal dose of insulin? Did you take supplemental Regular insulin if needed? Did you rest and stay warm during this sick day? All of these questions should be answered affirmatively in order for you to be able to handle future sick days. If you are a newly diagnosed diabetic person, you may have problems handling diabetes and illness for the first time. Observe the rules carefully and contact your doctor early.

As part of preplanning, keep a supply of certain medications at home. In this way, you will be prepared if illness strikes. These may include paregoric, Maalox, Milk of Magnesia. Medications such as glucagon and Regular insulin should be kept in the refrigerator. Have aspirin or acetaminophen at home as well as a fever thermometer. Non-prescription drugs, such as cough medicines, should not have a sugar base. Check with your pharmacist for advice concerning this.

Remember, you are attempting to balance diet, exercise and insulin in order to prevent diabetic ketoacidosis. You can never think to yourself: "I'm too ill to eat, so I won't take my insulin" or "I'm too ill to test, so I'll skip it today." You need to stay actively involved in diabetes self-management when you are ill or ask others for help.

We have found it helpful to preplan, problem-solve and role-play with patients in order to get them to react to different types of illnesses. Fear of the unknown and inadequate preparation will lead to difficulties in diabetes self-management.

It is to be hoped that illness will not occur and you will not need to fall back on sick-day rules. However, by preplanning what actions you could take and by role playing with family members and friends, the mystery of sick-day rules will disappear. These actions would include increasing testing, monitoring blood glucose and urine acetone levels, increasing communication with your doctor and taking medication as prescribed. You will be able to handle illness successfully. If you do become ill, take out this book and read about sick-day rules. Your education will allow you to manage your sick days along with your good days.

12

Pattern Control

The importance of controlling blood glucose to reduce or eliminate complications is emphasized throughout this book. In this chapter you will learn how to assess your diabetes control and make the necessary changes in your self-management program.

Pattern control refers to the use of diet, insulin and exercise to keep blood glucose as normal as possible at all times. It is the key to successful management of diabetes. A pattern may be seen from the results of your blood tests. The ideal pattern is normal blood glucose levels. However, it may not be possible for you to have a normal blood glucose all the time, particularly if you are newly diagnosed. Therefore, your goal is to have your blood glucose as close to normal as frequently as possible. Do not be frustrated by the occasional unexplained disruption in glucose control. It is realistic, though, to have capillary blood glucoses between 80 and 140 mg./dl. 85–90 percent of the time.

Pattern control will allow you to become skillful in assessing your pattern and any disruptions that may occur in it. Both hyperglycemia and hypoglycemia are considered disruptions in your pattern. In order to manage such disruptions, you need to use five tools: self-testing, diet, medication, exercise and special factors. Before looking at each of these, a discussion of how your pattern becomes established is necessary.

When you are diagnosed as having diabetes, your doctor prescribes a particular insulin dosage, a calorie-adjusted diet and a plan of exercise tailored for you. This plan is devised to lower your blood glucose. For the non-insulin-dependent person, diet and exercise alone may be prescribed. When weight loss occurs, your endogenous insulin supply may then take over in establishing diabetes control.

There are two aspects of blood glucose control in those who require insulin therapy: (1) keeping the blood glucose normal when fasting and (2) preventing the blood glucose from rising too high after eating (postprandial glycemia). These two goals are accomplished by separate phases of insulin secretion by the normal, non-diabetic pancreas. A small amount of insulin is always secreted by the normal pancreas, even during fasting. This "basal" insulin secretion is enough to control gluconeogenesis in the liver; it keeps blood glucose in the normal range between meals. Postprandial hyperglycemia is prevented in the non-diabetic person by having an adequate amount of basal insulin and by secretion of additional insulin in response to eating.

In some people with Type I diabetes, the pancreas still produces some insulin in response to eating. In this case, supplementing their endogenous basal insulin secretion with one injection of intermediate-acting insulin may be enough to maintain a normal blood glucose. (See Figures 11a and 11b.) However, the insulin reserve of the pancreas is lost with time. Most Type I individuals will have inadequate or no insulin secretion in response to eating. In this case, it is usually necessary to (a) provide basal insulin with two injections of an inter-mediate-acting insulin or one injection of a long-acting insulin and (b) add injections of a short-acting (Regular) insulin before meals. (See Figures 11c and 11d.) In this way, blood glucose is kept in the normal range after meals as well as when you are not eating. Thus, most people with Type I diabetes require multiple injections of insulin. Another way to accomplish this is with an insulin infusion pump. This provides a continuous infusion of Regular insulin (basal insulin) with extra amounts of Regular insulin added before meals.

There are factors that affect your pattern that are not under your control. These include the endogenous insulin supply, the pharmacology of the type of insulin you use and hormonal influences. If you have no endogenous insulin supply, you will surely need to carefully monitor your insulin dosage in order to become controlled. The pharmacology of insulin refers to how insulin works in your body. Some individuals have an earlier or later peaking of insulin than others. This, too, will determine your pattern. NPH insulin peaks at 6–12 hours. This is a wide range. Moreover, it may peak at 4–20 hours in some individuals. You must determine the peak and duration of insulin in your own body. This is an important early step in pattern control. Hormonal influences refer to the counterregulatory hormones that are present and work against the action of insulin. Pattern control recognizes the influence of these factors and then ma-nipulates the factors you can and must control, such as diet, insulin and exercise. You can then establish pattern control over a prolonged period of time. With changes such as illness, you may have periodic, unstable disruptions in your pattern. These will be detected through self-testing.

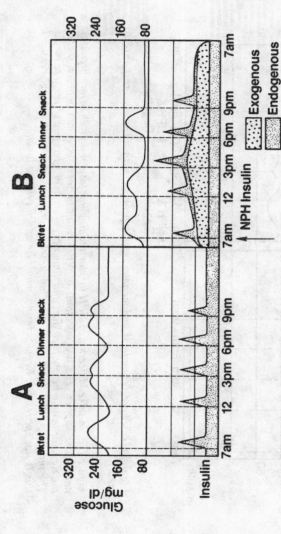

Figure 11a. In A there is decreased endogenous insulin reserve and basal insulin is low; the FBS (fasting blood sugar) is elevated and postprandial hyperglycemia is accentuated.

Figure 11b. In B a single injection of NPH insulin supplements the basal insulin supply, and endogenous insulin in response to meals prevents marked postprandial hyperglycemia. Note that the pharmacology of NPH results in high levels of insulin at 3–6 P.M., with the danger of hypoglycemia.

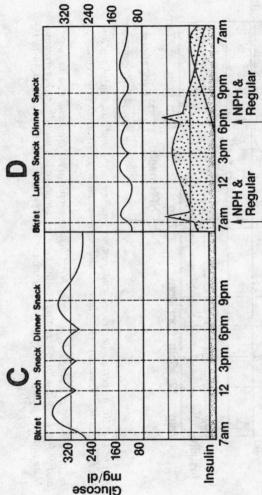

Figure 11c. There is minimal endogenous insulin present, with no insulin response to meals.

Figure 11d. A mixed injection of NPH insulin and Regular insulin is given before breakfast and before supper. The two injections of NPH result in normoglycemia between meals; the Regular insulin before breakfast and dinner prevents hyperglycemia after these meals. The morning NPH has its peak after lunch, which prevents post-lunch hyperglycemia. If this is not successful, Regular insulin would be added prior to lunch.

DETECTION OF A DISRUPTION

In order to detect a disruption in your pattern, choose a testing method that is right for you. Our emphasis on close control should lead you to choose blood glucose self-monitoring as the most accurate measure. Blood tests performed at various times of the day are essential in determining pattern control. The more often you test, the more information you will gather for pattern control. Remember to record test results along with particular situations such as increased mental stress, a cold, a flu, a virus or dietary indiscretion. Since your pattern should not change frequently, you will not observe disruptions on a daily basis. Recurring periods of elevated glucose or insulin reactions should alert you to the need for pattern control.

DIET ADJUSTMENT

How will you then establish pattern control? An important aspect of pattern control is dietary consistency. You cannot be controlled unless your diet is consistent. If you find consistently elevated test results during one time period, look at your dietary habits first. You can alter your meal plan, as your first step. If your pre-lunch glucose levels are quite high, look at the amount of breakfast or midmorning snack you are eating. If you find elevated glucose tests late in the evening or before breakfast, evaluate your dinner meal. Keep an eye on portion sizes and extra calories. When you have frequent insulin reactions, reevaluate your meal plan. You may need more food before the time at which a reaction occurs. Check with your dietitian or doctor about evaluating your food intake prior to hypoglycemia. These disruptions should not be occurring every few days if you are consistent in meal planning. If you have established a pattern and then find time periods of instability, check your diet first.

WHY DOES HYPOGLYCEMIA OCCUR?

Hypoglycemia	*Possible Causes*	*Possible Remedies*
Early morning	Exercise the night before	Eat more to compensate for exercise
	Alcohol the night before	Decrease alcohol intake
	Eliminated evening snack	Do not eliminate evening snack
	Delayed peaking of previous morning intermediate-acting insulin	Include late-evening snack

Hypoglycemia	*Possible Causes*	*Possible Remedies*
Midmorning	No time for breakfast	Attempt to eat some breakfast every day
	No midmorning snack planned	Include midmorning snack
	Peaking of Regular insulin	Include midmorning snack
	Early-morning exercise	Allow for extra food or decrease insulin dosage
Afternoon	Skipped lunch	Have meal consistency as goal
	No afternoon snack	Include afternoon snack
	Peaking of intermediate-acting insulin	Include afternoon snack and avoid exercise at this time
Bedtime	Skipped dinner	Continue meal consistency
	Eliminated evening snack	Include evening snack
	Peaking of Regular insulin	Reevaluate meal plan

WHY DOES HYPERGLYCEMIA OCCUR?

Hyperglycemia	*Possible Causes*	*Possible Remedies*
Early morning	Too little intermediate-acting insulin from the previous night	Include an evening injection
	Too little exercise	Incorporate more activity into daily routine
	Too many calories	Achieve dietary consistency
Midmorning	Early-morning intermediate-acting insulin was not adequate	An early-morning injection of a short-acting insulin
	Too many calories	Rearrange daily calorie intake; a midmorning snack would not be needed
Afternoon	Insufficient intermediate-acting insulin from the morning	Increase the amount of intermediate-acting insulin

Hyperglycemia	*Possible Causes*	*Possible Remedies*
	Too many calories at lunch	Reduce calories at lunch
	Not enough exercise	Incorporate more activity into your lifestyle
Bedtime	Not enough daily exercise	Reevaluate your day to fit in more activity
	Not enough insulin	Increase morning insulin dose
	Too many calories	Reevaluate your caloric intake
At any time	Possible underlying infection or unusual stress	Check glucose and acetone
	Problem with insulin absorption	Reevaluate injection technique

EXERCISE ADJUSTMENT

Review Chapter 9 before including exercise in pattern control. Maintaining a regular exercise program can lower blood glucose and help you establish pattern control. If you are quite active during the week, you may have glycosuria when you are sedentary on the weekend. The reverse may occur if you are quite active on the weekend. You may have blood glucose variations during different seasons, perhaps when you are more active in the summer. Because exercise lowers blood glucose, it may also cause hypoglycemia. If you take an intermediate-acting insulin and exercise at 4 P.M. (when the insulin may peak), hypoglycemia may occur if you do not properly prepare for exercise. This is a perfect example of the necessary balance of diet, exercise and insulin. We have already stressed the importance of consistency in diet. Consistency in exercise is necessary as well. Anticipation, or planning for situations in advance, results in eating more prior to vigorous exercise (or decreasing your insulin). Many patients, when finding an elevated blood glucose reading, will examine only their food intake or insulin dose. You can easily learn to use exercise for pattern control. Schedule regular exercise and observe your test results carefully. For some individuals, active exercise in the evening may substitute for a second injection. The effects of exercise are long-lasting. So if hypoglycemia occurs during the night or early in the morning, following an evening of exercise, consider exercise as a possible cause. Exercise consistently and anticipate problems by adjusting your diet and possibly your insulin.

MEDICATION ADJUSTMENT

In order to achieve pattern control, review the onset, peak and duration of different types of insulin. Individualized insulin programs are necessary. The process of pattern control is usually adjusted in three steps. At first, your doctor increases your morning intermediate-acting insulin until he sees a peak effect. A morning dose of NPH insulin will usually peak from 3 to 6 P.M., depending on the time you inject. Once this time period is controlled, the NPH insulin can't be increased further or you will have hypoglycemia in the afternoon. Next he watches your fasting blood glucose, and if it remains high, he may suggest a split dose of insulin. Finally, if you have postprandial hyperglycemia, he will add Regular insulin before meals to your insulin regimen.

Another insulin regimen is the use of an intermediate- or long-acting insulin with multiple injections of Regular insulin. This provides a basal insulin supply and prevents postprandial hyperglycemia. The intermediate-acting insulin is needed because Regular insulin doesn't last long enough to provide a continuous level of basal insulin. With this adjustment, meals and exercise may be varied within reason. For many individuals, this approach makes pattern control easier. It is an approach similar to that of the insulin infusion pump.

Insulin may also be adjusted according to other factors, such as exercise or illness. For example, insulin dosage may be lowered prior to a vigorous exercise program to prevent hypoglycemia. Insulin dosage may be increased during illness to prevent hyperglycemia. We do not recommend routinely adjusting your insulin dosage on a daily basis. But if you are following an intensive insulin regimen and monitoring blood glucose, you will make changes in your insulin doses. An example of this would be adjusting the amount of Regular insulin taken before meals based on pre-meal blood glucoses. Pattern control should become easier for you once you know how your insulin works. For example, NPH insulin has its onset within one hour. For this reason, take your insulin approximately thirty minutes prior to eating breakfast. Many patients have the misconception that insulin should be immediately followed with breakfast. That prevents the insulin from working properly with the food that you have eaten. One small change, such as eating at an appropriate time following your insulin injection, may regulate your pattern. Be aware of when your insulin peaks. This is when the possibility of hypoglycemia is greatest. You know that exercise helps to lower blood glucose and that delaying meals will also lead to hypoglycemia. Exercising prior to a delayed dinner, then, would be unwise.

SPECIAL FACTORS

Keep the general guidelines mentioned above in mind for pattern control. There are other special factors that will influence pattern control. These include illness, infection, stress, emotions, vacation, travel, menstruating and even weekends. The management of glucose control may be different during physical illness and stress. Special factors such as these should be included in the comments column of your record book so that you may accurately interpret your pattern. Have you been under a great deal of stress? Chapter 16 of this book is devoted to stress reduction. Stress, for some people, results in an increase in blood glucose. Emotional upsets or stresses in your life should be documented in the comments column. Vacation and travel may affect your pattern control. For vacations and travel, both anticipatory planning and record keeping are essential. Some women report difficulty with control during menstruation. Menstruation has not been shown to be directly related to the development of diabetic ketoacidosis, but many patients report elevated blood glucose during this time. Consult your doctor for an individual plan so that your pattern is not disrupted during your menstrual period. You may have problems with your pattern on weekends due to differences in sleeping hours, meal times, exercise routines or travel. Anticipation is the key factor in preventing problems in diabetes self-management at this time.

COMMON DISRUPTIONS IN PATTERN CONTROL

Your individual response to diabetes is unique. Yet there are some situations where pattern disruptions can be typically identified. If your blood glucose is well controlled, you will not see these patterns of instability. Let us look at four distinct situations where individual pattern control problems begin to emerge.

As you can see from the situation described in Table 11, this patient is experiencing hypoglycemia at 4:30 P.M. every day. A patient history revealed that this 21-year-old insulin-dependent female diabetic takes 24 units of NPH insulin and is crash-dieting in an effort to lose weight. She is having a limited breakfast of one piece of whole-wheat toast with diet margarine and half an orange. She is skipping lunch entirely. You should be familiar enough with the balance of diet, exercise and insulin to realize the effect of this diet on this patient's pattern.

First, observe the columns vertically. You will see a variety of results ranging from 40 mg./dl. to 180 mg./dl. Now look at the columns horizontally, and you will see that at 5 P.M., pre-dinner, this patient has blood glucoses of 40 mg./dl. Look at the comments column. The patient states that she is hypoglycemic

TABLE 11

	M	T	W	TH	F	SAT	SUN	COMMENTS
7A.M.	(150)	(150)	(150)	(150)	(180)	(150)	(150)	
11A.M.	(100)	(150)	(100)	(100)	(100)	(150)	(150)	
5P.M.	(40)	(40)	(40)	(40)	(40)	(40)	(40)	Hypogly-cemia at 4:30 PM each day this week.
10P.M.	(180)	(180)	(180)	(180)	(180)	(180)	(180)	

every day at 4:30 P.M. From the history, you learn that the patient is dieting extensively. Without the comments column, you might think that this patient's major problem is bouts of poor control in the evening and early morning. This is not true. This patient will need counseling regarding strict dieting. Why are the 10 P.M. glucose tests elevated? To answer this, you would need to know what occurred in the early evening. The patient says that because she has dieted all day, she eats a large meal at dinner. Since she had hypoglycemia at 4:30 P.M., she is hungry and overeats and snacks during the night. The first move in pattern adjustment here would be for the patient to eat regular, consistent meals. She should avoid eating excess food in the evening meal. She could also initiate a regular exercise program, which would help her lose weight and improve her blood glucose control. If she adjusted her diet accordingly and began an exercise program, pattern control could be established. If blood glucose test results were consistently high at 10 P.M. and in the early morning, how would the insulin be adjusted? This patient might be a candidate for a second injection prior to dinner. An intermediate-acting insulin would then control her blood glucose through the night and into the early morning.

In the situation described in Table 12, we see a pattern of poor control Monday through Friday with a dramatic increase in the amount of normal glucose results seen over the weekend. This is an 18-year-old insulin-dependent boy who takes 20 units of NPH insulin in the morning. The patient takes high school courses during the day and college preparatory courses in the evening, Monday through Friday. On Saturday and Sunday the patient "works out." Following breakfast on Saturday morning, he begins a program which can include two games of tennis, bicycling two miles and lap swimming in the late afternoon. The patient

TABLE 12

	M	T	W	TH	F	SAT	SUN	COMMENTS
7 A.M.	(210)	(210)	(210)	(180)	(210)	(180)	(100)	
11 A.M.	(210)	(210)	(210)	(210)	(210)	(180)	(180)	
5 P.M.	(100)	(110)	(100)	(90)	(100)	(100)	(100)	Exercising all day, Sat.& Sun.
10 P.M.	(180)	(180)	(180)	(180)	(180)	(100)	(100)	

has been taught how to compensate for exercise appropriately, so he does not experience hypoglycemia.

In the comments column there are no episodes of hypoglycemia listed. When you look at how this patient uses diet to help his pattern control, you can understand why no hypoglycemia occurs. The patient has learned how to properly prepare for exercise by increasing his food intake prior to exercise. The patient also keeps a supply of simple sugar with him at all times during the day to prevent the occurrence of hypoglycemia. Look at the columns vertically. You will notice that the patient is in poor control for the majority of the time. When you look at the columns horizontally, though, you will see normal blood glucoses may be attained by this patient every day at 5 P.M. Think back to what was presented to you when insulin adjustment was discussed. The NPH insulin has already shown its peak effect. His 10 P.M. and 7 A.M. glucose remain elevated, so the next step would be to split his dose of insulin. If the problems with the 11 A.M. and 10 P.M. blood glucose remain, the final step would be to add Regular insulin to the injections to reduce postprandial hyperglycemia. Here, insulin adjustment is an essential part of pattern control. Yet if these changes are made in his insulin regimen, he will have hypoglycemia on weekends unless he increases his diet or lowers his insulin. All diabetes-related activities have to be regulated in this manner and many diabetic persons are making such changes.

The situation discussed in Table 13 shows this patient in relatively good control on Monday, Tuesday, Thursday and Friday. By this time, your eye should go immediately to Tuesday night and all day Wednesday and you would question why the glucose rose so rapidly. Look at the comments section. The patient states that she was at a party Tuesday night. When asked about her diet,

TABLE 13

	M	T	W	TH	F	SAT	SUN	COMMENTS
7A.M.	(100)	(110)	N (320)	(120)	(120)	(40)	(40)	Early AM hypogly-cemia Sat. & Sun.
11A.M.	(100)	(100)	N (240)	(120)	(120)	(180)	(180)	Party Tues. night
5P.M.	(110)	(110)	N (180)	(110)	(110)	(110)	(120)	Dancing and drinking Fri. and Sat. nights.
10P.M.	(110)	(180)	(120)	(120)	(120)	(120)	(120)	

this 28-year-old insulin-dependent female, who takes 30 units of Lente insulin, stated that she went off her diet plan Tuesday evening and ate two pieces of birthday cake. Could that dietary change account for the glucose levels seen during Wednesday? It is important to note that when her blood glucose rose above 250 mg./dl., she checked for acetone. It is certainly possible that this could be corrected merely by not eating simple sugars. The patient has shown normal readings throughout the rest of the week. What is significant about Saturday and Sunday's early-morning low glucose reading? Look at the comments column. You will see that she experienced early-morning hypoglycemia on both Saturday and Sunday.

Under the comments section you will also see that she was out dancing and drinking alcohol Friday night and Saturday night. What is the effect of alcohol on the blood glucose? It lowers blood glucose. What is the effect of dancing, a vigorous form of exercise, on blood glucose? This also lowers blood glucose. The combination of these two activities resulted in hypoglycemia in this patient. She should be cautioned against drinking while exercising. She also needs dietary recommendations, such as taking additional snacks while out dancing. A late snack would be necessary when she arrives home. Here, exercise and diet had to be adjusted in order to achieve pattern control.

In Table 14, the situation involves a 42-year-old insulin-dependent male who takes 24 units of NPH insulin and 5 units of Regular insulin in the A.M. and 10 units of NPH in the P.M. He is testing for both glucose and acetone and begins to spill acetone in large quantities. As you can see, on Monday the patient is in good control. Check the comments column to see what may have happened on Monday night to cause acetonuria. The patient notes that he was nauseous

TABLE 14

	M	T	W	TH	F	SAT	SUN	COMMENTS
7A.M.	(100)	S (310)	M (250)	S (150)	(110)	(100)	(100)	Nauseous & vomiting Mon. & Tues. nights.
11A.M.	(120)	S (310)	M (180)	N (120)	(120)	(120)	(120)	
5P.M.	(180)	M (360)	S (180)	N (120)		(100)	(100)	
10P.M.	N (250)	L (310)	S (180)	N (120)	(120)	(120)	(120)	

and vomited. The nausea began Monday night; vomiting began Tuesday morning. As you can see, when the patient discovered his blood glucose was above 250 mg./dl., he checked his urine for acetone. As glucose increased and remained elevated, the acetone also increased. The patient demonstrates self-management skills by monitoring his acetone carefully, as well as using a meter to test his blood glucose. Between 10 P.M. Monday and Friday morning he continued to test for acetone. The disruption of his pattern represented by the nausea and vomiting was due to illness. He was wise to test for acetone and he was able to contact his doctor immediately. He used additional Regular insulin to help prevent potential diabetic ketoacidosis. The patient had to follow sick-day rules in order to successfully handle his situation. This situation involved insulin adjustment.

As you can see, all of these situations demand expertise in pattern control. In order to establish pattern control you must make necessary adjustments among insulin, exercise and diet.

COMMON MISTAKES WHEN ATTEMPTING PATTERN CONTROL

Common mistakes may occur as you attempt pattern control. One is attempting to correct a disruption in your pattern at the wrong time. You should not make a dietary or insulin adjustment at the time you noticed the problem. Instead, examine all your test results and correct them appropriately. For example, if your 4 P.M. glucose was elevated, would you increase your evening or morning injection of intermediate-acting insulin? You would not want to increase the injection that you are taking at the time that you just tested. The test result is showing you the action of your morning insulin, so you would need to increase your morning injection in the future. Keep in mind that test results show you what occurred in the past. If your glucose results are consistently high before dinner, you would not add an extra dose of NPH insulin at that time. That would begin to work after dinner and continue into the late evening and nighttime hours. To have an effect on your before-dinner glucose, you would have to increase your NPH insulin early in the morning, prior to breakfast, or take Regular insulin prior to dinner. Anticipation is the key to avoiding this pitfall of pattern control.

A second common mistake is not keeping a record. If you are testing four times a day and taking multiple injections of insulin and experiencing some hypoglycemic episodes, you will not be able to remember everything without a record. Do not trust something as important as pattern control to memory. Take an extra second to write down your test results. Another common mistake is to interpret results only in regard to medication changes. Don't forget about diet and exercise. Remember to look at the total picture of pattern control in regard to diet, exercise and insulin. Another common mistake in pattern control is analyzing each separate test. Remember to analyze your records only two to three times a week. In this way, you will stay on top of your diabetes control by looking at the total picture. You must analyze your whole self-management program, not just isolated tests. Two exceptions to this exist. When you are ill you will need to analyze each test result in order to prevent the development of diabetic ketoacidosis. Keep in close contact with your doctor and follow sick-day rules exactly. Increase your testing for glucose and acetone during this time. In addition, some individuals taking multiple injections will determine the dose of their pre-meal Regular insulin injection based on their blood glucose level at the time. Always bring your records with you when you visit your doctor, nurse or nutritionist.

Although the thrust of this chapter has been directed toward keeping your blood glucose pattern stable without making frequent changes, you should be aware that patients often use algorithms in order to control blood glucose changes. These algorithms, for example, might direct you to increase your Regular insulin dose by 1–2 units pre-lunch if your blood glucose two hours after lunch is greater than 150 mg./dl. for two or three days in a row. These adjustments are usually made over a time interval of two or three days. Some other patients may make daily adjustments in their insulin based on changes in their diet and insulin. For example, for an individual who takes an injection of long-acting insulin, varied doses of Regular insulin may be calculated to accommodate daily changes in diet or exercise.

Although it is difficult to commit yourself to frequent blood monitoring and multiple injections, it may be helpful to view this as an intermediate measure. Right now the tools for diabetes self-management are imperfect, but in the next five to ten years these will improve, as will self-management and control.

To conclude this chapter, look at your diabetes self-management carefully. Remember the words:

D   diet
I   insulin
A   activity
B   blood glucose
E   emotions
T   tests
E   exercise
S   special factors

In order to obtain pattern control, you must assess diet, insulin, activity, blood glucose readings, emotions, tests for urine, acetone, exercise and special factors, such as illness and infection. Pattern control pulls all the information together and it is you who will be gathering and interpreting this information. Here, your ability to self-manage diabetes can be proudly displayed.

13

Food Label Evaluation

You may find evaluating food labels a difficult task, for today's supermarkets contain anywhere from 8,000 to 10,000 items. Many of the foods found in a supermarket are appropriate in a meal plan for diabetic persons, with the exception of concentrated sweets. There are dietetic foods as well as many convenience foods which may be acceptable. To find out if foods are appropriate for your meal plan, you must evaluate the nutrition label.

The Food and Drug Administration (FDA) is the government agency responsible for enforcing specific regulations concerning food labels. The food label provides mandatory information on all products. This includes the name of the product and its net content or weight. The weight is usually expressed in metric terms as well as in household measurements. Also included are the name and address of the manufacturer or distributor. Additional information, such as a listing of ingredients, is also required on foods for which there is no standard of identity. A standard of identity is similar to a recipe. It includes ingredients that must be used for a product to be called by a specific name. There are over 300 items that have a standard of identity. Some of these are ketchup, tomato sauce and paste, jelly, cheddar cheese, mayonnaise and ice cream. If additional ingredients are added to products with a standard of identity, those items must appear on the label. The list of ingredients must state the ingredients in order of descending weight. The following shows the mandatory items on a food label.

MANDATORY INFORMATION ON ALL FOOD LABELS

Information	*Example*
1. Name of the product	1. Special Crackers
2. Net weight expressed in metric as well as avoirdupois (household) system; if the product is packed in a liquid, the weight of the liquid and solid must be given	2. Net weight: 1.5 lbs. (681 g.)
3. Name and address of the manufacturer or distributor	3. Special Cracker Company, Funtown, NY
4. Listing of ingredients in order of descending weight	4. Ingredients: flour, dry milk, sugar, salt

The type of food label is dependent on the manufacturer. The brand-name label is usually found on an item manufactured by a specific company. A private or house label is on a food manufactured by a large chain store that has products distributed under its own name. Generic labeling or no-frills labeling (the "no name" product) is found on certain items distributed in large chain stores. They are usually common foods packed in a plain wrapper. They may be less expensive, and may or may not differ in taste from brand-name items, but will not contain fewer nutrients.

THE NUTRITION LABEL

The nutrition label differs from the food label. Nutrition labeling was developed in 1973 to provide consumers with nutrition information on most foods. Nutrition labeling can be used to compare the nutritional aspects of similar products, to evaluate the nutritional composition of new products, to plan healthy, nutritious meals and to determine foods that are good sources of nutrients. Nutrition labeling is mandatory for food that is enriched (nutrients in the food that are lost in processing are put back) or fortified (nutrients that were never in the food are added to make the product more nutritious) with vitamins and minerals. A nutrition label must appear on a product if the food makes a nutritional claim such as "low in fat" or "a good source of iron." Finally, foods that claim to be beneficial for special dietary use must have a nutrition label.

ITEMS ON A LABEL

A nutrition label gives you information about the food item. The serving size is arbitrarily determined by the manufacturer. It is usually an amount suitable for consumption as part of a meal for an adult male who engages in light activity.

The remaining information on a label is based on that serving size. The servings per container indicates how many persons the food item will serve if each person is given the stated serving size. The nutrition label also gives the number of calories, or the value of food energy, provided in each serving. It then lists the grams of carbohydrate, protein and fat. This information becomes useful if you want to fit the food product into your Exchange Plan. You can easily change the grams of carbohydrate, protein and fat into calories. Remember that carbohydrate and protein provide 4 calories per gram and fat provides 9 calories per gram. Adding up the calories of the carbohydrate, protein and fat in the product should give you a figure equal to or close to that stated on the label.

You will find nutrients listed on the label as a percentage of the U.S. Recommended Daily Allowances (U.S. RDA). The percentage of U.S. RDA for vitamin A, vitamin C, thiamine, riboflavin, niacin, calcium and iron must be included. Other product labels may provide optional nutrient information for foods that are fortified. For example, the vitamin D and phosphorus content of some dairy products may be listed. The fiber and sodium content and the amount of polyunsaturated and saturated fats may be listed. Many food companies also list the cholesterol content of foods. The following depicts a typical nutrition label.

NUTRITION INFORMATION PER SERVING

Corn Flakes
Serving size: ¾ cup
Servings per container: 16

	¾ cup	With ½ cup whole milk	
Calories	80	160	(label may appear in
Protein	2 g.	6 g.	this manner for
Carbohydrate	17 g.	23 g.	foods eaten with
Fat	1 g.	6 g.	other foods)
Sodium	120 mg.	180 mg.	

Percentage of U.S. Recommended Daily Allowances (U.S. RDA)

		¾ cup	With milk
	Protein	4	10
	Vitamin A	*	2
Essential	Vitamin C	*	*
nutrients	Thiamine	4	6
to be	Riboflavin	*	8
listed	Niacin	8	8
	Calcium	*	15
	Iron	6	6

* Less than 2 percent of U.S. RDA.

Additional nutrient listing at manufacturer's option	Phosphorus	8	20
	Magnesium	8	10
	Zinc	4	4
	Copper	2	4

CALORIC SWEETENERS

It is virtually impossible in this day and age of modern processing to have a diet without caloric sweeteners or sugars. A caloric sweetener is one that provides 4 calories per gram. In general, caloric sweeteners are added to five different categories of food. These are canned and processed foods, jams, ice cream and other dairy products, beverages and cereals and baked goods. Sweeteners are added to foods to provide them with sweetness and texture and to preserve their freshness. Caloric sweeteners include sucrose, which is also known as beet sugar, brown sugar, cane sugar, confectioners' sugar, invert sugar (sucrose treated with an acid to break it into glucose and fructose). Invert sugar is found in candy and baked goods. Powdered sugar and table sugar are also caloric sweeteners, along with molasses, glucose syrup, corn syrup, sorghum syrup and cane syrup. Glucose may also be known as corn sugar, dextrose or grape sugar. Fructose is a caloric sweetener that is also known as fruit sugar or levulose. Other caloric sweeteners include sorbitol, mannitol, xylitol, mannose, lactose, high-fructose corn syrup, honey and maple syrup.

SUCROSE

Sucrose is a disaccharide formed by glucose and fructose. Approximately 99.9 percent of table sugar is pure sucrose. After ingestion and digestion, sucrose enters the small intestine, where it is broken down to glucose and fructose. Glucose and fructose then enter the bloodstream for transport to the liver. Sucrose is the major sugar found in candy, cakes, cookies, pies and jellies.

FRUCTOSE

Fructose is a monosaccharide that provides 20–40 percent of the sweetness in fruit. It is 1.5 times as sweet as sucrose. Approximately 80–90 percent is absorbed in the small intestine. Fructose is absorbed more slowly than glucose or sucrose. This sugar can enter the liver without the aid of insulin, but the final metabolism of fructose requires insulin. A small amount of fructose is converted to glucose during absorption. The glucose requires insulin in order to be used by body cells. In severe insulin deficiency, a rise in plasma glucose levels may occur after fructose ingestion because of this immediate need for insulin. If your diabetes is controlled, there may not be any reason to exclude fructose from your diet. However, keep in mind that fructose is a carbohydrate providing 4 calories per gram. In addition, in its refined state fructose lacks minerals, vitamins and fiber.

A number of weight-loss schemes and misleading ideas about the use of fructose in the diet of diabetics have developed. Advocates of fructose have claimed it is a safe sweetener for diabetic persons because it reduces the rise in blood glucose levels. While this is true, remember that in poorly controlled persons some fructose will be converted to glucose and the blood glucose level will rise. Some have also claimed that fructose is a helpful alternative to sucrose because it is "natural." As of yet, there is no legal definition for the word "natural." Moreover, sucrose is as "natural" as fructose. Sucrose and fructose both come from plants. There is no evidence to support claims that fructose is an appetite suppressant, burns off fat or aids in weight reduction. Advertisers have also claimed that fructose is better than sucrose because it is sweeter, so you use slightly less fructose. This is a minor advantage because the caloric content of the sugars is the same.

THE SUGAR ALCOHOLS

The sugar alcohols comprise another group of caloric sweeteners. They differ from the mono- and disaccharides in that part of their chemical molecule contains an alcohol group. However, the alcohol group is not the same as ethyl alcohol (in liquor). These are non-glucose-containing caloric sweeteners that are naturally occurring but may also be produced commercially for foods. They are incompletely absorbed and therefore may have a laxative effect. All sugar alcohols provide 4 calories per gram.

Xylitol is a five-carbon sugar alcohol found in plants, particularly in berries and mushrooms. It is produced commercially from the sugar xylose. Xylitol is slowly absorbed and does not raise the blood glucose as much as sucrose or glucose. It does not require as much insulin as sucrose to be metabolized. Xylitol is metabolized in the liver without the aid of insulin. However, like fructose, xylitol can be converted to glucose in the absence of insulin. An osmotic diarrhea can result if as much as 30–40 grams of xylitol are consumed in a food. (Osmotic diarrhea results from the pooling of fluids in the intestine due to the presence of a sugar.) Xylitol has been used in chewing gum because it does not cause dental caries. At present, all food uses for xylitol have been stopped until further research on the safety of xylitol can be performed.

Sorbitol is also a naturally occurring sugar alcohol found in fruits and vegetables. It is 50 percent as sweet as sucrose. Like other sugar alcohols, sorbitol is absorbed slowly and metabolized in the liver without insulin. However, sorbitol can be converted to glucose during insulin deficiency, and elevations in blood glucose may result. Osmotic diarrhea may also occur after the ingestion of sorbitol.

THE NEW SWEETENER

The newest high-potency sweetener and flavor enhancer is chemically known as aspartame. Aspartame is marketed by the G. D. Searle Company under the name of NutraSweet or Equal. Aspartame was approved for use by the FDA in 1981. It is made up of two amino acids: phenylalanine and aspartic acid. When these amino acids are chemically joined they produce an extremely sweet-tasting substance. Aspartame is 180 to 200 times as sweet as sucrose. Aspartame is not a carbohydrate; it is a protein providing 4 calories per gram. It also leaves a pleasant aftertaste, unlike many non-nutritive sweeteners. Due to the extreme sweetness of the product, only a small amount is necessary to produce a sweet flavor. You can see the caloric contribution in the following ratio:

$$\frac{0.1 \text{ calorie aspartame}}{16 \text{ calories granulated sugar}} = 1 \text{ teaspoon equivalent}$$

This means that one teaspoon of sugar, or 16 calories, can be replaced by an equally sweet amount of aspartame to provide only 1/10 of a calorie, with no bitter aftertaste.

Aspartame can be used in various ways. However, aspartame cannot be used in baking because the heat will chemically destroy it, causing the product to be less sweet. It can be added after the heating process. Recently, aspartame has been added to carbonated beverages. It will be used as a sweetener in cold cereals and chewing gum and as a dry base for beverages, instant coffee and tea, gelatins, puddings, dairy products and fillings. You will also see it as a dry, free-flowing substitute for table use, in packaged units, or as tablets for sweetening hot beverages. Due to its concentrated sweetness, foods will contain fewer calories. In addition, aspartame has not been shown to promote tooth decay, because it is not a carbohydrate.

You will be able to recognize aspartame on the food label by any of the following terms: L-asparto-L-phenylalanine methyl ester, phenylalanine and aspartic acid, or aspartame. In addition, all products containing phenylalanine must also have a warning on the label stating: "Phenylketonurics: contains phenylalanine." This is necessary for those individuals who for special health reasons must restrict their intake of phenylalanine.

NON-CALORIC SWEETENERS

Saccharin is a non-caloric sweetener that has been the source of much controversy for several years. This is because there are contradictions in both the experimental and the epidemiological studies for and against the safety of saccharin. You probably remember the saccharin scare which began in the late 1970s when Canadian researchers reported that large amounts of saccharin produced bladder cancer in rats. The Canadians were quick to remove saccharin from all of their foods. However, manufacturers in the United States were not so quick to follow suit. Saccharin has been used for over a hundred years. It sweetens foods and beverages without adding calories or nutrients. Saccharin is useful in the meal plan of those who have diabetes because it does not raise the blood glucose level or provide calories. The use of saccharin may, however, produce a psychological perception of an improved quality of life. In other words, you may not feel deprived following a meal plan as long as you are able to eat a sweet, saccharin-containing product. In terms of obesity there is no evidence that saccharin will cause weight reduction or help people lose weight. Saccharin, though, can be used to contribute to a reduced calorie intake, which is essential for weight loss.

While the Canadian studies with saccharin did arouse a lot of fear, many subsequent studies have been reported which conflict with the Canadian research. American researchers found that, as a group, those consuming artificial sweeteners are at little or no excessive risk of bladder cancer. There is no saccharin-induced epidemic of bladder cancer. In addition, there may be little evidence of bladder cancer occurring due to the consumption of artificial sweeteners in the doses and in the manner presently used. The American Diabetes Association realizes that there is such a lack of agreement between the results of animal and human studies that current food safety laws with respect to saccharin are inappropriate. The American Diabetes Association recognizes that there is a perceived benefit to saccharin use for patients with diabetes that is too great to warrant a ban on saccharin.

However, despite all the controversy, many doctors are still concerned about the use of saccharin in the United States in some groups. Women in childbearing years are heavy users of saccharin. Children are also consuming more artificial sweeteners than desirable. The American Diabetes Association suggests that saccharin intake should be limited in pregnant women and young children. It is also suggested that excessive use by anyone is ill-advised.

FOOD ADDITIVES

With today's hectic lifestyle and erratic eating patterns, it would be difficult to put a meal together without the presence of food additives. A food additive is any substance that becomes part of a food product when added directly or indirectly. There are over 2,800 substances added purposely to food. There are over 10,000 substances that may be added with processing, packaging or storage of food. Many commonplace items have been used as food additives for centuries. These include salt and sugar, which are used for food preservation. Today, more food additives are used because more convenience foods are served. Additives are used to increase the shelf life and reduce spoilage of foods. Food additives have been used to provide you with a year-round supply of foods that would ordinarily be in season only part of the year.

There are several reasons why food additives may be intentionally added to food. Manufacturers may want to maintain or improve the nutritive value of food. They may add vitamins such as B complex or a mineral such as iron that may otherwise be lacking. An example of this might be the addition of vitamin C to fruit drinks or the addition of vitamin D to dairy products. Food producers may want to maintain food appearance as well as taste. Here, food additives will be included to prevent spoilage and to preserve color. Examples of this would be the use of butylated hydroxyanisol (BHA) or butylated hydroxytoluene (BHT) to prevent changes in the color and flavor of foods. An additive may be used to help the food preparation process. It may give body or texture to foods by retaining moisture or preventing a cake-type buildup. An example of this would be an emulsifier which is used in mayonnaise to prevent the oil and egg yolk from separating. A humectant may be used to maintain moisture in foods such as shredded coconut. Finally, other additives may be used to add color or enhance flavor. Examples of these are artificial colors used in soft drinks or monosodium glutamate used as a flavor enhancer.

A manufacturer must go through a specific approval process before an additive may be used in a food. First, the manufacturer must subject the additive to experimental tests. The additive must be fed in large amounts to two types of animals over an extended period of time to determine whether it causes cancer or birth defects or to see if any other problems result. The manufacturer will then submit these results to the FDA, which will determine if it is safe. The FDA will then establish regulations for its use. Regulations for use dictate that only 1/100 of the maximum test amount of the food additive may be incorporated into food.

The FDA must also enforce the Delaney Clause, which is the amendment that prohibits the addition of substances to food that have been shown to cause cancer in animals. It is because of this clause, as well as the Canadian research, that the saccharin controversy developed. While manufacturers continue to experiment with food additives, there are already over 700 food additives in use that are considered harmless on the basis of extensive use in the past without harmful effects. These 700 items comprise the GRAS (generally recognized as safe) List. All 700 items are presently being retested to reevaluate their effect on humans.

LABEL TERMINOLOGY

The information you have just read can be used when purchasing food. Develop the habit of reading labels and become familiar with their terminology. While this task is difficult at first, being knowledgeable about food labels will enable you to add variety to your meal. It will be helpful to know the meaning of some general terms that appear on labels. For example, a "diet beverage," as defined by the FDA, must contain at least 50 percent fewer calories than the same product made without artificial sweeteners. No diet beverage can contain more than 6 calories per fluid ounce. The word "imitation" is used if the food resembles another food but differs in nutrient composition when compared with that food. For example, imitation mayonnaise does not have the same amount of fat as regular mayonnaise, as stated in its standard of identity. A "low-calorie" food may be called such only if a serving of the food supplies no more than 40 calories and the food does not provide more than 0.4 calorie per gram. The term "low-calorie" must precede the name of the food so that you will understand that the food has undergone some changes.

A "reduced-calorie" food has undergone a change so that it contains fewer calories than the similar food that did not undergo the change. It must have at least one-third fewer calories. The label on a reduced-calorie food must compare the calories of the reduced item and the calories of an equivalent serving of the similar food that has not undergone the change. For example, a nationally known brand of reduced-calorie salad dressing lists the calories per serving of the reduced dressing as well as the calories per serving of the same type of dressing not reduced in calories.

Reduced-calorie Italian salad dressing: 30 calories per tablespoon
Italian salad dressing: 70 calories per tablespoon

Terms such as "sugar-free," "sugarless" and "no sugar" can be very misleading. You might expect that when these words appear on the food label, the product is lower in or significantly reduced in calories. Oftentimes, however, sweeteners other than sugar may be used. Read the label carefully for ingredients. Foods that are sugar-free must also have a statement saying the food is "not a reduced-calorie food" or "not a low-calorie food" or "not for weight control" or "useful only in preventing tooth decay." This means that the food has a specific purpose other than weight control.

Also become familiar with words on the label that indicate fat or cholesterol, since you want to keep your blood lipids normal. The FDA states that no label may contain a claim suggesting that a product will prevent, mitigate or cure heart disease. A food label may include the amount of cholesterol in the food. The cholesterol content must be stated in the nearest 5 mg. increment per serving. The cholesterol section of the food label must be included under the information on fat.

You may see the word "shortening" on a label. Shortening usually means the fat is saturated. Shortening can be a vegetable oil that has been made solid through a chemical process called hydrogenation, or the shortening can originate as a saturated fat such as coconut or palm oil. These are used in food because they are inexpensive and help keep foods fresh longer. Whatever the shortening, it is probably not acceptable for your meal plan.

The words "hydrogenated fat" may also appear on labels. Stick-type margarines are an example of a hydrogenated fat. Therefore, the soft tub margarines are better choices. The FDA states that each individual fat or oil must be listed by its common name, such as lard or soybean oil. It must also be listed among the ingredients in the order of descending weight. Fats can be listed as a blend of vegetable or animal fats. Specific names of fats or oils do not have to be listed if the manufacturer uses varying mixtures of fats or oils or is unable to adhere to a constant pattern of use. "Partially hydrogenated oils" may also be included on food labels. Fats that are not in the product may be listed if they are sometimes used in the product. You will recognize this by the statement: "This product contains one or more of the following fats."

The nutrition part of the food label may provide additional information about the fat content of food. The total fat content is expressed as a percentage of the total calories provided by fat. The amount of fatty acids will be stated in grams per serving. The amount of polyunsaturated fatty acids will be expressed as "polyunsaturated" and the amount of saturated fatty acids will be stated as "saturated." In addition, the food label must say: "Information on fat and cholesterol content is provided for individuals who, on the advice of a physician, are modifying their dietary intake of fat and cholesterol," where appropriate.

When purchasing a liquid oil, make sure it is made from a vegetable source that is polyunsaturated, such as sunflower, safflower, corn or cottonseed oil. When purchasing a margarine, make sure it is a tub margarine with a liquid vegetable oil as the first ingredient. You also want to look for a p/s ratio on the label of the tub margarine. A p/s ratio is one way to express relative amounts of fatty acids in foods or diets. It refers to the amount of linoleic or polyunsaturated fats in relation to the amount of saturated fats. The higher the amount of polyunsaturated fat to saturated fat, the better the margarine is for cholesterol-lowering diets. An example of a margarine that has a p/s ratio of 3 follows. To determine the ratio, all you do is divide the amount of polyunsaturated fats by the saturated fats. Whichever brand of margarine you choose, try to obtain one with a p/s ratio of at least 2.

NUTRITION INFORMATION FOR TUB MARGARINE

Serving size	1 tbs.	Fat (100% of calories)	10 g.
Servings per pound	32	Polyunsaturated	3 g.
Calories	100	Saturated	1 g.
Protein	0 g.	Cholesterol (0 mg./100 g.)	0 g.
Carbohydrate	0 g.	P/S	3

Other words to become familiar with indicate different ways that salt is added to foods. Learn these words if you want to reduce your intake of salt to avoid or control hypertension. Sodium is present in all foods, but additional salt may be added to food during processing. You can determine whether salt is added by the words: salt, table salt, iodized salt, sodium benzoate, monosodium glutamate, sodium phosphate, sodium propionate, sodium citrate, sodium calcinate, sodium caseinate, sodium hydroxide or sodium nitrate. Soy sauce, spices with salt added to them and other additives that have sodium as their first word may also be avoided.

DIABETIC AND DIETETIC FOODS

What about dietetic and diabetic foods? You may be thinking that the word "dietetic" means sugar-free or sugarless. However, to millions of people around the country, the words "dietetic food" can mean a variety of things. Persons with hypertension may want a dietetic food low in salt. Those who are concerned with heart disease may want a dietetic food to be high in fiber as well as low in calories. In this country, most people are conscious of some aspect of their diet. You can no longer think that food manufacturers are concerned only with the sugar content of food. Therefore, look at the food product and make sure it is dietetic in the way you want.

There is really no such thing as a "diabetic" food. Foods that are called "diabetic" claim to have no sugar. That is usually a true statement. However, instead the manufacturer has added another type of sweetener. Make sure you read the label to determine this. Often a sugar alcohol is used instead of sugar. Remember, words that end in "tol" or "ose" connote a caloric sweetener.

You might be pleased to know that you do not have to spend extra money on dietetic foods. These foods are not an essential part of your plan and are usually more expensive. In addition, foods that are called "dietetic" or "diabetic" may in reality contain more saturated fat and more calories than the product's non-dietetic counterpart. Often, a food that is considered diabetic uses a sugar alcohol instead of sucrose to provide a sweet flavor. Foods that may be lower in calories are fruits packed in water, dietetic gelatin, dietetic hard candies and dietetic gum. These lower-calorie dietetic items usually contain sorbitol in an acceptable amount so as not to provide excessive calories. Dietetic or diabetic ice cream, puddings, cakes and cookies should not be used unless you can work these foods into your meal plan. Remember that these foods usually cost more, contain just as many calories and do not taste as good as the product's non-dietetic counterpart.

When doing your regular supermarket shopping, read the ingredients part of the label and use the following general information as a guide. If sugar is listed as the sixth ingredient or after on the list, then the product is acceptable for your use. The FDA has set up certain rules for manufacturers to follow in food labeling of special dietetic products. To help you avoid inadvertent use of a product, if a beverage contains a combination of caloric and non-caloric sweeteners, it must have the statement: "Contains sugar, not for use by diabetics without the advice of a physician." The label of a beverage containing a sugar alcohol must say: "Contains carbohydrate, not for use by diabetics without the advice of a physician." A label that suggests that the food may be useful for a diabetic must say: "Diabetics, this product may be useful in your diet on the advice of a physician. This food is not a reduced-calorie food." The second sentence may be eliminated if the food is useful in reducing caloric intake and is labeled in accordance with the FDA rules. The words "diabetic," "for diabetics" or anything similar to that should not be included as part of the food label other than as previously discussed.

USING FOOD LABELS FOR CONVENIENCE FOODS

A food label can be used to translate one serving of a convenience food into the exchanges. A convenience food is a food that is partially or completely prepared before the product is sold. Usually these foods are used to save time and/or work in food preparation. The nutritional value of convenience foods may be comparable with that of the same product prepared from scratch. Convenience foods can make eating interesting while offering you variety. When you eat convenience foods, make sure your choices are worth the calories and provide you with essential nutrients. When reading the labels of convenience foods, check to see if a sugar or a fat-containing substance is one of the first six ingredients. Next look at the list of ingredients to determine the exchange group. That is, would it be in the milk, fruit or vegetable group? If the product is primarily a complex carbohydrate, it is in the bread group. Then look for the next most predominant ingredient. If it is a protein, then it fits into the meat group. Carefully read the following directions and use the worksheet, which describes in detail how to convert convenience foods into the Exchange System.

The following information provides general guide rules for evaluating food labels.

1. Different dietitians and nutritionists use different techniques for calculating the exchange value of convenience foods. We feel this system is useful with practice.
2. You can round off fractions:
    a. if less than ½, drop it,
    b. if more than ½, round to the nearest whole,
    c. if equal to ½, count as ½.
3. If the product you're working with is made primarily of complex carbohydrate (CHO), you would start your calculations with the bread exchange. Foods with CHO coming from sugar may be counted as the fruit exchange. If the food you're working with is made primarily of protein (p), you would start your calculations with the meat exchange.
4. You can vary 2–3 grams of CHO, p and/or fat (f) per meal, or a total 5–20 calories.
5. To check yourself, add the total number of grams of CHO, p and f and calories in your calculations and compare them with the information listed on the label.

1. List the main ingredients and the appropriate exchange group for each.
2. List the grams of CHO, p and f from the label.
3. a. Divide the CHO in the product by 15 to get the number of bread exchanges.
    b. List the grams of CHO and p in the total number of bread exchanges.
    c. Subtract 3b from 2.
4. a. Divide the remaining grams of p in the product by 7 to get the number of meat exchanges.
    b. List the grams of p and f in the total number of meat exchanges.*
    c. Subtract 4b from 3c.
5. a. Divide the remaining grams of f in the product by 5 to get the number of fat exchanges.
    b. List the grams of f in the total number of fat exchanges.
    c. Subtract 5b from 4c.
6. List the number of exchanges for one serving.

* Remember that a lean meat choice has only 3 grams of f, the medium-fat meat has 5 grams and the high-fat meat has 8 grams.

Proceed slowly when first learning this. It can be confusing at first, but eventually the procedure becomes easier. It is also helpful if you do your calculations at home rather than in the supermarket. Become familiar with Table 15, which summarizes the nutrient and caloric composition of the Exchange List. Keep this list handy when making your calculations. You can keep Table 15 on a 3-by-5 index card so you will have the figures written down when shopping. Read on to see the calculations necessary for specific convenience foods. See if you can follow the calculations and end with the same results.

TABLE 15
SUMMARY OF NUTRIENT AND CALORIC COMPOSITION OF THE EXCHANGE LIST

EXCHANGE LIST	CARBOHYDRATE (CHO) 4 CALS/G	PROTEIN 4 CALS/G	FAT 9 CALS/ G.	CAL-ORIES
Non-Fat Milk	12	8		80
Low-Fat Milk	12	8	5	125
Whole Milk	12	8	10	170
Vegetables	5	2	—	25
Fruit	10	—	—	40
Bread	15	2	—	70
Lean Meat	—	7	3	55
Medium-Fat Meat	—	7	5	75
High-Fat Meat	—	7	8	100
Fat	—	—	5	45

PIZZA

Serving size	¼ pizza (2 slices)
Calories	410
Protein	18 g.
Carbohydrate	37 g.
Fat	21 g.

1. List the main ingredients and the appropriate exchange group for each.

flour, mozzarella cheese, olive oil, tomato sauce

flour: bread exchange
mozzarella cheese: high-fat meat exchange
olive oil: fat exchange

	CHO	p	f
2. List the grams of CHO, p and f from the label.	37	18	21

3. a. Divide the CHO in the product by 15 to get the number of bread exchanges: 37 ÷ 15 = 2.466 = 2½. This is done because 1 bread exchange has 15 g. CHO.

       2½ breads

	CHO	p	f
b. List the grams of CHO and p in the total number of bread exchanges. 1 bread exchange has 2 g. protein, so 2½ exchanges has 5 g. protein. Bread contains no fat.	37	5	0
c. Subtract 3b from 2 (37 − 37 = 0) (18 − 5 = 13).	0	13	21

4. a. Divide the remaining grams of p in the product by 7 to get the number of meat exchanges: 13 ÷ 7 = 1.857 = 2. Divide by 7 because each ounce of meat has 7 g. protein.

       2 high-fat meats
   You know it is a high-fat meat product because the cheeses used are on the high-fat meat list.

	CHO	p	f
b. List the grams of p and f in the total number of meat exchanges. 1 high-fat meat exchange is 7 g. protein and 8 g. fat, so 2 exchanges would be 14 g. protein and 16 g. fat.	0	14	16

       (2 × 7 = 14) (2 × 8 = 16)

	CHO	p	f
c. Subtract 4b from 3c.	0	−1	5

5. a. Divide the remaining grams of f in the product by 5 to get the number of fat exchanges: 5 ÷ 5 = 1.

       1 fat

	CHO	p	f
b. List the grams of f in the total number of fat exchanges. 1 fat exchange is 5 g. fat.	0	0	5
c. Subtract 5b from 4c (5 − 5 = 0).	0	0	0

6. List the number of exchanges for one serving or 2 slices.

       2½ breads
   2 high-fat meats
   1 fat

STUFFED SHELLS

Serving size   7 oz.
Calories   350
Protein   22 g.
Carbohydrate   34 g.
Fat   13 g.

1. List the main ingredients and the appropriate exchange group for each.

macaroni, ricotta cheese, tomato sauce, parmesan cheese

macaroni: bread exchange
tomato sauce: vegetable exchange
ricotta cheese: medium-fat meat exchange

	CHO	p	f
2. List the grams of CHO, p and f from the label.	34	22	13

3. a. Divide the CHO in the product by 15 to get the number of bread exchanges: $34 \div 15 = 2.266 = 2$ bread exchanges.

2 breads

b. List the grams of CHO and p in the total number of bread exchanges.

	30	4	0

c. Subtract 3b from 2.

	4	18	0

4. a. Divide the remaining grams of CHO by 5 to get the number of vegetable exchanges: $4 \div 5 = .8$ or 1. Two grams of p are also included in a vegetable exchange.

1 vegetable

b. List the total amount of grams of CHO, p and f in a vegetable exchange.

	5	2	0

c. Subtract 4b from 3c.

	-1	16	13

5. a. Divide the remaining grams of p in the product by 7 to get the number of meat exchanges: $16 \div 7 = 2.29 = 2\frac{1}{4}$ or 2 medium-fat meats

2 medium-fat meats

	CHO	p	f
b. List the grams of p and f in the total number of meat exchanges.	0	14	10
c. Subtract 5b from 4b.	0	2	3

6. List the number of exchanges for one serving.

    2 breads
    1 vegetable
    2 medium-fat meats

MACARONI AND CHEESE

Serving size   ¾ cup
Calories   240
Protein   10 g.
Carbohydrate 32 g.
Fat   7 g.

1. List the main ingredients and the appropriate exchange group for each.

    macaroni, cheddar cheese, non-fat dry milk

    macaroni: bread exchange
    cheddar cheese: high-fat meat exchange

	CHO	p	f
2. List the grams of CHO, p and f from the label.	32	10	7

3. a. Divide the CHO in the product by 15 to get the number of bread exchanges: $32 \div 15 = 2.133 = 2$.

    2 breads

	CHO	p	f
b. List the grams of CHO and p in the total number of bread exchanges.	30	4	0
c. Subtract 3b from 2.	2	6	7

4. a. Divide the remaining grams of p in the product by 7 to get the number of meat exchanges: $6 \div 7 = 0.857 = 1$.

    1 high-fat meat

	CHO	p	f
b. List the grams of p and f in the total number of meat exchanges.	0	7	8
c. Subtract 4b from 3c.	0	−1	−1

5. List the number of exchanges for one serving.

    2 breads
    1 high-fat meat

CROISSANTS

Serving size   1
Calories   110
Protein   2 g.
Carbohydrate   15 g.
Fat   7 g.

1. List the main ingredients and the appropriate exchange group for each.

flour, shortening, water

flour: bread exchange
shortening: fat exchange

	CHO	p	f
2. List the grams of CHO, p and f from the label.	15	2	7

3. a. Divide the CHO in the product by 15 to get the number of bread exchanges: $15 \div 15 = 1$.

1 bread

	CHO	p	f
b. List the CHO and p in the total number of bread exchanges.	15	2	0
c. Subtract 3b from 2.	0	0	7

4. a. Divide the remaining grams of f in the product by 5 to get the number of fat exchanges: $5 \div 7 = 0.714 = 1$.

1 fat

	CHO	p	f
b. List the grams of f in the total number of fat exchanges.	0	0	5
c. Subtract 4b from 3c.	0	0	2

5. List the number of exchanges for one serving.

1 bread
1 fat

A knowledge of food labeling can make you a wise consumer. It is particularly useful to know about ingredients in foods to avoid as well as those that will enhance your meal plan. Check the list of ingredients for words that end in "ose" or "tol" to determine the position of sweetness on the ingredient listing. Look out for words that mean fat. When purchasing dietetic foods, make sure the product has advantages which make it worth the extra money. Read the small print on foods claiming to be dietetic and check their ingredients carefully. Use the label to help you identify low-calorie foods. Evaluate all labels as you fit food into your meal plan. Finally, if you have any questions, make sure to check with your nutritionist regarding any new or dietetic foods on the market.

14

Recipe Modification, Restaurant Dining and Special Occasions

This chapter takes a look at how to modify recipes, how to dine in restaurants and how to enjoy yourself on special occasions. We hope you will realize that your cooking habits need only minor changes to allow many more foods to be included in your meal plan. With proper preplanning of meals you can have an enjoyable time in restaurants and on special occasions. Following a few guidelines can make your decisions about food choices easier.

RECIPE MODIFICATION

Life would be rather boring without the inclusion of special recipes, particularly those handed down through families. Unfortunately, many special recipes are loaded with calories, sugar and fat. They may play havoc with blood glucose levels and cause excessive weight gain.

We will now look at how recipes can be altered to fit into your meal plan. Many recipe ideas are suggested not only for weight control but also to help prevent cardiovascular problems. Recipes should be modified for calorie and glucose control. You will recall that simple sugars are digested and absorbed quite rapidly. Therefore, sugar should be used in recipes in minute amounts. A small amount of sugar used in an entire recipe will probably not be detrimental to your blood glucose. Also, the sugar represents only a small amount of carbohydrate. Many recipes include raw fruit to replace refined sugar and to provide extra sweetness as well as fiber.

Finally, recipes should be modified for fat. Remember that fats provide the greatest amount of calories. Therefore, using less fat or low-calorie fats would be beneficial. The quality of the fat can also be changed. Saturated fats like butter and shortenings are frequently used in recipes. Remember, these types of fats raise blood cholesterol levels. The saturated fats may be replaced with polyunsaturated fats (vegetable oil). Much of this section will provide specific examples of recipes that have been modified. Study these recipes to identify ingredient changes as well as changes in the nutrient value of the recipe.

You can change the fat content of recipes in many ways. For example, instead of using butter you can choose soft tub or imitation margarines. If you like the consistency of cream but not the calories, try evaporated skim milk or polyunsaturated coffee lightener. Sour cream can be replaced in most recipes with low-fat plain yogurt or uncreamed cottage cheese blenderized with a small amount of skim milk. Many people may use lard, bacon or chicken fat to flavor food. Here again, it may be wise for you to sacrifice that flavor by switching to a polyunsaturated margarine or oil. The cholesterol content of recipes can also be modified. If you eat a lot of eggs, you may find you can develop a taste for the frozen egg substitutes. In cooking, you can often reduce the number of egg yolks or use more egg whites. Before you reduce the egg content, make sure you know why the eggs were needed in the recipe, that is, whether for binding, for browning or to help the product rise. Finally, you may be successful in lowering the sugar content of the recipe by using a sugar substitute where appropriate. Here again, carefully evaluate the recipe to make sure you can use the substitute. For example, a non-caloric sugar substitute usually cannot be used in a cake. In other recipes, a mixture of cinnamon and sugar substitute may be an effective sweetener, as may dried fruit, such as raisins.

Utilizing the aforementioned ideas, you will be able to modify most of your recipes. For example, let's say lasagna calls for: lasagna noodles, ground chuck (chopped meat), mozzarella, ricotta cheese and tomato sauce. You can easily reduce the calories and fat content of this recipe. You may or may not want to keep the lasagna noodles. Some recipes replace lasagna noodles with eggplant or zucchini strips. You may consider eliminating the ground chuck and replacing it with ground round or ground veal. A vegetarian lasagna, using chopped spinach or chopped broccoli instead of meat, is quite tasty. Part-skim-milk mozzarella and ricotta can be substituted. A very healthy substitute is cottage cheese. Of course, the tomato sauce remains the same. However, if you make your own, use a polyunsaturated oil and keep it meatless.

With a few simple guidelines, you can also modify a quiche. Let's consider that a quiche recipe calls for: Swiss cheese, bacon, cream, eggs, ready-prepared pie crust. For convenience, you may use the ready-prepared pie crust. If you prefer to make your own crust, a polyunsaturated oil can easily replace solid shortening. You can try to use a low-fat cheese, such as St. Otho (mild Muenster-type flavor). Here again, keep in mind how you want the end product to taste. You would not be able to derive the same flavor from a low-fat sliced American cheese, but a mild-tasting, cholesterol-free cheese might be appropriate. The cream can be replaced with evaporated skim milk or whole milk. Egg substitutes can be employed instead of eggs without a significant change in taste. Finally, you may want to make a vegetable or seafood quiche, thus avoiding the bacon.

Other high-fat condiments can also be altered. For example, many people make chicken gravy using chicken fat. Instead, you can try using margarine and chicken stock. The stock will help give a chicken flavor. Finally, onion dip, a favorite at many parties, can be just as tasty using low-fat plain yogurt instead of sour cream.

From the previous recipes you can see that with a little thought and imagination you can prepare fantastic food.

The following recipes will show you how changes in specific ingredients can produce significant nutrient changes.* Crab fondue was modified by using a low-fat cheese, skim milk and an egg substitute. The result is fewer calories, grams of fat and milligrams of cholesterol and sodium per serving.

Crab Fondue	*Crab Fondue* (Modified)
4 slices bread	4 slices bread
8 oz. flaked crab meat	8 oz. flaked crab meat
6 oz. American cheese	6 oz. Weight Watchers cheese
3 eggs	¼ cup Egg Beaters
1 cup whole milk	1 cup skim milk
½ tsp. chopped onion	½ tsp. chopped onion
1 tsp. salt	
paprika, sprinkle	paprika, sprinkle
Serves 4	Serves 4
1 Serving = 357 calories	1 Serving = 221 calories
18 g. carbohydrate × 4 (72 cals.)	19 g. carbohydrate × 4 (76 cals.)
24 g. protein × 4 (96 cals.)	25 g. protein × 4 (100 cals.)
21 g. fat × 9 (189 cals.)	5 g. fat × 9 (45 cals.)
286 mg. cholesterol	44 mg. cholesterol
1,695 mg. sodium	1,213 mg. sodium

* Please note: The calories and nutrients listed here are exact measurements obtained from nutrient analysis books and should be differentiated from the calorie and nutrient allotments in the Exchange System, which is based on averages.

The first lasagna recipe was modified by using spinach instead of meat and part-skim-milk cheeses, instead of whole-milk cheeses. The result is fewer calories, grams of fat and milligrams of cholesterol per serving.

Lasagna #1

1 lb. lasagna noodles
1 lb. ground chuck
½ lb. whole-milk mozzarella
½ lb. whole-milk ricotta
16 oz. tomato sauce

Serves 8

1 Serving = 563 calories
   49 g. carbohydrate × 4 (196 cals.)
   31 g. protein × 4 (124 cals.)
   27 g. fat × 9 (243 cals.)
117 mg. cholesterol
643 mg. sodium

Lasagna #2 (Modified)

1 lb. lasagna noodles
10 oz. frozen spinach
½ lb. part-skim-milk mozzarella
½ lb. part-skim-milk ricotta
16 oz. tomato sauce

Serves 8

1 Serving = 343 calories
   51 g. carbohydrate × 4 (204 cals.)
   19 g. protein × 4 (76 cals.)
    7 g. fat × 9 (63 cals.)
 35 mg. cholesterol
692 mg. sodium

This recipe was altered by using a lean cut of meat and part-skim-milk cheeses. The result is slightly fewer calories and grams of fat per serving.

Lasagna #3 (Modified)

1 lb. lasagna noodles
1 lb. ground round
½ lb. part-skim-milk mozzarella
½ lb. part-skim-milk ricotta
16 oz. tomato sauce

Serves 8

1 Serving = 434 calories
   50 g. carbohydrates × 4 (200 cals.)
   36 g. protein × 4 (144 cals.)
   10 g. fat × 9 (90 cals.)
102 mg. cholesterol
723 mg. sodium

The ingredients in zucchini bread were changed to include diet margarine, an egg substitute, half the amount of sugar but more raisins. The new product has fewer calories, grams of carbohydrate, fat and milligrams of cholesterol per serving.

Zucchini Bread	Zucchini Bread (Modified)
1 cup corn oil	1 cup diet margarine
1 large zucchini, grated	1 large zucchini, grated
1½ cups flour (wheat), sifted	1½ cups flour (wheat), sifted
½ cup walnuts	½ cup walnuts
½ cup raisins (not packed)	¾ cup raisins
1 tsp. baking soda	1 tsp. baking soda
1 tsp. baking powder	1 tsp. baking powder
½ cup sugar	¼ cup sugar
2 eggs (medium)	½ cup Egg Beaters
Serves 10	Serves 10
1 Serving = 387 calories	1 Serving = 244 calories
31 g. carbohydrate × 4 (124 cals.)	29 g. carbohydrate × 4 (116 cals.)
5 g. protein × 4 (20 cals.)	5 g. protein × 4 (20 cals.)
27 g. fat × 9 (243 cals.)	12 g. fat × 9 (108 cals.)
50 mg. cholesterol	0 cholesterol
131 mg. sodium	360 mg. sodium

Instead of using a high-fat cheddar cheese, whole milk and butter, the recipe below employs a low-fat cheese, diet margarine and skim milk. The result is fewer calories, grams of fat and milligrams of cholesterol. Unfortunately, the low-fat cheese in this and the other recipes contributes to a higher sodium content in the total dish. However, the benefits of a product lower in calories and fat can still be advantageous to those without hypertension, despite the high sodium content.

Macaroni and Cheese	Macaroni and Cheese (Modified)
½ lb. macaroni	½ lb. macaroni
½ lb. sharp cheddar cheese	½ lb. Fisher cheese (Countdown Chunk)*
1 cup whole milk	1 cup skim milk
2 tbs. butter	2 tbs. diet margarine
½ cup bread crumbs	½ cup bread crumbs
Serves 4	Serves 4
1 Serving = 474 calories	1 Serving = 313 calories
39 g. carbohydrate × 4 (156 cals.)	44 g. carbohydrate × 4 (176 cals.)
21 g. protein × 4 (84 cals.)	23 g. protein × 4 (92 cals.)
26 g. fat × 9 (234 cals.)	5 g. fat × 9 (45 cals.)
84 mg. cholesterol	1 mg. cholesterol
527 mg. sodium	1,088 mg. sodium

* Fisher cheese available by mail from: Diet & Health Products, Inc., P.O. Box 18865, Lima, OH 45801 *or* from some specialty cheese shops.

The following recipe was modified using margarine and evaporated skim milk. The result is a reduction in calories, grams of total fat and milligrams of cholesterol per serving.

Cream Sauce

2 tbs. flour
2 tbs. butter
½ cup heavy cream
½ cup whole milk

Serves 8 (1 to 2 tbs. each)

1 Serving = 97 calories
  3 g. carbohydrates × 4 (12 cals.)
  1 g. protein × 4 (4 cals.)
  9 g. fat × 9 (81 cals.)
  22 mg. cholesterol
  62 mg. sodium

Cream Sauce (Modified)

2 tbs. flour
2 tbs. soft tub margarine
1 cup evaporated skim milk

Serves 8 (1 to 2 tbs. each)

1 Serving = 59 calories
  5 g. carbohydrate × 4 (20 cals.)
  3 g. protein × 4 (12 cals.)
  3 g. fat × 9 (27 cals.)
  1 mg. cholesterol
  72 mg. sodium

This recipe was modified by using D-Zerta pudding and skim milk. The outcome is fewer calories and grams of carbohydrate per serving.

Banana Cream Pie

1 package vanilla pudding
2 ripe bananas
2 cups whole milk
pie shell

Serves 8

1 Serving = 218 calories
  29 g. carbohydrate × 4 (116 cals.)
   3 g. protein × 4 (12 cals.)
  10 g. fat × 9 (90 cals.)
   8 mg. cholesterol
  229 mg. sodium

Banana Cream Pie (Modified)

1 package vanilla D-Zerta pudding
2 ripe bananas
2 cups skim milk
pie shell

Serves 8

1 Serving = 154 calories
  21 g. carbohydrate × 4 (84 cals.)
   4 g. protein × 4 (16 cals.)
   6 g. fat × 9 (54 cals.)
   2 mg. cholesterol
  122 mg. sodium

This recipe was altered by using low-fat yogurt instead of sour cream. The product has fewer calories, grams of fat and milligrams of cholesterol per serving. Most of the sodium comes from the dry soup mix.

Vegetable Dip

1 cup sour cream
1 package dry onion soup mix

1 Serving = 2 tbs.

1 Serving = 78 calories
    4 g. carbohydrate × 4 (16 cals.)
    2 g. protein × 4 (8 cals.)
    6 g. fat × 9 (54 cals.)
  13 mg. cholesterol
374 mg. sodium

Vegetable Dip (Modified)

1 cup low-fat yogurt
1 package dry onion soup mix

1 Serving = 2 tbs.

1 Serving = 32.5 calories
    5 g. carbohydrate × 4 (20 cals.)
    2 g. protein × 4 (8 cals.)
    0.5 g. fat × 9 (4.5 cals.)
    2 mg. cholesterol
379 mg. sodium

The previous recipes show that a few simple modifications can dramatically change the nutrient composition of the recipe. With some practice and creativity, you will be able to modify many of your favorite recipes.

Recipes can easily be modified and calculated to fit into your specific meal plan. Most recipes can be changed into the Exchange System. To begin this procedure: (1) Itemize each ingredient and determine the exchange group it belongs in. (2) Calculate the number of exchanges per item in the recipe. (3) Add together all numbers in each column. (4) Divide by the total number of servings in the recipe. (5) Use the chart in Table 16 and the Exchange System from Chapter 8 to determine the correct exchanges and the correct amounts. Keep several copies of the chart for future use.

For example, if your recipe calls for 2 cups (16 ounces) of skim milk, you would enter the number 2 under milk. This is because 2 cups is equal to two

TABLE 16

INGREDIENT	MILK	VEGETABLE	FRUIT	BREAD	MEAT	FAT
TOTAL						
TOTAL/SERVING						

milk exchanges. However, if the recipe calls for 1 pound of meat, you would enter 12. While there are 16 ounces in 1 pound, cooked meat loses one-quarter of its weight. So 1 pound of meat would lose 4 ounces. You would add together all the numbers in each column and divide by the total number of servings in the recipe. It might be difficult to determine the number of exchanges of several recipe ingredients. These include: flour, 1½ cups = 10 bread exchanges; shortening, 1 cup = 16 tablespoons = 48 fat exchanges; sugar, 1 cup = 20 fruit exchanges.

If the exchange totals are fractions, you can round them off as follows: if a total is ¼ or less than ½, you can eliminate the fraction. If the total is ½, count it as is. If the total is more than ½, round it up to the next exchange.

For this chapter, all recipes containing meat are calculated as a lean meat exchange. If the protein source is a medium-fat meat, ½ a fat exchange is added into the fat column for each exchange. If a high-fat meat is used, one fat exchange is added. Refer to the following tables for specific examples (Tables 17a–b, 18a–c, 19a–b, 20a–b and 21a–b). If whole milk is used as an ingredient, it is calculated as a milk and a fat exchange. If skim milk is indicated, it is counted only as a milk exchange.

The crab fondue recipe in Table 17a was modified to make it lower in calories and fat. Each ingredient fits into the Exchange System as stated in the directions for that procedure. After the recipe is modified, it provides you with one bread and four meat exchanges. However, the fat exchanges are omitted.

The lasagna recipe in Table 18a was changed to make it lower in calories and fat. When you fit the modified recipe into the Exchange System, you see that you need not count as many fat or meat exchanges with the vegetable lasagna as with the ground chuck lasagna.

The lasagna recipe in Table 18c shows you another way to modify the original recipe. You can use a leaner cut of meat along with part-skim-milk cheeses. When you fit the modified recipe into the Exchange System, you see again that you need not have as many fat exchanges.

The zucchini bread recipe in Table 19a was modified to be lower in carbohydrates, calories and fat. When you fit the modified recipe into the Exchange System, you see that it provides you with half the fat exchanges. Less sugar is used in the modified recipe.

The macaroni and cheese recipe in Table 20a was changed to be lower in fat. When you fit the new recipe into the Exchange System, you see that it provides you with fewer fat exchanges.

The cream sauce recipe in Table 21a was modified to be lower in fat in order to provide half the amount of fat exchanges.

Read on to find out how to order appropriate food choices in restaurants.

TABLE 17a
CRAB FONDUE

INGREDIENTS:	MILK	VEGETABLE	FRUIT	BREAD	MEAT	FAT
4 slices bread				4		
8 ounces crab meat					4	
6 ounces American cheese					6	6
3 eggs					3	1½
1 cup whole milk	1					2
TOTAL: 4 servings	1			4	13	9½
1 serving	¼			1	3¼	2⅓

1 serving of Crab Fondue = 1 Bread Exchange
                         3 Meat Exchanges
                         2 Fat Exchanges

TABLE 17b
CRAB FONDUE (MODIFIED)

INGREDIENTS:	MILK	VEGETABLE	FRUIT	BREAD	MEAT	FAT
4 slices bread				4		
8 ounces crab meat					4	
6 ounces Weight Watchers cheese					6	
¾ c. egg substitute					3	
1 cup skim milk	1					
TOTAL: 4 serving	1			4	13	
1 serving	¼			1	3¼	

1 serving of Crab Fondue (Modified) = 1 Bread Exchange
                                      3 Meat Exchanges

TABLE 18a
LASAGNA #1

INGREDIENTS:	MILK	VEGETABLE	FRUIT	BREAD	MEAT	FAT
1 lb. lasagna noodles				16		
1 lb. ground chuck					12	12
½ lb. whole-milk mozzarella		4				
½ lb. whole-milk ricotta					8	4
16 oz. tomato sauce					8	4
TOTAL: 8 servings		4		16	28	20
1 serving		½		2	3½	2½

1 serving of Lasagna = ½ Vegetable Exchange   3½ Meat Exchanges
2 Bread Exchanges   2½ Fat Exchanges

TABLE 18b
LASAGNA #2 (MODIFIED)

INGREDIENTS:	MILK	VEGETABLE	FRUIT	BREAD	MEAT	FAT
1 lb. lasagna noodles				16		
10 oz. spinach		2¾				
½ lb. part-skim mozzarella					8	4
½ lb. part-skim ricotta					8	
16 oz. tomato sauce		4				
TOTAL: 8 servings		6¾		16	16	4
1 serving		.8		2	2	½

1 serving of Lasagna = 1 Vegetable Exchange   2 Meat Exchanges
2 Bread Exchanges   ½ Fat Exchange

TABLE 18c
LASAGNA #3 (MODIFIED)

INGREDIENTS:	MILK	VEGETABLE	FRUIT	BREAD	MEAT	FAT
1 lb. lasagna noodles				16		
1 lb. ground round					12	
½ lb. part-skim mozzarella					8	4
½ lb. part-skim ricotta					8	
16 oz. tomato sauce		4				
TOTAL: 8 servings		4		16	28	4
1 serving		½		2	3½	½

1 serving of Lasagna = ½ Vegetable Exchange   3½ Meat Exchanges
2 Bread Exchanges   ½ Fat Exchange

TABLE 19a
ZUCCHINI BREAD

INGREDIENTS:	MILK	VEGETABLE	FRUIT	BREAD	MEAT	FAT
1 cup corn oil						48
1 lb. zucchini		4				
1½ cup wheat flour				10		
½ cup walnuts						8
½ cup raisins			5			
1 tsp. baking soda						
1 tsp. baking powder						
½ cup sugar			10			
2 eggs					2	1
TOTAL: 10 servings		4	15	10	2	57
1 serving		.4	1½	1	.2	5 ⁷⁄₁₀

1 serving of Zucchini Bread = ½ Vegetable Exchange   0 Meat Exchange
                           1½ Fruit Exchange   6 Fat Exchanges
                           1 Bread Exchange

TABLE 19b
ZUCCHINI BREAD (MODIFIED)

INGREDIENTS:	MILK	VEGETABLE	FRUIT	BREAD	MEAT	FAT
1 cup diet margarine						16
1 lb. zucchini		4				
1½ cup wheat flour				10		
½ cup walnuts						8
¾ cup raisins			7.5			
1 tsp. baking soda						
1 tsp. baking powder						
¼ cup sugar			5			
½ cup Egg Beaters					2	
TOTAL: 10 servings		4	12.5	10	2	24
1 serving		.5	1¼	1		2²⁄₅

1 serving of Zucchini Bread (Modified) = ½ Vegetable Exchange   0 Meat Exchange
                                      1 Fruit Exchange   2 Fat Exchanges
                                      1 Bread Exchange

TABLE 20a
MACARONI & CHEESE

INGREDIENTS:	MILK	VEGETABLE	FRUIT	BREAD	MEAT	FAT
½ lb. macaroni				8		
½ lb. sharp cheddar					8	8
1 cup whole milk	1					2
2 tbs. butter						6
½ cup bread crumbs				2		
TOTAL: 4 servings	1			10	8	16
1 serving	¼			2½	2	4

1 serving of Macaroni & Cheese = 2½ Bread Exchanges
2 Meat Exchanges
4 Fat Exchanges

TABLE 20b
MACARONI & CHEESE (MODIFIED)

INGREDIENTS:	MILK	VEGETABLE	FRUIT	BREAD	MEAT	FAT
½ lb. macaroni				8		
½ lb. Fisher cheese (Countdown Chunk)					8	
1 cup skim milk	1					
2 tbs. diet margarine						2
½ cup bread crumbs				2		
TOTAL: 4 servings	1			10	8	2
1 serving	¼			2½	2	½

1 serving of Macaroni & Cheese (Modified) = 2½ Bread Exchanges
2 Meat Exchanges
½ Fat Exchange

TABLE 21a
CREAM SAUCE

INGREDIENTS:	MILK	VEGETABLE	FRUIT	BREAD	MEAT	FAT
2 tbs. flour				1		
2 tbs. butter						6
½ cup heavy cream						8
½ cup whole milk	½					1
TOTAL: 8 servings	½			1		15
1 serving (1 oz.)	¹/₁₆			⅛		1⅞

1 serving of Cream sauce = 2 Fat Exchanges
0 Milk Exchange
0 Bread Exchange

TABLE 21b
CREAM SAUCE (MODIFIED)

INGREDIENTS:	MILK	VEGETABLE	FRUIT	BREAD	MEAT	FAT
2 tbs. flour				1		
2 tbs. margarine						6
1 cup evaporated skim milk	2					
TOTAL: 8 servings	2			1		6
1 serving (1 oz.)	¼			¼		¾

1 serving of Cream Sauce (Modified) = 1 Fat Exchange
0 Milk Exchange
0 Bread Exchange

RESTAURANT DINING

Dining out in a restaurant is an activity to which everyone looks forward. What are some reasons you dine out? You may enjoy dining out to avoid cooking, to change your usual environment and/or routine or simply to get out of the house. Others dine out to visit with friends or to try new foods. Many important plans are made while dining in restaurants, including financial arrangements or lifestyle changes, such as proposals of marriage.

Dining in a restaurant may be a stressful experience for a person with diabetes. You may be torn between eating what you desire as opposed to what your intellect dictates. However, some people think dining in a restaurant is actually easier than cooking at home. When dining out, the main goal for the obese non-insulin-dependent person is to avoid excess calories. For the insulin-dependent person, consistency in the composition of the meal and staying as close to the usual meal plan as possible are important goals. You can balance dining out with good nutrition by following a few suggestions. There are specific techniques that you can use to avoid excess calories yet retain the pleasure of dining out.

You may be interested in avoiding excess calories either to prevent weight gain or to achieve blood glucose control. To start, you can order foods that are broiled, baked, steamed or boiled. Foods fried in fat provide more calories than foods that do not have fat added to them. Stay away from foods that are prepared with cream sauces to avoid excess calories. Most cream sauces are made with heavy or light cream and butter. In this case, the fat in these dishes adds the extra calories, not the starch. Other items that contain fat are gravies and salad dressings. Order these on the side so you can control the amount you put on food. Ordering lower-calorie foods is an excellent way to enjoy a complete dinner and eliminate extra calories.

Become an expert in estimating portion sizes. Even if all else fails, portion control is the next-best method to avoid taking in excess calories. In a previous chapter it was recommended that you weigh and measure all the food you eat for at least a week. This activity should be repeated periodically. Knowledge gained while weighing and measuring foods at home can be used when dining in restaurants. A useful guide to remember is that the size of an average woman's palm is approximately three inches by three inches by three-quarters of an inch. If your palm is that size, it resembles a portion of meat equivalent to approximately 3 ounces.

If you become knowledgeable in avoiding the pitfalls of restaurant dining, you can eat in any restaurant. This includes delis, coffee shops and seafood, Chinese, Italian and Indian restaurants. Experimenting with new food flavors is always interesting. Therefore, you may enjoy dining out in restaurants serving foreign cuisine. French cuisines may be more difficult to choose from because many foods are prepared with cream and butter sauces. You can still make a good choice by ordering foods broiled without butter or foods cooked in wine. You can always use portion control techniques and choose entrées from the lean meat exchange.

If you dine in a Chinese restaurant, remember calorie control. The Chinese use cornstarch as a thickening agent. One tablespoon of cornstarch is equivalent to one-half bread exchange. It is doubtful that you would consume more than that in a Chinese dish. In addition, the Chinese usually use polyunsaturated or monounsaturated fats in cooking, such as soybean, sunflower and peanut oil. This being so, Chinese food makes a nice choice, in that saturated fats are not used with great frequency. Food is usually stir-fried quickly in hot oil. Foods to avoid in a Chinese restaurant are those that are deep-fat fried or prepared in a sweet and sour sauce.

Many people would order an entrée such as chicken chow mein and try to itemize all components of it, to fit it into their Exchange System. While this is an admirable task, it is one that may be quite frustrating. Since dining in restaurants should be a pleasurable experience, this frustration should be eliminated. You can easily approximate the exchange groups. For example, you can estimate that a typical serving of chicken chow mein contains about 2 ounces of chicken. This is equivalent to two lean meat exchanges. In addition, there may be a cup of vegetables, which is equal to two vegetable exchanges. About two fat exchanges may be used in the cooking process. If this seems rather difficult to you, you can always use portion control. In order to do this, however, you would have to know what a half cup or a cup of chicken chow mein looks like. You would be able to estimate this accurately only if you had practiced with a measuring cup at home.

While dining in an Italian restaurant, there are a few specific strategies to follow in addition to avoiding the pitfalls already mentioned. As in any restaurant, fried foods and cream sauces should be avoided. Refrain from ordering Italian entrées that are deep-fried or prepared with high-fat cheese. This includes eggplant Parmigiana, chicken cutlet and veal Parmigiana. You may be thinking, what can you have in an Italian restaurant? Any type of pasta prepared with tomato sauce, vegetable or seafood is an appropriate choice. You may choose any veal, fish, beef or chicken dish that is lightly sautéed, baked or broiled. Sautéed entrées will have more calories than those not sautéed, but less than those fried. Entrées such as veal scaloppine alla Marsala, chicken cacciatore, calamari and red snapper marinara are excellent choices. See the following to determine foods to order and foods to avoid.

Foods to Order

You can order the following items as part of your meal in delis, coffee shops or American restaurants:

Appetizer	fresh vegetable tray (free choice or 1 vegetable exchange)
	fresh fruit (1 fruit exchange)
	tomato juice (1 vegetable exchange)
	clam cocktail (approx. 1 meat exchange)
Soup	clear broths or bouillon or tomato-base soups
Salad	tossed (order dressing on the side); tomato and onion; spinach (estimate 2 fat exchanges)
Vegetable	any kind, boiled, baked, stewed, steamed, without any added fat (½ cup equals 1 vegetable exchange)
Potato	boiled, baked, parsleyed (one small equals 1 bread exchange)
Bread	half hard or soft roll (1 bread exchange)
	small, plain muffin (1 bread exchange)
	breadsticks (3 sticks equal 1 bread exchange)
Entrée	meat, chicken or fish: broiled, boiled, roasted, baked (one serving 3″ × 3″ × ¼″ equals 3 ounces) (choose lean meats and trim off excess fat)
Sandwich	lean, boiled ham, roast beef, sliced turkey or chicken (1 ounce equals 1 lean meat exchange)
	tuna, salmon, chicken or shrimp salad (allow 2 tsp. fat per ½ cup) (½ cup equals 2 fat exchanges and 2–3 lean meat exchanges)
Dessert	fresh fruit (1 fruit exchange)
	angel food cake (1 bread exchange)
	sherbet (once in a while—2 fruit exchanges)
	cheese and crackers (1–2 bread and 1–2 high-fat meat exchanges)
Beverage	sugar-free soda
	coffee, tea
	skim milk (1 milk exchange)
	wine (3½ ounces equals 1½ fat exchanges)

Foods to Avoid

Appetizer	sweetened juices
	creamed soups
	canned fruit in syrup
	antipasto
Entrée	fatty and fried foods
	entrées prepared with cheese or cream sauce
	stews or casseroles with unknown ingredients
Potato	fried
	creamed
	scalloped
	au gratin
Fats	gravy
	fried foods
	creamed foods
	cheese-type salad dressings
Bread	sweet rolls
	coffee cake
Vegetable	creamed
	scalloped
	au gratin
	fried
Dessert	puddings
	custards
	pastry
	cakes
	sweetened fruit
Beverage	chocolate milk
	shakes
	regular soda

Dining out with friends may need special planning. At this time you must gather all your assertive tips and take control of difficult situations. For example, when planning to dine out with friends, it may be appropriate for you to suggest the restaurant and choose the cuisine. In this way, you can preplan for any food-related problems. Many people feel that it is not essential to do this. However, if you find yourself in a restaurant that makes choosing appropriate food difficult, the next time you will want to dine in one that makes your choices easy. If you have a friend who is constantly coaxing you to eat foods you do not want, learn to say "no." Be convincing at this. Practice saying "no" by using a tape recorder. Listen to your responses to hear whether or not you sound convincing. Non-verbal expressions that you convey are important as an accompaniment to your verbal statement of "no." So speak firmly and with confidence. Look directly at the person and maintain a convincing facial expression.

Most restaurant employees are very accommodating to their patrons. Waiters usually enjoy answering your questions and can be very helpful in describing the best choices for the evening. You should be somewhat assertive when speaking with waiters. Do not be afraid to ask how an entrée or sauce is prepared. Also, be careful when wording your questions. For example, if you ask whether sugar is added to a food, the answer may be "no." However, the food may be sweetened with honey or jam. Most restaurants allow you to make special requests. For example, you can ask for fish broiled without butter or oil. You can ask that your salad be served immediately if you are hungry. You can also ask for the bread to be removed from the table. Remember, an assertive person is one who takes appropriate action and gets the desired results. There is no room for either aggressive or passive behavior at this time.

There are a few things that you can do before you dine out. Preplan what you will eat. If you have non-insulin-dependent diabetes, you may save exchanges from snacks or calories from other times during the day to allow for extra calories in the restaurant. However, try to avoid starving yourself before a restaurant meal. If you enter the restaurant ravenous, you may be unable to exert self-control. So eat a preplanned snack such as fruit or raw vegetables or drink a glass of skim milk. Preplan what to eat to avoid extra calories. Preplanning can help you avoid using the menu, which may act as a cue to entice you to order what you might not have ordered had you not looked at the menu. You can fill up on vegetables first or on other foods that are low in calories. Leave a small amount of food on your plate. You do not have to finish everything that is served, even though you are paying for it. Many people feel they have to leave a clean plate to help "the starving children in Africa." The starving children in Africa will not benefit if you finish everything. So a good behavioral technique is to leave a small amount on your plate. This breaks the association between a clean plate and feelings of fullness. Therefore, you can enjoy restaurant dining even though you may be counting calories to control your weight.

Below are examples of breakfast, lunch and dinner eaten in a restaurant. Meal A contains foods that are very high in fat, prepared with fat or contain much sugar and therefore lots of extra calories. Meal B shows approximately the same amount of food but much better choices. It demonstrates the use of portion control techniques (5 ounces of steak vs. 9 ounces of steak) and low-fat food choices (skim milk vs. whole milk). The point here is that with a few modifications in restaurant ordering, you can still have an enjoyable meal.

Meal A	Calories	Meal B	Calories
2 eggs, scrambled in butter	205	½ grapefruit	41
brown-and-serve sausage (1 oz.)	118	½ cup oatmeal	75
½ cup hash browns	130	½ cup skim milk	40
8 oz. whole milk	160	1 slice whole-wheat toast	70
	613	1 tsp. margarine	45
		1 poached egg	80
			351
3 oz. ground chuck	300	¾ cup tomato juice	35
½ cup cottage cheese	120	3 oz. white meat turkey	176
2 peach halves	78	2 slices rye bread	140
½ cup Jell-O	97	1 tsp. mayonnaise	45
2 packs melba toast	70	celery sticks	25
	665	¼ cantaloupe	40
			455
2 martinis	240	3 oz. wine	85
salad with blue cheese		salad with lemon and vinegar	0
dressing (1 oz.)	141	1 slice whole-wheat bread	70
2 slices French bread	116	2 pats butter	90
2 pats butter	90	1 baked potato	95
1 baked potato	95	5 oz. filet mignon	275
9 oz. porterhouse steak	726		605
	1,408		
Total	2,686	Total	1,410

To help you practice meal planning, look at the following Italian menu. Think of foods you would choose and read on.

Here is an example of a menu from an Italian restaurant. See if you can determine the appropriate choices.

Appetizers

Scungilli Salad
Stuffed Mushrooms
Cold Antipasto
Melon and Prosciutto
Clam Cocktail
Clams Oreganata
Mussels Posilippo

Veal

Veal Parmigiana
Veal alla Marsala with Mushrooms
Veal Scaloppine with Mushrooms
Veal Pizzaiola in Red Sauce
Veal Piccata with Lemon Sauce
Veal and Peppers
Veal Française
Veal Sorrentino, eggplant, mozzarella cheese, topped with sauce

Salad

Mixed green with house dressing

Soups

Chicken Escarole
Onion
Minestrone

Italian Specialties

Chicken Cacciatore
Eggplant Parmigiana
Sausage and Peppers
Pork Chops Pizzaiola

Vegetables

Sautéed Escarole
Sautéed Mushrooms
Fried Zucchini

Home-Style Pasta

Fresh-Made Ravioli (Cheese)
Fresh-Made Lasagna
Baked Manicotti
Spaghetti with Sausage
Spaghetti with Shrimp
Spaghetti with Mushrooms
Linguine with Clam Sauce (Red or White)
Pasta e Fagioli

Seafood

Shrimp Scampi, Marinara or Fra Diavolo
Calamari Marinara or Fra Diavolo
Lobster Tail Marinara or Fra Diavolo

Desserts

Spumoni, Tortoni, Sherbet
Italian Cheesecake, Ice Cream

You probably will still question the waiter regarding ingredients and food preparation techniques. However, the following choices would be appropriate. You could order scungilli salad, mussels Posilippo, clam cocktail or melon (without the prosciutto) for an appetizer. Soup might include minestrone, chicken escarole or onion. A salad with dressing on the side is fine, along with spaghetti with mushrooms, linguine with clam sauce, spaghetti with shrimp or pasta e fagioli as a pasta choice. Your entrée might include chicken cacciatore, pork chops pizzaiola, veal pizzaiola, broiled entrées, veal alla Marsala, veal piccata, shrimp marinara or Fra Diavolo, calamari marinara or Fra Diavolo, mussels Posilippo or Fra Diavolo, lobster tail marinara or Fra Diavolo. All vegetables prepared without fat (unless you can afford the calories or exchanges) would be O.K. Finally, dessert might include melon or, once in a while, sherbet or ice cream.

If you are insulin-dependent you may find your friends dining at different times than you are used to. Remember, your most important goal is consistency in the timing and nutrient composition of your meals. However, in our society we are accustomed to dining out late, particularly on the weekends. You can preplan in order to enjoy the late dinner hour. While switching around your mealtime is not recommended on a daily basis, it may occur once in a while. If you are eating dinner later than usual, try to have part of your dinner or your evening snack at the usual dinner hour. For example, if you normally eat dinner at 6 P.M. but tonight dinner will not be until 9 P.M., try to have a fruit and a bread exchange or a milk and a bread exchange at 6 P.M., then eat the rest of your dinner at 9 P.M. The following two examples will illustrate this:

This is your typical meal plan:

> 3 P.M.: snack; 6 P.M.: evening meal; 9 P.M.: snack

You are dining out this evening and will not eat dinner until 9 P.M. Take appropriate measures to prevent problems such as hypoglycemia. Many patients feel the best step would be to have the 9 P.M. snack at 6 P.M. and the evening meal at 9 P.M. So the new plan would be as follows:

> 3 P.M.: snack; 6 P.M.: snack; 9 P.M.: evening meal

If you are not scheduled to have a 9 P.M. snack, do not have your 3 P.M. snack at 6 P.M. This must be avoided because you may be taking an insulin that peaks in the late afternoon. So you need that afternoon snack to prevent hypoglycemia. Instead, the best thing to do would be to divide the allowed servings of food for the evening meal into two small snacks.

> 3 P.M.: snack; 6 P.M.: ¼–½ of evening meal;
> 9 P.M.: remaining serving from evening meal

If dinner is very late and you will not be able to have your bedtime snack, the snack can be included in your dinner meal.

Use of the Exchange System when dining in a restaurant can be very helpful. For the person who has practiced using the Exchange System, it will be easy to dine in restaurants. The only prerequisite is that you know how many choices from each food group you are allowed. Many people take their Exchange booklet to the restaurant until they are proficient in ordering from a menu. This is a useful technique and one that need only be done a few times until you know your food exchanges.

ALCOHOL AND COCKTAIL PARTIES

How do you handle cocktail parties? Undoubtedly, you have specific tips to help you. This is the type of party filled with much gaiety as well as food and drink. A myriad of ideas exist to deal with alcohol and food. If you do take an alcoholic beverage, remember to count exchanges or calories. Alcohol, in excess, can provide excess calories, so limit your intake to one drink. When you drink, stay with dry wines or mixed drinks without added sugar. Remember that sparkling water (e.g., Perrier) or wine spritzers are very refreshing. Review Chapter 2 for additional tips. Remember that alcohol lowers your blood glucose. The blood-glucose-lowering effect may be dangerous if you take medication for diabetes. The calories contained in some alcoholic beverages are listed here. Drinking too much may cause you to eat too much food or the wrong kind of food.

CALORIC CONTENT OF ALCOHOLIC BEVERAGES

Beverage	Amount	Calories
beer	12 oz.	150
beer, light	12 oz.	90–100
gin, rum, vodka, scotch	1½ oz.	112–135 (depending on the proof)
martini	3½ oz.	140
tom collins	10 oz.	180
champagne	4 oz.	84
wine, table	3½ oz.	84
wine, dessert	3½ oz.	137
rum and Coke	4 oz. Coke and 1½ oz. rum	164

Finally, if you have insulin-dependent diabetes, you must eat on a regular time schedule. A long cocktail party may delay your dinner hour. If this is the case, remember to preplan your meals accordingly.

What about the food at cocktail parties? Usually you are faced with a wide array of food choices. Make sure you do not attend the party hungry. In this way you will be able to control your intake. Position yourself away from the food to avoid food cues. Before deciding what to eat, survey all your choices. Avoid foods that are fried or cooked with sugar. Choose foods that contain the fewest calories. It is advantageous to adhere to the Exchange System; however, if you cannot, always remember to use portion control. Prior to each party, review the fundamental principles you have read in this chapter to help you to maintain control.

FAST FOODS

Fast foods have become a part of our society and will probably continue to be so. Therefore, you should know how to choose foods in a fast-food restaurant should the need arise. If you have insulin-dependent diabetes, again the main objective is to stay within your allotted exchanges. If you have non-insulin-dependent diabetes, your main objective is calorie control. Always remember to order the smallest serving size possible. Avoid sweetened beverages and desserts. If you order fried chicken or fish, remove the calorie-laden breading.

Try fast-food restaurants that offer a salad bar. You can often fill up with salad while your friends are having other items. Some newer fast-food restaurants offer lettuce and tomato along with the hamburgers. Other restaurants serve leaner meats. You can write to the individual companies to get a nutritional analysis of their products or refer to the "Fast-Food Guide" in the back of this book. The addition of milk and/or juice will also increase the nutritional value of your meal. Continue reading to learn how you can best deal with special events in your life.

FOOD AND SPECIAL OCCASIONS

Special occasions, such as birthdays or holidays, can present unwanted signals that can easily trigger overeating. The following general guidelines should help you to handle special times.

Anticipate each situation and plan a strategy to prevent overeating. Some factors to anticipate are delayed meals, the use of alcoholic beverages and the presence of an overabundance of food. Preplanning can eliminate the element of surprise. When preplanning you can mentally rehearse or imagine yourself at a party. Pretend you are making appropriate food choices and focus on the special aspect of the party rather than the food. Remember, anticipation plus knowledge equals control. Not only can you achieve blood glucose control but also self-control, or the ability to make proper decisions.

Reward yourself if you follow prearranged plans. For example, if you have club soda instead of scotch, reward yourself for that with something not related to food. A reward can be something nice you do for yourself. You may treat yourself to a movie, take a bubble bath or save some money for yourself. Whatever you choose, make sure you like it and that it is something that makes you feel good about yourself.

Assertiveness in a restaurant or in a friend's home is only one small part of any social event. Learn to be assertive with friends and relatives. Enlist the support of family and friends when dealing with special occasions. There are a variety of social norms in our society that make eating a part of almost every social occasion. Social norms may include feelings or statements such as "You are not a good hostess if you do not offer a guest something to eat or drink"; "If you refuse an offer of food you will personally reject the giver"; "You cannot celebrate without food or drink"; and "Holidays must have an abundance of food." Think of ways to challenge these social norms. Praise yourself and indulge in positive self-talk when you have handled situations appropriately.

Each week could conceivably include a special event, such as a family member's birthday or anniversary, Mother's Day, Father's Day or Valentine's Day. Each holiday or occasion is usually accompanied by a gift. You may have been taught from childhood that these occasions must be enjoyed with food. You also learn to use gifts of food as tokens of appreciation or expressions of caring. For example, you may wonder what Valentine's Day would be without a box of chocolates. Retrain your mind so that the focus of the special occasion is not food but enjoying the occasion. Gifts should be something you cannot eat. These may include books, records, flowers, games, money, donations to a favorite charity, golf clubs, even a kitchen or living-room knickknack. With the proper planning you can think of hundreds of gift-giving ideas that have nothing to do with food. You can also enlist the support of family and friends simply by asking them to bring flowers instead of candy. Ask for help around the house rather than frequent dinners out.

Entertaining in your home may be easier than in someone else's home. Here, you have total control over what is served. A successful party may revolve around a creative and entertaining presentation of food rather than fancy, high-calorie foods. Try to be creative when reviewing your cookbooks. Experiment with exotic cuisines. Use your best china and crystal and have flowers as a centerpiece on the table. Provide your guests with pleasant music and a relaxing atmosphere. You do not have to use diet foods excessively. You may have favorite recipes you enjoy using when entertaining. If some items are going to be particularly rich and high in calories, remember to use portion control techniques.

Take a chance and try new and different recipe ideas. Modify your recipes so that they are low in fat. Use yogurt instead of sour cream in dips. Make a quiche with an egg substitute instead of eggs. Have a meatless meal or salad party just to be different. Friends will be interested in new tastes and enjoy fewer calories. For more ideas, see the section on recipe modification in the early part of this chapter.

Many "accepted" social rules influence you when dining at a friend's home. Carefully think about how you will handle situations by planning ahead. Obtaining information from the hostess before the event can help. Find out if it will be a sit-down dinner or a buffet. Buffets offer the advantage of allowing you to control portion size. If you know the hostess well, you may even find out what is being served so you can determine what you will eat. If this kind of preplanning is unfeasible, then a few general rules prevail. Plan to use portion control techniques throughout the meal. Prepare yourself for an insistent hostess. This is the hostess who becomes offended if you refuse seconds or if you do not finish everything on your plate. Be ready to give appropriate responses, such as "No, thank you, I've had enough" or "Everything is so good I couldn't possibly eat any more." Some people feel comfortable telling the hostess they have diabetes and cannot eat certain foods. Remember that not eating food does not mean "I don't like you." Sit away from the snack foods or buffet table. You may want to keep a small amount of food on your plate so it appears as if you are still eating. If you have non-insulin-dependent diabetes, you may save extra calories from the day to allow for more calories at the party. If you develop a strong urge to eat, sit down, eat slowly, choose wisely and enjoy what you eat. If you have insulin-dependent diabetes, try to stay within your allotted exchanges and avoid foods with simple sugars.

Buffets as well as cocktail and hors d'oeuvre parties can pose special problems. When you attend these occasions you are confronted with free food. Preplan to eat only a specific amount. If there will be a variety of foods to choose from, decide in advance to have one taste of new or different foods. Try to avoid foods prepared with excess sugar or fat. Finally, since these parties lend themselves to eating a lot of food, remember to eat small, predetermined portion sizes. When you finish eating, stay away from the food table.

Finally, never accept food from anyone. Don't allow someone else to bring you a plate with buffet food piled high or a bowl filled with snack foods. You should be the one to go to the buffet or party table or ask for food to be passed to you. This way you cannot blame excessive eating on someone else. Engage in positive self-talk when you have successfully adhered to your plan.

You may find holidays a particularly difficult time. If you have diabetes, you are often confronted with many delicious-looking foods that may not be appropriate for blood glucose control. When planning holiday meals, it is sometimes helpful for you to decide on a few traditional foods that would satisfy everyone's gastronomic desires. Plan a few dishes that are low in calories. Preparing food in small quantities may also be a good idea. Remember, the festivity of a holiday should not be dampened by the absence of traditional holiday food. If someone offers to help in food preparation, suggest a low-calorie dish. If special foods are prepared, decide in advance the portion sizes you will allow yourself. Don't overdo it. Remember to listen to your stomach for feelings of fullness and ask friends to take leftovers home.

Special occasions and holidays are filled with many environmental cues. The sight and smell of food may become overwhelming at these times. You may find that you have used every trick you can think of, yet your desire for something rich and fattening continues to grow. Remember that this is a special occasion. It may be appropriate for you to have a cookie or a piece of pie at Christmas or other holidays. This is the time when you may have to give in to your appetite because you might feel deprived if you don't. A rare dietary treat such as this should not create guilt feelings. Sometimes a feeling of deprivation can last several weeks, causing you to overeat constantly. This would disrupt your blood glucose control; therefore, it would be acceptable for you to give in to the cues on one occasion only.

Prior to a vacation, try to rethink past vacations. Did you gain weight? What factors were responsible for the weight gain? How did you resolve the problem? How could you improve upon those solutions? Is it reasonable for you to expect weight gain again? Since all three meals for several days will be eaten away from home, some control over meals will be lost. A vacation can be a happy time filled with enjoying new sights. Food is only one component of the vacation. Here again, being prepared for situations is a necessity. If you find you have no desire to adhere to your meal plan, try to enlist support from your companions. Engage in positive self-talk and try to encourage yourself to do the best you can. If you feel overwhelmed because all your meals are eaten in restaurants, use restaurant-eating techniques and try to purchase your own low-calorie snacks.

Eating has an important place in your life. If you have diabetes, you must give extra thought to changing recipes, dining out in restaurants and how you will deal with food on special occasions. We hope this chapter has given you some insight into how to modify recipes for weight control and blood glucose control and to aid in preventing blood lipid elevations. While it may require a little arithmetic, you can take any recipe and calculate the ingredients to fit into your meal plan. Modifying recipes and fitting them into your meal plan may prevent you from feeling deprived and can allow you to enjoy homemade specialty items. We also hope you now have added confidence to enter any restaurant, or attend any special social event, knowing how to order appropriately. Restaurant dining is part of your social life. If you are attempting to lose weight, try to become accurate in estimating portion sizes, choose low-calorie entrées, avoid excess fats from salad dressings, fried foods, gravies and butter. Also ask questions about food preparation. Order à la carte rather than complete dinners. Eat a preplanned snack before going out to avoid being overhungry.

Avoid ordering from a menu. At a buffet, view the entire array of foods before deciding. Avoid long periods of food deprivation prior to a restaurant meal.

If you are overweight yet you are insulin-dependent, become consistent in the timing of meals, snacks and insulin injections when dining out. Become knowledgeable in using the Exchange System. All persons with diabetes will benefit from being aware of appropriate food choices to order as well as from assertive techniques to use with friends and waiters. Dining out should be a pleasant experience. With information about calorie control, portion sizes, fats, alcohol limitations and dining times, you can enjoy the social experience of restaurant dining.

Remember to anticipate special events and be consistent in your food choices and caloric intake. During special occasions, enlist the support of family and friends. Engage in positive self-talk. Preplan for unexpected events and reward yourself when you have adhered to your plan. *Bon appétit!*

15

Psychosocial Adjustment

There is no other chronic illness in which health behavior must be as continuously and rigidly controlled as diabetes. You must acquire skills and knowledge in areas of psychology, pharmacology, laboratory testing, nursing, nutrition and medicine. You must use your knowledge to control blood glucose with diet, insulin and exercise. As a diabetic person, you are expected to learn all about self-management. Adjusting your diet, performing self-testing, establishing an exercise program and taking medication are examples of such requirements. Sometimes, the less technical requirements, such as the psychological adjustment to diabetes, are forgotten. A major adjustment is the necessary change in lifestyle. You must now develop self-control in situations that ordinarily·do not require such control. The demands of diabetes are constantly with you. In this chapter, we will offer some guidance so that you can more easily adjust to these demands. Diabetes will be viewed as a crisis. How do you cope with this crisis? What coping strategies are available? How does diabetes affect individuals differently? What role does the family play in diabetes? These questions are answered so that you can adjust to diabetes.

Psychological adjustment is an essential part of self-management. You must make the difficult adjustment to a chronic and incurable disease. The news that you have diabetes always comes as a shock. Adjustment is defined as settling into a comfortable state. This may be a more realistic way of looking at how you handle diabetes, rather than using the word "acceptance." "Acceptance" is often used when discussing psychosocial aspects of diabetes. Acceptance can be defined as the act of favorably receiving something. Quite often, people are told to "accept your diabetes and go on with life." You may not be able to favorably *accept* your diabetes, but through *adjustment* you may certainly "go on with life."

DIABETES AS A CRISIS

Being told that you have diabetes creates a crisis. The crisis involves not only you but your family as well. What is a crisis? A crisis is defined as an overwhelming, threatening event. Your normal way of solving problems may not be adequate for this difficult situation. You may respond to a crisis with feelings of anxiety, confusion and helplessness. Other reactions to a crisis include shock, disbelief, fear, anger, denial, panic, guilt, anxiety and depression. Think back to the time you were first told you had diabetes. What kinds of emotions came to the surface? Did you feel angry, depressed, fearful? Did you feel unable to believe you had diabetes and chose to ignore it? Did you feel that if you bargained you might have obtained freedom from diabetes?

DEFENSE MECHANISMS

You may use a variety of defense mechanisms to help control anxiety and reduce the stress that results from a crisis. Defense mechanisms allow you to cope temporarily with a crisis until you can adjust. Adjustment to diabetes involves a coping process. "Coping" is defined as struggling with something, usually with a certain degree of success. Defense mechanisms are used by everyone in varying degrees. They allow you to distort reality so that you are not overwhelmed. However, they are only temporarily useful. Overuse of defense mechanisms eventually slows adjustment. If you continue to use defense mechanisms in response to diabetes, you may not obtain emotional control. Common reactions to diabetes such as denial, anxiety, anger, bargaining, guilt and shame will now be discussed.

Many people attempt to cope with diabetes by using denial. Denial is the disregard of the existence of diabetes in your life. Denial may be manifested by neglecting to take your insulin injections, not following a diet or not keeping doctor's appointments. Other examples of denial are refusing to wear an identification bracelet and not carrying a simple carbohydrate to prevent hypoglycemia. You may deny diabetes by refusing to participate in diabetes clubs or education programs. Examine some of your actions to see if you are denying that you have diabetes. Denial should be a temporary coping mechanism. For some individuals who are upset and shocked, denying diabetes for a short time may be the only way of coping with the illness.

Some diseases are more difficult to deny than others. Unfortunately, diabetes is easy to deny because its physical effects may not be experienced on a daily basis. Many diabetics with elevated blood glucose levels have no symptoms of diabetes. If each time the blood glucose became elevated you experienced a pain, rash or some physical symptom that warned you that your blood glucose was out of control, diabetes would seem more real. Control over your behavior might then be easier.

Presently, you may blame others for much of what is happening to your own diabetes control. For example, you may say that "other people" bring cakes and cookies to your home, which tempt you to go off your diet. This is known as rationalization. Education about your role in diabetes self-management may help you to become more aware of your own responsibility. The following are four commonly used defense mechanisms.

DEFENSE MECHANISMS COMMONLY SEEN IN DIABETES

Denial	Blocking out aspects of reality that cause pain or fear
Rationalization	A false explanation of behavior that you do not wish to acknowledge; it prevents guilt
Displacement	Placing emotions or feelings upon a person other than the one to which the feelings belong
Regression	Unconsciously returning to an earlier level of emotional adjustment

DO YOU RECOGNIZE YOURSELF?

1. "My blood sugar is only 200. I'm sure I don't have diabetes." (*Denial*)

2. "I know I should exercise but the doctor told me that getting proper rest is important too." (*Rationalization*)

3. "The doctor told me to lose weight today. Tonight my husband is driving me crazy." (*Displacement*)

4. "I can't give my insulin; only my husband should give it to me." (*Regression*)

Diabetes is a complex disease. Information about diabetes may seem confusing. It is difficult to learn the difference between low and high glucose as well as all the other details needed for self-management. Therefore, you may become quite anxious in response to receiving the shocking diagnosis of diabetes. As your anxiety level rises, your learning capacity will decrease. Therefore, the overwhelming amount of information you receive when diagnosed is often of limited value. You will need to have this information repeated in the future. It may help to look at experiences you may have had with people who have diabetes. If your contact with the disease was unpleasant, this will certainly have an effect on how you now feel about having diabetes. For example, if a close relative was blind or had an amputation as a result of diabetes, you may become very anxious. Anxiety is worsened by the unknown and your own lack of control over diabetes. Comprehensive education may reduce anxiety by providing accurate information. Communication systems with psychological support from health-care professionals or family members will also decrease anxiety. Often, just talking about your feelings will decrease anxiety. This is especially true if you talk with people who share your concerns, that is, others who have adjusted to having diabetes.

Anger develops in response to diabetes because now you may be asked to follow certain restrictions to control the disease. Patients become so angry they frequently ask, "Why me? Why has this occurred to me?" There is no answer to "Why me?" You may become more angry when others tell you, "Be glad that you have diabetes. It could be worse; it could be something more serious." In a way, they are telling you to be glad that you have diabetes. This is unfair. It robs you of the right to become angry over the diagnosis. *Your* individual problem cannot be compared with any other problem. It is unique and specific to you. Try to realize that your anger is justified when you hear you are "lucky" to have diabetes. Problems may arise when you remain angry and the anger interferes with self-management. Express your anger rather than trying to withhold it. If anger is held inward and not expressed, you may find yourself depressed and unable to cope with the demands of diabetes self-management. Discuss your anger with friends, family members or groups that act as support systems for you.

The term "bargaining" describes a situation in which a person may attempt to negotiate in order to have a problem taken away or reduced in severity. For example, if you had just been diagnosed as diabetic, you might have promised that you would never eat sweets again as long as you could avoid taking insulin. Of course, if you are insulin-dependent, this would not be possible. Although the bargaining is unrealistic, it may be a necessary step in adjustment. If you continue to use bargaining, it will hinder successful adjustment to diabetes. However, bargaining can be turned into a constructive device for dealing with diabetes by using it to form contracts. Goal setting can be used as a positive form of bargaining. For example, you can set a goal of losing two pounds per week and include a reward if you follow through. You may involve your spouse or other family members in the contracting process. You may contract that your two-pound weight loss would require your spouse to share household responsibilities.

You may feel guilty about having diabetes for a variety of reasons. If your diabetes is obesity-related, you may feel guilty that you ignored previous warnings to lose weight. You may feel you brought diabetes on yourself. You may feel that if you had taken better care of yourself, you would not have developed diabetes. Since there is a hereditary nature to diabetes, family members often experience guilt. Family members may place guilt on one side of the family versus the other. A mother may experience guilt if her child is diagnosed as having diabetes. She may look at her maternal role differently since her child is not in perfect health. This may become a source of conflict for husbands and wives. Some people feel shame after the diagnosis of a chronic illness and are unwilling to tell others they have diabetes. Guilt and shame have little value in assisting you to cope with diabetes. If allowed to continue, the adjustment process will become more prolonged and difficult. These feelings are often caused by ignorance about the disease or misconceptions about its treatment. It is most important, though, not to repress feelings of guilt or shame. These feelings should be shared with a health-care provider, a family member or a friend.

At the Diabetes Education Center we have often seen patients react to diabetes by feeling guilty. They describe themselves as "bad" people. This is typified by the use of what we call the "ugly words of diabetes." These "ugly words" include "cheating" and "bad." Often patients describe how they cheat on their diet. Cheating implies dishonest behavior. Cheating on your diet may not involve dishonesty at all, but rather a lack of knowledge about food choices. Try not to put yourself in a childlike position by saying you are "bad" or that you "cheat." "Good" and "bad" are moral judgments and are not appropriate in discussing diabetes self-management. If you choose not to follow a prescribed diabetes self-management program, it is a decision that you have made based on your own responsibility for self-care. Another word often used to describe a diabetic person's activity is "non-compliance." Non-compliance implies that you could comply with diabetic self-management but you refuse to do so. It does not leave room for the possibility that there are some barriers preventing you from complying with diabetes self-management, such as a lack of information. We hope to see those words banished from the vocabulary of health-care professionals and diabetic persons.

Another important reaction that occurs after the shock of diabetes is your awareness of your own vulnerability. If you have been healthy prior to the diagnosis, you may now feel vulnerable to chronic illness. Because of the threat of diabetes' complications you may begin to question your current lifestyle as well as your future. Let these questions surface instead of hiding them and becoming afraid of the future. Our imagination is usually worse than reality.

LIFE CHANGES

We have discussed how diabetes is a crisis and how some people react to crisis. There are also changes that occur in your life. These include the transitions of going through adolescence, getting married and having children. Important life changes involve making choices with regard to careers and education.

Adolescence is a time of transition and conflict. When diabetes is super-imposed on the conflicts that occur in adolescence, problems may develop. During adolescence you begin to make choices about friends, dating, sex and careers. Problems specific to the teen-age years revolve around peer groups, dating, sex, physical appearance, participation in sports, use of alcohol, drugs or cigarettes. Adolescents have many problems with which to cope. Some also have the added burden of diabetes. These adolescents should undergo com-prehensive diabetes education in classes with their peers. The educational setting should provide emotional support, which is as essential as the education itself. If you are an adolescent, seek out and actively participate in an education pro-gram.

Marriage can be seen as another development in life that may present a crisis. In marriage, serious questions are raised about the future. A chronic illness may be seen as a threat to future plans. Fears and concerns of a partner should be openly expressed. Marriage will also provide you with a major emotional sup-port. Both partners will share in future plans. You might discuss future com-plications of diabetes, childbearing decisions and the economics of possible hospitalizations. The discussion does not have to dwell only on serious aspects of the future. It can also focus on the mutual sharing necessary to work diabetes into your lives together. Such things as exercise plans, travel arrangements or special nutrition planning can be discussed. You may work together to strengthen your marriage, and diabetes does not have to be a barrier. At the Diabetes Education Center family members are invited to attend classes so that these problems can be discussed.

Pregnancy produces physical as well as emotional changes as a woman pre-pares for her new role as a mother. Diabetes must be given special attention during this time. The expectant mother must handle two roles, as a person with diabetes and as a future mother. An excellent resource for the pregnant diabetic woman is *The Baby Team*, by Sheila Garvey, R.N., and Donald Coustan, M.D., available through the Monoject Company.

Diabetes may present a problem in the area of employment. You may have doubts about your ability to hold a job and manage diabetes. These doubts may prevent you from making a commitment to a career choice. Doubts about work and diabetes self-management can often be erased through education. Diabetes' effect on life crises may be modified through the use of group support from professionals, peers and family members.

THE IMPACT OF DIABETES

Certain aspects of diabetes are stressful. We have already discussed the strong reaction usually seen at the time of diagnosis. Changes in your diabetes self-management may also be stressful. For example, many diabetic persons find that they are able to cope with diabetes until insulin therapy is initiated. Initiation of insulin therapy may make the disease more real. This requires an emotional adjustment. Profound episodes of hypoglycemia or hospitalization for diabetic ketoacidosis are also examples of stressful medical events. The development of complications of diabetes may also be a crisis. Be aware that your adjustments to diabetes may not be easy and continuous. Often diabetic persons are hard on themselves, thinking that because they have had diabetes for several years, they should have made a total adjustment. This is not always true. There are particular times in your life and your diabetes management when crises will occur. At those times, you may need extra support. You may regress to the use of defense mechanisms such as denial.

Certain factors in your life affect how you react to the diagnosis of diabetes. One factor is your basic personality. It is the sum total of your physical, mental, emotional and social characteristics. Basic personality traits such as independence, perseverance and strong emotional ties to others may help you to meet the demands of diabetes. Age is another factor that will influence how you react to diabetes. Young people may adapt more readily to the changes needed for diabetes self-management. It is often more difficult for the adolescent or the elderly to react to crisis. Previous experience with illness will also affect how you react to diabetes. If you have always been healthy, you may feel that you are able to handle diabetes self-management. You may not feel as crushed by the diagnosis as someone who has had other illnesses and now feels unable to cope with the demands of diabetes self-management. Socioeconomic, cultural and educational factors are important in your adjustment to diabetes. Health professionals carefully look at each of these areas when helping you to cope. A final factor that has a great influence on how you react to diabetes is support systems.

SUPPORT SYSTEMS

A support system is an individual or group that you become attached to for a variety of reasons. The best example of support systems for your purpose is diabetes clubs. Other examples of support systems are health-care professionals, family members, friends, clergy and other people with diabetes. Support systems help to offer guidance and give feedback on the actions you are now taking to cope with diabetes. They help you to adjust emotionally to diabetes. They may boost your self-confidence in diabetes self-management.

The family is an important support system. Family members are often required to make decisions that affect diabetes self-management. In families with young diabetic children, the parents must take over the management of diabetes. This may also occur in families where adult members have diabetes. A wife may have to learn how to cook proper meals for her husband, or a husband may have to be alert to the signs and symptoms of hypoglycemia and diabetic ketoacidosis in order to aid his wife. Also, diabetes' routines may interfere with established family activities. This can be seen in the area of meal planning, where consistency in the timing and composition of the meal may alter family routines. If a family has never eaten at specific times, diabetes self-management can conflict with family patterns.

Diabetes has an impact on families and family members in very specific areas. Family members take on specific roles over a period of years. These roles may change due to the diagnosis of diabetes. Diabetes also has an impact on a family by producing financial stress. The financial burden of diabetes self-management is a reality. People are generally concerned with finances, and the expense of diabetes-related equipment and medical care adds to this stress. Diabetes has an impact on parent-child relationships. In an effort to achieve control in children, parents may try to insist on perfection in all areas of self-management. Children may rebel or be unhappy. Usually, a flexible but consistent approach to diabetes self-management will result in fewer problems in parent-child relationships. Marital and family interactions can be affected by diabetes. Parents of diabetic children may experience marital stress. In all of these areas, we can see that diabetes has an impact on the family.

Some family members react to diabetes with depression and resentment. Referral for special counseling before family interactions become disruptive is imperative. Your entire family unit has many adjustments to make regarding the diagnosis of diabetes. Ask your family members to read this book so they may acquire an understanding of diabetes. Include your family members in any education you receive.

The elderly have well-established habits and routines, and diabetes may intrude on these. If you are in this age group you may find it difficult to change long-standing routines. You may feel socially detached due to the death of a spouse. You may be geographically isolated from family members and support systems that could help you adapt to diabetes. The elderly may be financially dependent. You may be concerned with the financial needs of day-to-day living plus diabetes self-management. If you experience diabetes in the later years of your life or have an older family member with diabetes, seek out education that is paced according to learning needs and abilities. Support systems will be particularly helpful.

We have discussed how diabetes is a crisis and how some people react to this crisis. All individuals have the potential to develop adverse coping patterns (behaviors that negatively affect coping). Jay Skyler, M.D., has identified the following eight potential adverse coping patterns in those with diabetes.

POTENTIAL ADVERSE COPING PATTERNS

Seclusiveness

Aggressiveness

Bravado (boastfulness, devil-may-care attitudes)

Shame, leading to concealment of feelings

Guilt feelings, depression

Open resentment, rebellion, subversiveness (e.g., faking urine tests, omitting insulin, disregarding diet)

Meticulousness, conscientiousness, perfectionism and other obsessive-compulsive reactions

Submissiveness (especially in those who developed diabetes early in childhood)

Reprinted with permission from J. Skyler, M.D., "Living with Complications of Diabetes," *Behavioral and Psychosocial Issues in Diabetes,* Proceedings of the National Conference on Behavioral and Psychosocial Issues in Diabetes, 1979.

It may be difficult for you to obtain the proper balance between being involved with diabetes and not being overwhelmed. You must be conscious of your role as a person with diabetes, but avoid labeling yourself as a "diabetic." In fact, "diabetic" is another ugly word of diabetes that we have attempted not to use in this book. When "diabetic" is used as a noun, it implies that your entire personality centers on diabetes. Rather, "diabetic" should be used as an adjective to describe a diabetic person. If you think of yourself as an individual with diabetes, rather than a diabetic, you can avoid overinvolvement with the disease. You need to self-manage your diabetes without relying on others, yet avoid becoming seclusive or ashamed of the disease. The most difficult task is probably becoming conscientious about diabetes self-management without becoming perfectionistic about every minute detail.

Some persons react negatively to diabetes, while others seem to have no reaction at all. They do not progress to adapt positively, nor do they cope negatively. They are in a state of psychological immobility. They become almost paralyzed in other aspects of their lives. This occurs because of the threat of future complications as well as denying diabetes. They may have the sustained hope that diabetes will be cured and they may resist allowing diabetes into their lives. Try to recognize and guard against psychological immobility. Fear of the future can cause you to waste important times in your life. You may be unable to make career choices or social decisions or improve your health because you feel threatened or fearful of the future.

Some people react positively and others negatively to diabetes. How do you cope with diabetes? What are some strategies that will aid you in coping with diabetes?

The most important strategy is for you to seek information. Education will allow you to feel better about yourself and your ability to control diabetes. If you know little about diabetes, you will feel that you cannot cope. You will feel insecure in recognizing signs and symptoms of impending problems. You will not feel protected by the fact that you have the ability to prevent certain complications. Thus, education is an important tool in psychological adjustment.

Another coping strategy is taking positive action to improve your health. Health-related behaviors such as scheduling doctor's visits, attending a diabetes education center and establishing a regular exercise program are examples of such actions. You can begin to set priorities for your health in an effort to cope with the disease. Concrete steps such as avoiding simple sugars and quitting cigarette smoking are also coping behaviors. Other coping efforts may be directed at controlling emotional distress through stress-reducing exercises.

SELF-MANAGEMENT

The establishment of a self-management program is another coping behavior. In a study performed at Rockefeller University, patients were evaluated in respect to depression as well as diabetes control prior to entering an intensive blood glucose self-monitoring program. Insulin-dependent patients were found to have high depression scores and high hemoglobin A_{1C} levels. They exhibited feelings of helplessness, hopelessness, worthlessness, sadness and low self-esteem. They blamed others rather than themselves for problems in their lives. At the end of eight months of intensive training in home blood glucose monitoring as well as education regarding their disease, they were retested. Their depression and hemoglobin A_{1C} scores were decreased by half. They were more enthusiastic and had increased feelings of well-being. They increased their own problem-solving skills.

The development of your own problem-solving skills is an important part of your coping with diabetes. Problem-solving skills involve *your* actively finding solutions to your own problems. In order to solve problems successfully you must be able to identify them. Next, you must establish priorities. Look at which problems need immediate attention. Set goals for yourself and see what is available to help you meet these goals. Be realistic about the scope and time involved in the solution of such problems. Look, too, at how you can evaluate whether or not meeting the goals helped you to solve the problem. As with other kinds of self-management presented to you, evaluation is important. Problem solving involves your identification of a problem, setting priorities to deal with the problem and identifying the factors that either support or hinder you in your attempt to reach your goal.

Let's look at the following as an exercise in problem solving. A 17-year-old girl has had insulin-dependent diabetes for two years. She has several problems, including (1) diabetes being out of control, (2) too little money, (3) difficult school work, (4) fights with her boyfriend. Although she has multiple problems, in order to set priorities she chooses to focus on diabetes control. The next step is setting goals to bring diabetes under control. These would include (a) remaining on a diet, (b) becoming more consistent in the timing of meals, (c) beginning home blood testing, (d) checking for urinary acetone daily. Factors that hinder successful problem solving would be (a) a late dinner due to class schedule, (b) fear of using the fingerstick necessary for self-monitoring, (c) her boyfriend likes eating sweets and does not like hearing about diabetes, (d) she feels that thinking about diabetes is a bore. Factors that can help her problem solving include (a) her mother cooks according to her meal plan, (b) her doctor is in favor of home blood testing, (c) she wants to prevent hospitalization for DKA, (d) other diabetes club members who are in control say that they feel better; she wants to feel better.

Now a choice must be made to pick possible solutions. She should identify the positives that were listed, such as the support from her mother, her doctor and the diabetes club. She needs to look at the negatives and try to make the appropriate changes. She can change her class schedule, receive education on self-monitoring and invite her boyfriend to the diabetes club. It will take time to complete this process of problem solving. The next step is the evaluation process. How will she know when she gets her diabetes under control? She should be able to evaluate this through home blood testing, avoidance of hypoglycemia, the absence of urinary acetone or signs and symptoms of diabetic ketoacidosis. Review these problem-solving steps.

PROBLEM-SOLVING STEPS

1. Identify problems.
2. Set priorities.
3. Identify factors that hinder success.
4. Identify factors that foster success.
5. Decide on solutions.
6. Evaluate.

Another important aspect of coping is your need for a support system. You may have to deliberately seek out a support system. Your family members may be willing to help you cope with the disease but may not be able to give you the kind of help that you need. You may find help in the unfamiliar setting of a diabetes club where you can meet people with similar problems. For some, a diabetes club and a group approach may not offer significant help. Seeking out a clergy member or health-team member may better assist you to cope. If you have no support systems available to you, then you must actively try to find an appropriate support group. The "Community Resources" section at the end of this book may help you with this. It is realistic that you will need help in coping with the disease. Be assertive in searching for such help.

Another way of increasing your skill in adjusting to diabetes is to use anticipatory coping. Role playing or rehearsing possible stressful situations often strengthens individual coping abilities in the event these stressful situations become reality. This is further discussed in Chapter 16.

Another coping strategy involves your relationship with your health-care provider. This may be a doctor, nurse, nutritionist or other member of the health-care team. Try to develop the best possible relationship with this individual. Make sure that you feel comfortable in expressing your feelings. Ask as many questions as necessary. Look for and accept encouragement for tasks that you have mastered as well as direction for those that need further work. Your health-care provider should give you the feeling that he or she is prepared to *share* the responsibility of diabetes management with you. Together, both of you will be able to look upon diabetes and its psychosocial adjustment as a challenge.

Feelings of anger, depression or fear may arise at various times in your life. If you feel you have adjusted to diabetes, try not to become discouraged when you are unhappy about the demands of diabetes self-management. Realize that these may be temporary occurrences, and reflect back to the ways in which you successfully coped with diabetes in the past. Try to relax, take a break, or do some of the stress-reducing exercises described in Chapter 16.

If you feel you have a problem in adjusting to the changes that diabetes has caused in your life, or if you are frequently unhappy because of diabetes, you may need professional help. People usually do not hesitate to ask a nutritionist for more details regarding diet, or a nurse for extra help with insulin administration. Yet they often feel that psychological adjustment must be accomplished without help. This is not true. Do not be afraid to seek out professional help from a psychologist, social worker, psychiatrist or any other member of the health-care team who is prepared to meet your emotional needs. You *alone* will be able to have control over your diabetes, but you will not have to achieve this *alone*.

If you have a chronic illness such as diabetes, you must acquire a variety of self-management skills. However, you must also adjust to a major change in your lifestyle. Receiving the diagnosis of diabetes is a crisis. Adjusting to the crisis can be quite difficult. You may react to the crisis with shock, disbelief, fear, anger, denial, anxiety. These reactions arise out of your struggle to cope. Defense mechanisms are useful initially, but prolonged use may prevent you from self-managing the disease. Psychosocial adjustment to diabetes becomes more of a crisis when other changes in your life occur, such as adolescence, marriage or pregnancy. Diabetes affects you and your family. Oftentimes your family can be used as a support system to help you through your crisis. You can cope with the crisis of diabetes through education and self-management. Developing problem-solving skills is also important. When you have made a psychosocial adjustment to diabetes, you have made diabetes an important part of your life but not its central focus. If you are having difficulty with this adjustment, do not hesitate to seek help. See the "Community Resources" section at the end of this book.

16

Stress

What is stress? How does it affect you? Does it affect your glucose control? How can you recognize stressors and improve your coping skills? All these questions will be answered in this chapter.

Stress is your body's mental, physical and chemical reactions to circumstances that frighten, excite, confuse or delight you. Life without stress is impossible. Think of stress as having two meanings: danger and opportunity. If you handle stress well, it will strengthen you for the next challenge. If you handle it poorly, it may endanger your health. Hans Selye was the first physician to look at the impact of stress on man's life, recognizing it as a common response to several diseases. Changes may occur in many parts of the body to protect it from harm. These changes are unconscious and often not under mental or physical control. This concept is similar to your balance of blood glucose control. You have no conscious control over the counterregulatory hormones released during hypoglycemia. Yet those hormones help to raise blood glucose. You unconsciously respond to hypoglycemia and you can also unconsciously respond to other conditions.

A condition which causes stress is known as a stressor. Stressors can come from the physical, psychosocial or internal environment. The stressor can be either real or perceived, conscious or unconscious. The stress response occurs even if the stressor is not real, but imagined. For example, something may not actually be placing you in danger, but if you think it is, this becomes a stressor for you. Stressors may be perceived on a conscious or subconscious level. Your past exposure to stress and your health will affect how you learn to accept stress. How you cope with stress is another part of the stress response. There are mental and physical activities that can help you to adapt constructively to stress.

Stress is a response that has been part of human existence since primitive man. Primitive man lived in a hostile world where physical confrontation was part of everyday life. The "fight or flight" mechanism was and still is part of the body's defense system. "Fight or flight" refers to the quickened pulse, keyed-up feeling, increase in breathing, circulation and strength of muscles that occur when people are faced with immediate danger. In prehistoric times, man had to have the physical capacity that enabled him to remain to fight or to flee from danger. Unfortunately, physical confrontation remains in many areas of the world today. However, stress occurs more frequently in a mental way today, as evidenced by arguments or tension, not by physical outlets. Yet the "fight or flight" mechanism remains as a response. If you overrespond to stress, you may harm yourself, physically and mentally.

A certain amount of stress in life is necessary. Change and progress usually produce some stress. Uncertainty and strangeness can lead you to devise a way to handle situations better in the future. For example, a stressor of a desire to get ahead, perhaps to obtain a better job, will lead to the acquisition of new skills. You will then grow and change. This can be considered a positive aspect of stress.

Very positive as well as very negative experiences or situations are stressors in your life and need to be identified. Look at what makes you uncomfortable, anxious, depressed, as well as what makes you excited or happy, in order to identify areas of your life filled with stress. Identification of stressors may be difficult, since some of them occur on an unconscious level. One way of identifying such stressors is to notice how you feel and how you behave when you are under stress. Watch for these behaviors and look at their cause. Some people find it useful to keep a stress diary similar to a headache diary used to help people identify the cause of chronic headaches. By listing such behaviors, you may identify stressors in your life.

What are some stressors in the environment? In the general physical environment, stressors may appear as increased noise levels, traffic jams and fears for personal security. In your personal physical environment, stressors may appear as chronic illnesses, fevers, infections, cuts, wounds and burns. In the psychosocial environment, stressors may appear as job pressures, family interactions and financial worries.

A useful tool in the identification of general stressors is the following Social Readjustment Rating Scale. This scale evaluates recent life events and their relative impact on a person's life. It measures the amount of readjustment needed to respond to such events. It is a good indicator of the level of stress present in your life. "Stress" is also an overused term and may be incorrectly applied to any feeling of vague discomfort. Through tools such as the Social Readjustment Rating Scale you can begin to accurately identify stress. This tool can help you to become familiar with certain life events. The number of points indicates the amount of change needed to readjust. The more changes you have, the more likely you are to become ill. Almost 80 percent of the people who have over 300 life-change units in a year become ill in the near future. This can be compared with only 30 percent who become ill in the near future following a year with fewer than 150 life-change units. If your score is high, you have to be alert to staying healthy. By knowing this, you can anticipate life changes and do advance planning.

SOCIAL READJUSTMENT RATING SCALE

Life Event	Mean Value
1. Death of spouse	100
2. Divorce	73
3. Marital separation from mate	65
4. Detention in jail or other institution	63
5. Death of a close family member	63
6. Major personal injury or illness	53
7. Marriage	50
8. Being fired at work	47
9. Marital reconciliation with mate	45
10. Retirement from work	45
11. Major change in the health or behavior of a family member	44
12. Pregnancy	40
13. Sexual difficulties	39
14. Gaining a new family member (e.g., through birth, adoption, oldster moving in, etc.)	39
15. Major business readjustment (e.g., merger, reorganization, bankruptcy, etc.)	39
16. Major change in financial state (e.g., a lot worse off or a lot better off than usual)	38
17. Death of a close friend	37
18. Changing to a different line of work	36
19. Major change in the number of arguments with spouse (e.g., either a lot more or a lot less than usual regarding child rearing, personal habits, etc.)	35
20. Taking out a mortgage or loan for a major purpose (e.g., for a home, business, etc.)	31
21. Foreclosure on a mortgage or loan	30
22. Major change in responsibilities at work (e.g., promotion, demotion, lateral transfer)	29
23. Son or daughter leaving home (e.g., marriage, attending college, etc.)	29

Life Event	Mean Value
24. Trouble with in-laws	29
25. Outstanding personal achievement	28
26. Wife beginning or ceasing work outside the home	26
27. Beginning or ceasing formal schooling	26
28. Major change in living conditions (e.g., building a new home, remodeling, deterioration of home or neighborhood)	25
29. Revision of personal habits (dress, manners, association, etc.)	24
30. Troubles with the boss	23
31. Major change in working hours or conditions	20
32. Change in residence	20
33. Changing to a new school	20
34. Major change in usual type and/or amount of recreation	19
35. Major change in church activities (i.e., a lot more or a lot less than usual)	19
36. Major change in social activities (e.g., clubs, dancing, movies, visiting, etc.)	18
37. Taking out a mortgage or loan for a lesser purchase (e.g., for a car, TV, freezer, etc.)	17
38. Major change in sleeping habits (a lot more or a lot less sleep, or change in part of day when asleep)	16
39. Major change in number of family get-togethers (e.g., a lot more or a lot less than usual)	15
40. Major change in eating habits (a lot more or a lot less food intake, or very different meal hours or surroundings)	15
41. Vacation	13
42. Christmas	12
43. Minor violations of the law (e.g., traffic tickets, jaywalking, disturbing the peace, etc.)	11

From T. H. Holmes and R. H. Rahe, "The Social Readjustment Rating Scale," *Journal of Psychosomatic Research*, 11:213–18, 1967. Reprinted with permission from Pergamon Press, Inc.

DIABETES-RELATED STRESSORS

Are there diabetes-related stressors? Diabetes itself is a stressor. The diagnosis of a chronic illness is difficult to handle. The media portray television doctors with instant cures and "miracle" drugs that prevent illness from lasting more than thirty minutes. The public is generally unaware that there are few total cures in medicine. When you receive the diagnosis of diabetes, you are told that you have a chronic illness. After hearing that diabetes can be controlled but cannot be cured, you may enter a crisis state while adjusting to the diagnosis. Daily activities of self-management may also be stressors. Daily urine testing, dietary restrictions, insulin self-administration and regular exercise are stressful changes in lifestyle.

Much of how you perceive and adjust to stress is related to your general personality and your past exposure to stressors. If you have been exposed to stressors in the past and have been able to handle them, future stressors may not be so difficult. Your reaction to stress will be influenced by your basic personality and your previous handling of stress. People under stress often react by clenching their teeth, tensing their bodies and breathing rapidly. Other people may have emotional reactions to stress, such as crying, sobbing, shouting or becoming angry. Still other people may develop stress-related disorders such as hypertension, chronic backache, stomachaches, headaches and chronic fatigue. Learn to identify how you respond to stress in order to improve your ability to cope with stress.

The stress response may lead to a rise in blood glucose. This occurs because counterregulatory hormones which are released from your adrenal glands as part of the stress response (cortisol and epinephrine ["adrenaline"]) increase blood glucose. Stress may affect your self-management program by making you reluctant to fulfill the demands of the program. Stress may stop you from following your diet, taking medication as prescribed and exercising regularly. Learn how to cope with stress effectively as part of your total diabetes self-management program.

You must consider the effect of your reaction to stress on the members of your family. They are an essential part of your self-management system. Stress affects the family in many areas. The intimacy between couples and the interpersonal communication between family members may be affected by stress. Financial worries or a decrease in leisure time can create more stress. Because family members are closely involved with diabetes, they will also be involved with and respond to the stress of diabetes. The members of your family need time to discuss their own fears and concerns. This chapter is intended for all family members, not just the individual with diabetes.

Some non-helpful means of coping with stress include the use of alcohol, drugs, cigarette smoking and food. Alcoholism and drug abuse are widespread in society today. Is this a response to stressors in our environment? Many people use cigarette smoking to cope with pressures of everyday life. Food is known as a natural tranquilizer. Many people overeat in response to stress. Other people find that they behave aggressively when under stress. Still others decide to abandon their diabetes regimen. When exposed to stressors, some may omit insulin injections or decide that testing is not valuable. They may go off their diet. A person may also develop hypoglycemia under stress due to a loss of appetite or skipped meals.

Group settings are useful to discuss the stressors present in your life. Family, financial, work and health problems are often mentioned. It is difficult to remove such stressors as family finances and work problems from your life. For this reason, it is important that you learn to handle stress properly. Look at the following list for appropriate ways to cope with stress.

DO COPE WITH STRESS THROUGH

Education
Priority setting
Assertiveness
Communication
Progressive relaxation
Visualization
Breathing exercises
Yoga, meditation
Exercise
Recreation
Hobbies
Worship

DON'T COPE WITH STRESS THROUGH

Overeating
Drugs
Alcohol
Cigarette smoking
Aggression
Neglect of diabetes self-management

The first coping mechanism for effective stress reduction is education. Read and learn as much as you can about diabetes and self-management. Often, diabetic persons are plagued by a fear of the unknown. Imagination is usually worse than reality; therefore, obtain facts about diabetes. As a result of a lack of knowledge about your disease, feelings of hopelessness and helplessness may emerge. Education concerning diabetes will help you battle this. People with diabetes often feel frustrated due to the expectations placed upon them for their own self-care. You may lack the education needed to meet such expectations. A comprehensive education program will aid in stress reduction.

Although you may not realize it, another stress-reducing activity is anticipating and preparing for the worst. You should be able to think about future fearful occurrences and to anticipate how you would handle such situations. Anticipatory coping involves preparing to solve future problems. For example, if you are concerned about unexpected hypoglycemia disrupting your work setting or if you are anxious about diabetic ketoacidosis developing during an illness, role-play with a family member or health professional. This can prepare you for necessary actions to handle unexpected emergencies. If you learn how to prepare yourself to avoid acute complications of diabetes, stress will be reduced. At the Diabetes Education Center, anticipatory coping is used. Patients are taught to wear identification and carry a short-acting carbohydrate to combat hypoglycemia. They are taught how to avoid, treat, recognize and evaluate hypoglycemic episodes. They are instructed in self-care during sick days, with specific directions. Patients are also taught how to recognize signs and symptoms of impending diabetic ketoacidosis and how to gain access to the health-care system quickly. This information and education helps you to organize for an emergency. If you use anticipatory coping, you will not feel out of control or helpless. You will have the necessary information to treat a diabetes-related emergency.

Another way of coping effectively with stress is to maintain a high level of general health and physical fitness. Keep strong in order to face stress which may accompany diabetes. It is unrealistic to expect that someone who is poorly nourished or physically unfit would have the energy to cope effectively with stress. General health and fitness, then, will aid in combating stress.

Certain concrete goals may be set to cope with work-related stress. Be realistic about the kind of employment you choose. Very few employment opportunities are not open to people with diabetes; those that are not open, such as airplane piloting, are realistic limitations. Even so, there are some occupations which may not be suitable for an individual who is not coping effectively with stress. For example, work in an advertising firm may demand specific weekly quotas of new accounts to be opened. This would be demanding and time-oriented, and might be overwhelming for someone who is experiencing great life stress outside the work setting. It is important to set realistic work-related goals. Some people may refuse a promotion (although this is not usually the "American way"). Yet they are able to analyze what their goals are and what gratification they need from the work setting. As long as goals are being met and gratification is received, it is possible to set limits and avoid work stress. It is useful for all workers to relax at least once a day by doing some of the stress-reducing exercises that will be listed later in this chapter. For the person with diabetes, this release from the mental drain and pressures of the work setting will be beneficial in aiding blood glucose control.

Family pressures often affect your response to stress. Often, family members are not aware of the demands of diabetes self-management. They find diabetes difficult to understand. You must be realistic about the members of your family and their reaction to your diabetes. Because one family member has diabetes does not mean that the family must be subjected to unhappiness or tension. Nor does it mean that the family will be perfect and free of friction. Family crises will occur and must be realistically viewed in light of the entire family structure. The use of open communication between all family members is important. Family members will not be able to read your mind if you are having specific problems. Develop the confidence to verbalize these feelings. Positive stress-reducing activities for family members include the use of self-help groups, family education classes and the diabetes clubs affiliated with the American Diabetes Association.

Another sign of difficulty in coping with stress is sleep disorders. Hans Selye states that "it is during the whole day that you must prepare for your dreams." It is unrealistic to think that if you are feeling overly stressed and attempt to sleep, sleep will come just because you have gone to bed. Prior to this, you must gradually reduce the amount of external stimuli (noise, heat, excessive light) in order to have a profitable night's sleep. A good night's sleep will have a soothing effect on the nerves and enable you to handle stress more effectively. If you go without sleep because you are under stress, a vicious cycle—stress → sleep disorder → decreased ability to handle stress → sleep disorder—will persist. By attempting to relax frequently throughout the day, sleep may come more easily at night.

Another way of effectively coping with stress can be seen in the use of assertiveness. Many patients have stated that they felt more stressed when they were not able to communicate effectively. People who are hesitant to question prices of self-monitoring materials or insulin in drugstores, or are afraid to take a health professional's time for questions, experience stress by not appropriately asserting themselves. The use of assertiveness-training techniques helps in improving communication and reduces stress. See Chapter 23 for more details on assertiveness.

If you try to separate yourself from the normal day-to-day demands of life and examine areas of beauty and magnificence, both in nature and in everyday occurrences, you may reduce stress. You may feel relaxed when listening to music, reading literature or attending a play. Knowing that you have love, friendship, security, a place in society and in a family can minimize some of the stress-producing events that may occur.

Another positive way of coping with stress is the use of prayer and meditation. An escape from the demands of everyday living into the spiritual world may lead to a reduction in stress. Activities involving prayer, meditation and worship can be personally helpful as well as stress-reducing.

Learn how to set appropriate priorities in your life. Setting objectives and goals for certain periods of time can be quite helpful in giving definition and direction to your life. After setting your objectives, next choose which ones are of the greatest importance and plan to meet those first. Many people set too many priorities and give themselves too little time to complete goals. Begin to set priorities relating to your diabetes, family life, work setting and leisure time.

Parents and teachers are often concerned about children's opportunity to play. Play increases a child's socialization skills. Children are encouraged to play with others and to enjoy this time together. As the child grows older, the concept of play and its importance diminishes. Addiction to work is sometimes seen as virtuous in American society. In adulthood, play must once more be actively pursued. This need can be transferred to recreation. The use of hobbies as a way of relaxing is an excellent stress reducer. Hobbies have a creative element intertwined with the activity. This can be stress-reducing and produce desirable results. Do not expect the same returns from a hobby as those from a work setting. Don't try to overachieve when engaging in a hobby and expect to excel as you would in your work setting. Developing an appreciation for socialization and recreation can help to reduce stress.

Selye has stated: "Either remove yourself from stress or learn to relax." The idea of learning to relax may seem strange, but through psychological as well as physical methods, you can learn to relax. You may have to learn to relax physically because you are accustomed to tensing your body. You may no longer be aware of the difference between a tense and a relaxed muscle. Progressive relaxation can be used to help you relax. Here is an example of progressive relaxation.

You would sit in an easy chair in a comfortable position and slowly stretch out both arms and legs. The relaxation begins at the feet and progresses upward. You would be instructed in soft tones to relax the toes and feet and concentrate on a feeling of warmth, heaviness and relaxation in the feet. This warmth works gradually up to the legs, torso, arms and neck. Even facial structures such as the eyes, tongue and mouth can be relaxed. Very slowly, you would become aware of your body's change toward relaxation. You would be instructed to come gradually out of the state of relaxation. It will take time for you to learn to relax physically if you have grown accustomed to tensing your body.

The second physical stress-reducing method that is used is deep breathing. Progressive relaxation can be used as a daily stress reducer but is not useful during a time of acute stress. Deep breathing can be used as an acute-stress stopper. A deep, cleansing breath can often short-circuit a stress response. You can easily learn to do this anywhere. You take a cleansing breath when you put your hands on your stomach and feel your stomach swell as you draw a deep breath down to the bottom of your lungs, filling the middle of your lungs and then the top of your lungs, as if you are filling a glass of water. When you exhale, the air will come out of the top of your lungs first, then the middle, and then the stomach will constrict as the lower part of the lungs empties out. One or two deep breaths during a stressful situation may help to alleviate tension.

The third method for relaxation is guided imagery. You use a particular scene that you imagine in your mind and allow it to unfold in order to reduce stress. You can sit and slowly clear your mind and allow a pleasant image to develop. Guide and follow the image as it begins to unfold. Certain examples that can be used are an image of a perfect rosebud unfolding into a blooming flower, and a vacation spot which has pleasant memories for you. This helps because you are totally concentrating on complete stress reduction for at least five minutes. This also allows you to be removed temporarily from your harried life and reminds you that there are other activities going on in other settings. You are not alone in a pressured, tense environment. This image can be practiced at least once a day in order to build up a reserve against stress. You would not want to overdo the use of imagery. Your goal is not to escape from stressors but face them and cope with them.

Active participation in stress reduction is as important for you as accurate insulin administration. When priority setting for diabetes self-management, begin to value stress reduction to achieve diabetes control. Evaluate your ability to cope with stress by looking at the following guide.

EVALUATE YOUR ABILITY TO COPE WITH STRESS

1. Identify stressors in your present life.
2. Identify your own response to stress.
3. Change or eliminate, when possible, the stressor.
4. Change your own response to stress by
     a. incorporating daily stress-reducing exercises into your lifestyle,
     b. practicing acute-stress alleviators when necessary.
5. Use *stress* to *progress* through life situations.

Stress is your body's reaction to certain situations. A stressor can be anything that causes stress. Try to identify stressors in your personal, psychosocial or physical environment. Diabetes is a stressor in and of itself because you are faced with the fact that your disease can be controlled but not cured. Stress affects your blood glucose control, your diabetes self-management program and your family. Try not to cope with stress through overeating, alcohol, drugs, cigarette smoking or ignoring self-management. Instead cope with stress by obtaining education, anticipating problems, maintaining good health, communicating openly with others and engaging in relaxation exercises.

17

Cardiovascular Disease and Its Prevention

This chapter will deal with a serious topic of great importance to diabetic persons, cardiovascular disease: diseases of the heart and blood vessels. You will read about high blood pressure, heart attacks, stroke and peripheral vascular disease. These constitute the number-one health problem in the United States today, accounting for over 50 percent of all deaths each year. It is estimated that 30 million Americans have cardiovascular disease. These diseases are caused by atherosclerosis ("hardening of the arteries"). All people get atherosclerosis as they get older, but diabetic persons get it more frequently and at a younger age. Because diabetic individuals are at greater risk for the development of these conditions, you may be frightened or overwhelmed by the following information. It is presented so you will know exactly what these conditions are, how you can recognize them and, most importantly, how you can prevent them. Risk factors for the development of cardiovascular disease have been identified and will be discussed later. For now, it is important for you to know that diabetes is considered a risk factor in the development of cardiovascular disease. You play a role in preventing cardiovascular disease; it is not an inevitable occurrence.

The purpose of the circulatory system is to transport blood. The blood carries oxygen, nutrients and hormones to the tissues and returns carbon dioxide and cell wastes from the tissues to the heart. Think of the circulatory system as having two "sides," arterial and venous. Arteries are blood vessels that carry blood away from the heart to the tissues. The largest artery is known as the aorta. The smallest arteries are known as arterioles. Veins are blood vessels that carry blood back to the heart. Inside veins, small valves work to push oxygen-poor blood on its return trip to the heart and lungs. The largest veins are known as the superior and inferior vena cavae. The smallest veins are known as venules. Capillaries are the tiniest blood vessels. These blood vessels connect the arterioles and venules. The capillaries consist of a single layer of cells lined by a membrane, known as the basement membrane. The exchange of waste materials, nutrients and gases within cells takes place as blood passes through capillaries. The heart also has its own circulatory system. Blood supply to the cardiac muscle (myocardium) is obtained from the coronary arteries. These arteries branch off the aorta and provide oxygen and nutrients to the heart itself. Read more about the cardiovascular system in the "More Useful Information" section at the end of this book.

DIABETES AND CARDIOVASCULAR DISEASE

In the United States, diabetic persons are twice as prone to coronary heart disease, twice as prone to stroke and five times as prone to the development of arterial disease of the limbs. Approximately 75 percent of the deaths among diabetic persons are due to cardiovascular disease. In fact, diabetes is characterized by accelerated vascular disease.

Diabetes' main effect on the cardiovascular system is to cause angiopathy (disease of the blood vessels). There are two forms of angiopathy, microangiopathy and macroangiopathy. Microangiopathy refers to diseases of the small blood vessels, the capillaries, and it affects organs such as the eyes and kidneys. This form of vascular disease (microvascular disease) is discussed in Chapter 18. Macroangiopathy refers to diseases of the large blood vessels of the body, the arteries. Atherosclerosis is responsible for this. In diabetes, atherosclerosis seems to be more severe in the arteries of the heart, causing chest pain or heart attacks; the arteries of the head, causing strokes; or the arteries of the legs, causing poor circulation to the extremities.

How does diabetes cause atherosclerosis? This cannot be simply explained. It may be due to excess blood glucose or to other metabolic defects. Although how diabetes causes atherosclerosis is not entirely certain, there is much information available concerning atherosclerosis.

The commonly known name for atherosclerosis is "hardening of the arteries." The atherosclerotic process is the same in diabetic and non-diabetic individuals. Fats are deposited in the lining (lumen) of the arteries. This fat deposition is known as plaque. Plaque is composed of cholesterol, triglyceride, protein and some calcium. As their linings become thickened, arteries become inflexible.

Because fat deposition is involved in plaque development, elevated cholesterol and triglycerides can lead to atherosclerosis. A normal cholesterol level is 220 milligrams per deciliter or less. Persons who have higher levels than this have had a greater incidence of heart disease. A normal fasting triglyceride level is 65–150 mg./dl. An abnormal triglyceride level is common in obese diabetic persons. To understand the development of atherosclerosis, you must first understand how fats are carried in the blood.

Fats cannot be dissolved in watery solutions such as the blood. In order to be transported in the blood, they must be attached to a protein molecule. This combination is then known as a lipoprotein. Lipoproteins include the chylomicrons, the very low-density lipoproteins (VLDL), the low-density lipoproteins (LDL) and the high-density lipoproteins (HDL). The lipoproteins differ from each other with respect to chemical composition, size and function in the body.

The chylomicrons and the VLDL are the chief transporters of triglycerides in the blood. Chylomicrons are formed in the intestine after a fatty meal and carry dietary fat (as triglycerides) to various body storage sites. The small VLDL are made in the liver and small intestine. These carry triglycerides that are manufactured in the body. The VLDL are broken down by enzymes to form the LDL. The LDL are the chief transporters of cholesterol, and are a major culprit in the development of atherosclerosis. They can deposit cholesterol in the linings of blood vessels. The level of LDL should be less than 190 mg./dl. The HDL is a small molecule which is thought to clear excess cholesterol from the blood vessels. Therefore, it may play a role in the prevention of atherosclerosis. A normal HDL is 45 mg./dl. or greater. Here, interestingly, an elevated blood value can be beneficial.

Elevated lipid levels with an increased LDL and decreased HDL levels may indicate fat is being deposited in the linings of the blood vessels. The plaque formed from this fat clogs the vessel, preventing the adequate flow of oxygen-rich blood. Arteries become narrow and lose their ability to contract or expand. If blood flow through an artery is difficult, a clot may easily form, further blocking important organs from receiving blood. If there isn't enough oxygenated blood reaching a tissue, ischemia occurs. This refers to a local deficiency of blood supply. This temporary lack of blood supply may cause some changes that are reversible. For example, certain conditions of the heart (angina), brain (transient ischemic attacks), legs (intermittent claudication) are caused by ischemia. Ischemia may produce uncomfortable, painful symptoms as cells do not receive enough oxygen, but does not cause cell death.

If blood supply to an organ is further decreased, actual tissue death may occur. This is known as an infarction. An infarct refers to an area of an organ which dies as a result of inadequate blood supply. For example, myocardial infarct (heart), stroke (brain) and gangrene (legs) are all caused by infarction. Although these changes are not as reversible as those caused by ischemia, treatments are available for these conditions.

Atherosclerosis does not develop simply from a buildup of plaque. Other important factors, such as blood flow through arteries and platelet clumping on a part of the artery as well as the actual development of a blood clot, are all under investigation at the present time. Many of the conditions already mentioned will now be described. Their description and treatment will be noted. Later, your role in their prevention will be detailed.

Angina pectoris is chest pain that results from cardiac ischemia. At times, due to emotional excitement or exercise, the heart requires more oxygen. If the coronary arteries are narrowed, there may not be enough blood available to meet the increased needs of the heart. This results in chest pain. The heart is a muscle; this pain results from the same process that makes your muscles hurt when you exercise for a long time. The pain lasts for five minutes or less and is usually described as pressure or tightness behind the breastbone. Sometimes the pain spreads to the arms, neck or jaw. Anginal pain is treated with nitroglycerin, beta blockers, calcium-channel blocking agents and other medications. Some patients can also experience coronary spasm. Spasm may lead to reduced coronary blood flow, ischemia or infarction. Most people with coronary spasm do have atherosclerotic narrowing of their coronary arteries.

What is a heart attack? A heart attack is known as a myocardial infarction (MI). A blood clot may form in an artery supplying the heart, causing a blockage of blood supply (coronary occlusion or coronary thrombosis). Without enough oxygen and nutrients, the area of heart muscle supplied by the blocked artery may die. Blood vessels may develop around the blocked area. This blood supply is known as collateral circulation. Collateral circulation may develop before a heart attack occurs. This may prevent the progression of ischemia to infarction.

Signs of a heart attack include uncomfortable pressure, fullness, squeezing or pain in the center of the chest lasting for more than a few minutes. This pain, unlike angina, is not usually related to exercise or emotional excitement. The pain may spread to the shoulders, neck or arms. Other signs may include severe pain, dizziness, fainting, sweating, nausea and shortness of breath. Commit these symptoms to memory. If you experience them, seek help immediately. Call an ambulance to take you directly to the hospital. The actual diagnosis of a heart attack will be made at the hospital when your electrocardiogram is interpreted as abnormal. Your levels of blood enzymes that rise after a heart attack occurs will also be assessed. Diabetic individuals also may have "silent" myocardial infarctions (heart attacks that occur without pain). This is discussed in Chapter 18.

A heart attack occurs acutely (suddenly) and is a serious emergency. Heart attacks claim over 600,000 lives each year and are the leading cause of death in America. If a heart attack causes the heart to stop beating, cardiopulmonary resuscitation (CPR) is required. This is a life-saving technique that combines mouth-to-mouth breathing with closed chest massage. In this way, blood is still circulated to the brain while the heart has stopped. Many people, including all emergency workers, have learned to do CPR in order to save lives. You and your family members should know how to participate in this important procedure. Courses are offered from your local Heart Association and Red Cross.

A person who has experienced a heart attack must be hospitalized for several weeks while his or her condition is stabilized. Drugs, oxygen and rest are used to accomplish this. Rehabilitation after a heart attack involves a physical exercise program, dietary changes, weight loss, if necessary, and the cessation of cigarette smoking. The blood supply to the heart, following an MI, may be evaluated through coronary arteriography (X rays of the coronary arteries). If necessary, blood supply to the heart can be improved by coronary bypass surgery. This involves taking a vein from the leg and using it to bypass a blocked area of a coronary artery.

Arrhythmias (also known as dysrhythmias) are irregular heartbeats. They may occur following a heart attack. The heart's natural pacemaker may not work properly, causing an irregular rhythm or a fast or slow rate. Most arrhythmias are signs of irritability in the atria or ventricles of the heart. This irritability can be treated with medication. If the heart's rate of beating slows too much, an artificial pacemaker may be necessary to keep the heart functioning properly.

Blood pressure is the force with which blood is pushed through the circulation to the various tissues. This force is created by the pumping of the heart and the tension in the walls of the blood vessels. If the arterioles (small arteries) are narrowed, blood cannot easily pass through them. The heart pumps harder in order to push the blood through. The heart's forceful push and the resistance of the blood vessels increases the blood pressure in the arteries. If your blood pressure remains elevated, you are said to have hypertension (high blood pressure).

Blood pressure is measured with a sphygmomanometer (an inflatable rubber cuff with a gauge) and a stethoscope. The cuff is placed around your arm and inflated. The cuff compresses an artery in your arm and blood flow stops for a moment. Air is then slowly released from the cuff and blood flow begins again. The doctor or nurse taking the blood pressure can listen as the blood begins to flow through the artery. Two readings are taken while listening and watching the gauge. The first reading is the systolic pressure, the pressure when the heart beats; the second reading is the diastolic pressure, the pressure in the artery when the heart relaxes. Both numbers are recorded as blood pressure measurement. Normal blood pressure can range from about 110/70 to 140/90. However, a lower blood pressure is not necessarily associated with a disease state. Many people live healthy, normal lives with a lower blood pressure level. A blood pressure level higher than 140/90 indicates the presence of hypertension. Over 35 million Americans have high blood pressure; it is responsible for over 30,000 deaths a year.

Congestive heart failure (CHF) occurs when there has been damage to the heart muscle. This damage is most commonly due to atherosclerosis or high blood pressure. The damage causes the heart muscle to pump less effectively, so circulation becomes inadequate. The blood flow back to the heart slows, resulting in congestion in the tissues. Swelling or edema may then occur in the legs and ankles. Edema is excess fluid in tissues. Shortness of breath often occurs because of edema in the lungs. Heart failure may also affect the kidneys' ability to eliminate sodium and water; edema then increases.

Treatment of CHF includes a combination of rest, diet and medication. Dietary restriction of salt is necessary. Drugs such as diuretics will help to eliminate excess salt and water. The drug digitalis is used to strengthen the pumping action of the heart. Vasodilators are often used to reduce the pressure in the blood vessels and allow the heart to pump more effectively. Many people confuse congestive heart failure with having a heart attack. These are two separate conditions, although CHF may occur as a result of a heart attack. Remember, in CHF the heart is having difficulty pumping blood whereas in a heart attack an area of the heart has become infarcted.

VASCULAR DISEASE

Vascular disease includes both stroke and peripheral vascular disease. These topics will now be discussed.

If you review the nervous system as discussed in the section entitled "How Your Body Works," in the back of this book, you will see that the brain is a complex organ. Arteries are responsible for providing important fuels to the brain such as oxygen and glucose. If the brain is deprived of blood, due to a blockage in the vascular system, a stroke results. Each year there are over 170,000 deaths due to strokes and 500,000 new stroke victims. There are three different types of strokes that may occur. When blood supply to an artery is blocked by a clot (thrombus), a cerebral thrombosis is said to have occurred. Usually clots form in arteries with atherosclerosis. Another form of stroke is called a cerebral embolus. This is caused by a wandering blood clot (embolus) that has traveled to a part of an artery leading to the brain and blocked it. The third type of stroke is called a cerebral hemorrhage, caused by a rupture in the wall of an artery. Strokes are also known as cerebrovascular accidents (CVA).

There are certain warning signs of a stroke that can be recognized. These include temporary numbness or weakness of one side of the face, an arm or a leg. Temporary loss of speech or difficulty in speaking or understanding speech are other signs. Dimness, or loss of vision, especially in one eye, dizziness, unsteadiness and sudden falls can be signs of a stroke. Become aware of these symptoms that often precede a stroke. Identification of "small strokes" can help prevent a major stroke. A "small stroke" is also known as a transient ischemic attack (TIA). TIAs last from ten to twenty minutes to twenty-four hours. They may include temporary blindness, confusion, dizziness, memory lapse and weakness of body parts. Symptoms of a TIA may be caused by ischemia. Although these symptoms may last only a few minutes, they should be treated as a medical emergency and help should be obtained immediately. Much research is now being done on preventing stroke from developing. Part of the research is the investigation of the use of aspirin and other drugs to prevent the development of blood clots.

A stroke is diagnosed by physical examination and several tests. Arterial angiography (X-ray studies with injected dye) will assess obstruction in the arteries. Recently some centers in the country have begun to offer a new, safer procedure developed as an alternative to angiography. It is called Digital Subtraction Angiography. It can be performed on an outpatient basis using a simple intravenous injection placed in the vein of the arm. A CAT scan (computerized axial tomography) is a safe, painless way to assess any damaged area to the brain and evaluate the stroke victim.

If a stroke occurs, the patient may become disabled. The disability may be a difficulty in speaking or inability to move one side of the body. Strokes usually affect only a small area of the brain. Because of this, rehabilitation is possible. Rehabilitation and treatment for a stroke usually involve hospitalization. Anticlotting medication may be used to prevent further clots from occurring. If necessary, surgery may be performed to relieve the blockage. This process is similar to coronary artery bypass surgery. A surgical procedure called carotid endarterectomy may be performed. Atherosclerotic plaque is removed from the carotid artery during this procedure. Rehabilitation after a stroke includes the professional assistance of many health-team members and the help of family members. You have a role in preventing stroke by controlling your diabetes, diet and blood pressure.

Diabetic persons are at risk for the development of peripheral vascular disease (blood vessel disease of the lower extremities). Most of this blood vessel disease occurs in the small arteries of the foot. These small blood vessels narrow due to atherosclerosis. Less oxygenated blood becomes available to tissues. How can you recognize peripheral vascular disease? Pain in the legs while walking is a common symptom of peripheral disease. The pain is usually temporary, occurring in the calves during exertion, and is relieved by resting. This condition is also known as intermittent claudication and results from an inadequate blood supply (ischemia). During exercise, such as walking, the leg muscles need more oxygen. If peripheral vascular disease is present, narrowed blood vessels cannot supply enough oxygen and pain occurs. This is similar to ischemic pain that occurs in heart muscle during exercise (angina). This condition may be controlled by vasodilators (drugs that open blood vessels) or by surgery that bypasses the narrowed area of circulation.

Other symptoms of peripheral vascular disease include cold feet and continuous severe aching in the extremities during sleep or rest. Dangling the legs may help this condition, but often medication is necessary. Weak or absent pulses in the extremities, small cracks in the skin of the foot, hair loss on the feet and toes are other signs of peripheral vascular disease. Dependent rubor is another symptom of partially blocked vessels. "Dependent" refers to dangling and "rubor" to redness. This symptom involves the foot becoming reddish purple when it hangs down. This occurs because the blood is not correctly pumped back up the legs. Additional trouble signs include paleness of the foot when it is raised with a delayed return of color when the foot is then dangled.

Aside from less blood being available, small blood clots often form in the vessels of the feet when an infection is present. These clots are made up of platelets that attach to the wall of the blood vessel. This further prevents oxygen from reaching infected tissues. Blockage of this type can lead to infarction, in this case gangrene. Gangrene is usually accompanied by an infection. It is a serious complication of peripheral vascular disease and accounts for many of the amputations that occur in people with diabetes.

The Doppler technique is used to evaluate peripheral vascular diseases. The Doppler is a device which sends out sound signals that bounce off moving red cells in blood vessels. The Doppler will give off specific signals where the vessel is narrowed or blood flow is reduced.

Patients with diabetes may be referred to a vascular surgeon. This is a doctor who specializes in operative procedures on blood vessels. If surgery is indicated, arterial angiography may first be performed. Digital Subtraction Angiography can also be used to diagnose peripheral vascular disease. Either technique may be used if you experience pain at rest, since this may be a sign of impending gangrene. They may also be indicated if an ulcer or infection is not responding to bed rest or antibiotics. They will help determine the extent of the disease and the feasibility of vascular reconstruction.

Angiography may help the surgeon determine which surgical procedure to perform. Vascular reconstruction involves a "bypass" procedure. Blood is rerouted around the blocked artery using a synthetic vessel or a healthy blood vessel from another part of the body. An endarterectomy involves removing clots from inside the artery. Transcutaneous angioplasty may also be performed. Here, a collapsed balloon is passed into the artery, and inflated, to increase the space in the blood vessel.

People with diabetes are seventeen times more likely to develop gangrene than those without diabetes. Gangrene may develop after a foot injury. A cardinal danger sign is a reddish color in the foot of someone with peripheral vascular disease. Amputations are performed because of severe infection, gangrene or uncontrolled pain. Amputations remove dead or unhealing body parts. Part of a toe or the entire foot may be removed. An amputation of the lower extremity may be performed below or above the knee. The level of amputation is determined by the site and amount of gangrene. After an amputation, physical therapy and the use of an artificial limb can help to restore a normal, healthy life. These complications are not inevitable. Read on to learn how to prevent them.

PREVENTION OF CARDIOVASCULAR DISEASE

Through education and self-control you have the opportunity to prevent the cardiovascular complications noted in the preceding section. Embracing the philosophy of active intervention to promote health can place you less at risk for the development of atherosclerosis than the uninformed diabetic person. As always, the decision to choose health is yours and requires self-control. In this section, the risk factors for the development of atherosclerosis will be identified. Recommendations will be made for specific intervention to help you combat atherosclerosis.

Several risk factors interact to determine the development of atherosclerosis. A risk factor is a trait, habit or condition in an individual that increases the chance of developing a disease. The causes of cardiovascular disease are multifactorial, meaning there are many risk factors. Heredity, sex, race and age play a role in its development. There is a family predisposition to atherosclerosis. Men have a greater risk of heart attack than women. Black Americans have a 50 percent greater chance of developing hypertension than do whites. One in every four heart attacks occurs after the age of 65. These risk factors cannot be changed. Other risk factors can be changed. These include blood cholesterol and triglyceride levels, high blood pressure, cigarette smoking and diabetic control. These risk factors have a cumulative effect. Having more than one will increase your chances of developing cardiovascular disease, so each one must be reduced. Obesity, lack of exercise and stress may also be contributing factors. Each of them is addressed in other chapters of this book. See Chapter 4 for guidelines on weight reduction and the prevention of obesity. Review Chapter 9 for guidelines on obtaining regular exercise. Chapter 16 will give you details on managing stress effectively.

Risk factors for the development of a stroke are similar to those previously described. Two risk factors that cannot be changed are sex and race. Men have a greater risk of stroke than women. Women who use oral contraceptives have a greater risk of stroke than women who do not. This is compounded if they smoke cigarettes. Some risk factors for stroke can be changed. They include hypertension, atherosclerosis and diabetes control.

Risk factors for peripheral vascular disease include heredity and age. Cigarette smoking is a risk factor for peripheral vascular disease. The longer you have diabetes, the greater your risk of developing peripheral vascular disease becomes. Controlling your blood pressure, cholesterol level and diabetes can reduce your risk of peripheral vascular disease.

The Framingham Study was the first long-term study to identify risk factors associated with the development of coronary heart disease. Information was obtained by annual physical examination performed on 5,000 men and women in the small town of Framingham, Massachusetts. Three specific risk factors were shown to have a direct relationship to cardiovascular disease. These were cigarette smoking, elevated blood pressure and high serum lipid levels. These three major changeable risk factors will now be discussed.

Cessation of Cigarette Smoking

In 1964, the U.S. Surgeon General issued the first warning that cigarette smoking is harmful to your health. Evidence concerning the hazards of cigarette smoking has continued to accumulate. There are several reasons why cigarette smoking is harmful. Two dangerous chemicals, nicotine and carbon monoxide, cause immediate and long-term harm to your coronary arteries. Nicotine increases the heart's demand for oxygen, causing the heart muscle to contract harder and faster. This increases blood pressure. Hemoglobin carries oxygen to every cell. Carbon monoxide interferes with oxygen delivery to tissues, including the heart. Nicotine raises the demand of the heart for oxygen while carbon monoxide decreases the ability of blood to furnish oxygen. They both work against you, the smoker. This is especially dangerous for individuals with coronary heart disease.

In men, the death rate from coronary heart disease is much greater for smokers than for non-smokers. Men and women smokers between the ages of 45 and 74 have a higher death rate from stroke. Cigarette smoking worsens peripheral vascular disease. Besides macroangiopathy, smoking has been implicated as a risk factor in the microangiopathy of diabetes. One study of insulin-dependent persons showed that the incidence of kidney disease, as evidenced by proteinuria, was increased in those who smoked ten or more cigarettes a day. There is an association between cigarette smoking and retinopathy (diabetic eye disease) as the duration of diabetes increases. Carbon-monoxide-induced hypoxia may be toxic to blood vessels of the eyes. Diabetic persons should not smoke because of the effect of cigarette smoking on the coronary arteries, peripheral circulation and the capillaries of the eyes and kidneys.

Smoking also affects the respiratory and digestive systems. Lung cancer is caused by the chemicals in tobacco and was responsible for 105,000 deaths in 1981. Peptic ulcer disease is more common in both men and women who smoke.

Before you begin to stop smoking, it is helpful to examine why you have been smoking. There are many reasons why you may smoke. You may feel addicted to cigarettes, although researchers do not feel tobacco smoking is a true addiction. You may associate your smoking habit with other activities, such as drinking coffee or alcoholic beverages or "lighting up" after a meal. You may use smoking to deal with difficult social situations. You may smoke because others around you smoke and you never really thought about quitting.

It is never too late to quit. Some damage to your lungs can be reversed. Within twelve hours after you stop smoking, your lungs start healing. Within five to nine years after you quit, your chance of developing heart disease is cut in half Many people who wish to quit are afraid of weight gain. You would have to gain much weight before the excess pounds outweighed the health benefits of smoking cessation. You can guard against weight gain when you stop smoking by using these food substitutes.

FOOD SUBSTITUTES FOR CIGARETTES

diet soda
½ cup fruit juice mixed with club soda
tomato juice
pretzel sticks
popcorn, unbuttered
saltines
rye wafers
blueberries
strawberries
melon balls
carrot and celery sticks
cucumber coins
radish flowerets
zucchini sticks
cherry tomatoes
sugarless gum
sugarless mints
rice or wheat puffs

There are two ways you can stop smoking. One way is "cold turkey," which many people find successful as a quick final break. The other way is tapering. Tapering gives you a chance to prepare yourself for quitting by gradually decreasing your use of cigarettes. Here are a few helpful hints.

Begin to decrease the number of cigarettes you smoke by choosing one time during the day that you will least miss a cigarette. Reduce the number of cigarettes that you smoke by increasing the time between each cigarette. Buy cigarettes by the pack and not by the carton. Avoid carrying cigarettes with you and decide before hand how many cigarettes you will smoke each day. Review your list of reasons to quit and keep them available to give you motivation. Try not to smoke in association with other activities. Plan a special "quit day." Break all associations with cigarettes from the beginning of that day. For example, if you usually sit at the breakfast table for morning coffee and your first cigarette of the day, plan to have coffee in another part of your home. This may help break your association between the breakfast table, coffee and cigarettes. Enlist the support of others for reinforcement. Use substitute activities such as exercise, reading and hobbies to take your mind off smoking. Engage in positive self-talk. Tell yourself what you are doing is great for your health. There are many types of self-help groups (commercial and non-profit) for those who would like to stop smoking. Look for group therapy programs such as those sponsored by the American Heart Association or the American Cancer Association.

In summary, avoid smoking cigarettes. Try to have substitutions for cigarette smoking and use behavioral strategies for cigarette cessation. As difficult as these activities may be in the beginning, if you stop smoking you are improving your health and well-being as well as preventing the complications of diabetes.

Hypertension

Diabetes is in itself a risk factor for cardiovascular disease. When diabetic individuals have another risk factor such as hypertension, aggressive efforts have to be made to eliminate the additional risk. Risk factors will add up to increase the danger of developing cardiovascular disease, so hypertension needs special attention in diabetic persons.

Hypertension can be treated with diet and medication. Many medications are available, but most fall into three broad categories. These include drugs that eliminate excess fluid and salt (diuretics), drugs that widen the blood vessels (vasodilators) and drugs that block certain stimulation to the heart and blood vessels (beta-adrenergic blocking agents). There is usually a trial period during which patients and their doctors attempt to find the right combination of drugs for the treatment of hypertension. Certain diuretics may cause your kidneys to excrete excessive amounts of potassium. Therefore you may have to increase your intake of dietary potassium to prevent hypokalemia (low blood potassium). Refer to the "More Useful Information" section at the end of this book for a list of foods high in potassium.

Hypertension usually produces no symptoms. Because of this, people with hypertension may fail to take medication as prescribed. Antihypertensive medications may have unpleasant side effects, such as chronic fatigue or impotence. These prevent people from taking medication on a daily basis. It is essential that if antihypertensive medication is prescribed, you take it as directed. Discuss the medication's side effects with your doctor. A large variety of antihypertensive medications are available today and your doctor may easily switch you to another drug. Never stop taking your blood pressure medication on your own.

Because an elevated blood pressure often causes *no* symptoms, have your blood pressure checked regularly. For some individuals, weekly checks are necessary. Self-monitoring of blood pressure can be done with the use of special equipment. Often, family members and friends can check each other's blood pressure. If your blood pressure is not checked during a routine visit to your doctor, speak up and ask that this be done.

Nutrition intervention is necessary in treating hypertension. There is a relationship between diet and hypertension, although the exact mechanism remains unclear. Your weight and sodium intake are the most significant dietary factors. Weight loss alone helps to control hypertension, even if your ideal body weight is not attained. Review Chapter 4 for guidelines on safe weight loss.

A reduction in blood pressure occurs following a mild sodium-reduced diet. The diet does not have to be tasteless, but simply involves avoiding an excessive intake of salt. Therefore, you may want to consider reducing your sodium intake as recommended by the dietary guidelines (Chapter 2). Most Americans consume an average of 8 to 18 grams of salt per day. This is far above the guideline of under 5 grams. Most dietary sodium is found in table salt. Table salt is 40 percent sodium and 60 percent chloride by weight. Approximately one teaspoon of table salt is equivalent to 2,000 milligrams of sodium. A moderate sodium restriction should be considered which includes the elimination of salt used in cooking and at the table. But if you are overweight, do not hesitate to choose low-calorie foods such as celery. Although celery may be higher in salt than other vegetables (160 mg. per half cup) it may help in your weight-reduction program by enabling you to avoid high-calorie snacks. The "More Useful Information" section lists foods that are high and low in salt.

Taking antihypertensive medication and checking your blood pressure frequently will combat hypertension. Nutrition intervention through weight loss and a reduced sodium diet can decrease the risk of hypertension. Next, the third changeable risk factor will be discussed.

High Blood Lipid Levels

The risk of high blood lipid (cholesterol and triglyceride) levels can also be reduced through nutrition. This section of the chapter will provide you with information on how to make necessary diet changes that will prevent atherosclerosis. Many of the changes advised here have already been given in other chapters but bear repeating.

If overweight, lose weight. You have already learned that obesity is a contributing factor to the development of atherosclerosis. Chapter 4 is devoted to safe weight loss. Follow its guidelines while reducing. If you are not overweight, maintain your ideal body weight in order to control cholesterol and triglyceride levels.

Reduce your intake of cholesterol. Cholesterol is found only in animals, although many people mistakenly believe cholesterol is found in vegetables or plants. It provides no calories, yet it is found in every animal product from egg yolks to breakfast meats to cheeses. Dietary cholesterol raises blood cholesterol levels. Eggs contain the largest amount of cholesterol: 250 mg. per yolk. Reduce your intake of cholesterol by eating only two eggs per week. Organ meats such as liver provide about 125 mg. of cholesterol per ounce and should be avoided. Many people mistakenly believe shellfish is also high in cholesterol, but several years ago shellfish was reanalyzed and found to contain acceptable amounts. Most Americans consume 500 to 1,000 mg. of cholesterol each day. The American Heart Association recommends that you reduce your daily intake of cholesterol to 300 mg. or less. Refer to the "More Useful Information" section for the cholesterol content of common foods and begin to reduce your intake of these foods.

Combat atherosclerosis by reducing triglyceride levels. If you have high triglycerides and are overweight, lose weight. Reduce your intake of simple sugars, particularly dietary sucrose. Alcohol intake should be curtailed because alcohol plays a role in elevating triglycerides. Exercise has been shown to reduce triglycerides. So, by reducing your calories, simple carbohydrates and alcohol you can reduce your triglycerides.

Reduce the total fat content of your meals. Because the intake of dietary fat affects your blood cholesterol level, changes can be made in the type and amount of fat you eat. Americans consume approximately 40 to 45 percent of their total calories from fat. This amount should be reduced to 30 to 35 percent. This can be achieved by consuming less than 10 percent of your total calories from saturated fat, 10 percent from polyunsaturated fat and the remainder from monounsaturated fat sources. These changes may not only lower cholesterol levels but may also reduce your total caloric intake. This helps fight obesity as well as atherosclerosis.

Reduce your intake of saturated fats. Saturated fats provide 9 calories per gram and tend to raise blood cholesterol levels. Although they are found primarily in animal sources, some plants provide saturated fats, such as palm oil and coconut oil. These fats are often used in convenience and chip-type foods to help the product stay fresh longer. Foods that contain saturated fats include commercially prepared baked goods, high-fat dairy products such as whole milk and hard cheese, chocolate candy bars, breakfast meats such as bacon, sausage, lard and chicken skin. Avoid these foods. Review your meal plan to determine how often you eat foods with saturated fats. Start making changes in your food choices by concentrating on one food group, such as the dairy group, switching from whole milk to low-fat milk to skim milk. Slowly switch from butter to margarine. Gradually reduce your intake of high-fat luncheon meats and choose leaner cuts of red meat. Review this list of types of fats in foods. All foods contain a mixture of fatty acids. This list shows the primary fatty acid in each fat or oil.

TYPES OF FATS IN FOODS

Saturated Fat	*Monounsaturated Fat*	*Polyunsaturated Fat*
coconut	olives	safflower oil and seeds
coconut oil	olive oil	sunflower oil and seeds
palm hearts	peanuts	corn oil
palm oil	peanut oil	soybean oil
lard	avocado	cottonseed oil
chicken fat		sesame oil
beef fat		walnuts
cocoa		fish oils

Increase the use of polyunsaturated fats in your diet. These are fats from vegetables or plants which are liquid at room temperature. They provide 9 calories per gram and tend to lower blood cholesterol levels. Although helpful in reducing cholesterol, they are not a magical cure for atherosclerosis. Polyunsaturated fats are just one component of your diet to help lower serum cholesterol levels. Choose sources of polyunsaturated fats which include oils or soft tub margarines made of safflower, sunflower, corn, soybean, cottonseed or sesame oil. Gradually switch from butter to stick margarine, then to a soft tub margarine. Certain nuts and lean fish are also excellent sources. Monounsaturated fats have no effect on raising or lowering cholesterol levels. This type of fat is found primarily in avocados, peanuts, peanut oil, olives and olive oil.

Increase the fiber content of your food choices. Certain patients, after following a high-fiber, low-fat, high-complex-carbohydrate diet, show reductions in blood cholesterol and triglyceride levels. Initial studies also show that oat bran may effectively lower LDL levels. Oat bran is similar to oatmeal in that it may be used as cereal or in baking. Choose foods high in fiber (raw vegetables, fruits, bran cereals, whole-wheat breads and pastas) daily, in your meal plan.

Change your eating and cooking habits to keep your cardiovascular system healthy. Changing food habits to prevent elevations of blood cholesterol begins when shopping for food. Purchase lean meats instead of high-fat meats. Lean meats have the least amount of marbling and include round, flank and shoulder cuts of beef, pork or lamb, as well as all types of poultry and fish. Avoid high-fat cuts of meat such as T-bone and porterhouse steaks, breast of veal, luncheon and breakfast meats. These are high in saturated fat, cholesterol and calories. Purchase beans or legumes for use as protein substitutes along with tofu. Tofu is soybean curd which is frequently used in Oriental cooking; it is now readily available in the produce section of supermarkets. Switch to non-fat or low-fat dairy products. Use cheeses made with part skim milk and other cheeses that are low in fat. Replace animal fats, such as butter, lard or bacon, with polyunsaturated margarines and oils. Skim milk or evaporated skim milk can replace non-dairy powdered coffee lighteners. Avoid rich desserts or dishes made with butter or cream, as well as snack foods such as chips, and crackers made with palm or coconut oil. Gradually reduce your portions of meat, fish, poultry or cheese to a total of 6 to 10 ounces per day. Read the following for more specific ideas of categories of foods that contain excessive cholesterol and saturated fat and the appropriate foods to replace them.

INSTEAD OF	TRY
Dairy Products	
whole milk	skim, low-fat, evaporated skim milk
eggs	egg substitutes
high-fat, hard cheeses	Lite Line, Weight Watchers, St. Otho,* Sapsago,* Chol-free Fisher,† Hoop
high-fat cottage cheese	low-fat cottage cheese
sour cream	low-fat yogurt, blenderized cottage cheese
Meat Products	
cold cuts	packaged meats like: Carl Buddig, Louis Rich; Swanson chicken; tuna, shrimp
hot dogs	vegetable franks by Loma Linda Foods
sausage	Morningstar Farms breakfast meats
Porterhouse, Delmonico club steak	sirloin, flank, round
Fats and Oils	
solid shortening	safflower, soybean, sunflower, corn oil
butter, bacon fat, chicken fat	safflower, soybean, sunflower, corn oil
coffee lighteners (solid or liquid)	Poly Perx, evaporated skim milk

Change your food-preparation habits. Before cooking meat or poultry, remove all visible fat and skin. Skim the fat off broths, soups and gravies. Prepare foods by baking, broiling, boiling or poaching. These suggested dietary interventions can significantly reduce cholesterol and triglyceride levels. If diet does not effectively lower these levels, medication may be used to treat them.

Cardiovascular complications are not inevitable. You can do many things to prevent them from developing. The following guidelines are designed to protect

* Available in specialty cheese shops
† Available by mail: Diet and Health Products, Inc., P.O. Box 1886, Lima, OH 45802

your heart and blood vessels. Note that nine of these ten guidelines apply to all Americans. Only one is specific for diabetes. (1) Learn about diabetes and maintain good control. (2) Lose weight if you are overweight. (3) Stop smoking, or never start. (4) Control high blood pressure, if present, and have your blood pressure checked regularly. (5) Limit your intake of cholesterol and saturated fats. (6) Exercise on a regular basis. (7) Avoid stress and enjoy life. (8) Have regular checkups with your doctor. (9) Drink alcohol only in moderation. (10) Keep in mind the warning signs of strokes and heart attacks and seek help immediately if they develop.

Following these ten guidelines will allow you to combat the number-one killer in America today, cardiovascular disease. More information about cardiovascular disease can be obtained from the American Heart Association.

18

Avoiding Long-Term Complications

In this chapter, you will learn about the long-term microvascular complications that may develop in diabetes. These complications occur in the eyes (retinopathy), kidneys (nephropathy) and nerves (neuropathy) and have been called diabetic "triopathy." They are caused by the metabolic abnormalities of diabetes and may be avoided by glucose control. Their avoidance is the reason for trying to be normoglycemic as often as possible.

For a number of years, there was great debate among scientists concerning the relationship of glucose control to microvascular complications. Thickening of the capillary basement membrane had been shown to be characteristic of diabetes. This abnormality in the capillary membrane leads to leakage of substances from blood into the tissues of the kidneys and eyes and reduces blood supply to these organs. Early research studies claimed that newly diagnosed diabetic individuals already had thickened capillary basement membranes. This suggested that microvascular complications might be unavoidable. However, more recent studies have clearly shown that this is not the case. Capillary basement membrane thickening has been shown to increase with the duration of diabetes. There is an overwhelming amount of recent evidence that diabetic triopathy is related to poor glucose control and can be prevented by good glucose control. In 1976, the American Diabetes Association issued a policy statement on this subject. It was concluded that "microvascular complications of diabetes are decreased by reduction of blood glucose." In the 1980s, there is no longer room for debate. Blood glucose levels must be kept as normal as possible. This is your difficult challenge as a self-manager. To help you meet this challenge, in the last few years glucose-monitoring materials and insulin infusion systems have been developed. The necessity of comprehensive patient education in self-management is now widely recognized.

When it was incorrectly believed that microvascular complications could not be avoided, it was felt by many that the reality of complications should be hidden from individuals with diabetes. Why should we speak of "gloom and doom"? People with diabetes would ask, "If I am healthy now, do I have to know about future kidney or eye problems?" We realize that complications can be considered a "gloomy" topic, but that feeling of gloom may be lifted when you realize that you have a definite role in preventing them. Full understanding of the consequences of poor glucose control should be an incentive to make the daily sacrifices necessary to keep healthy in the future. When serious complications (such as renal failure) occur, the most frequently heard complaints are "Why didn't anyone tell me this happens with diabetes?" and "No one told me I could prevent this from happening with good glucose control." We believe that many of the statistics quoted in this chapter about how frequently complications occur will be reduced in the future as more diabetic persons attain good glucose control.

Thus far, we have stressed hyperglycemia as a risk factor for diabetic triopathy. Hyperglycemia, indeed, is the major changeable risk factor. The length of time you have diabetes is a risk factor that cannot be changed. Other changeable risk factors include cigarette smoking and uncontrolled hypertension. For individuals with diabetes, there are many reasons to stop smoking, to keep blood pressure normalized and to strive for normoglycemia.

In the remainder of this chapter, we will discuss specific organs that are affected by diabetes and how these complications occur. Prevention of complications will be addressed with an emphasis on your role in diabetes self-management.

DIABETES AND YOUR EYES

The Eyes

The parts of the eye are seen in Figure 12. Their functions are outlined in the following list.

Part of the Eye	Function
Cornea	Transparent covering at the front of the eye
Sclera	Tough, white protective coat of the eye
Conjunctiva	Mucous membrane that lines the eyelids

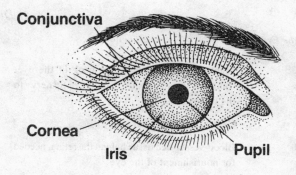

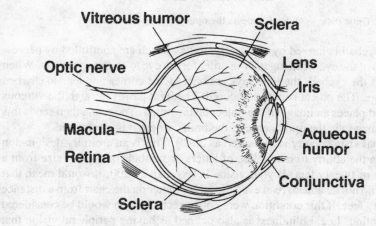

Figure 12. Front and side view of the normal human eye

Part of the Eye	Function
Iris	Colored part; regulates light entering the eye
Pupil	Adjustable opening at the center of the iris that allows light to enter
Aqueous humor	Watery liquid that flows below the lens and the cornea
Lens	Transparent area behind the iris which allows light to pass through
Vitreous humor	Transparent, colorless mass of soft, jelly-like material

Part of the Eye	*Function*
Retina	Light-sensitive tissue at the back of the eye; transmits visual impulse from the optic nerve to the brain
Macula	Central area of vision
Choroid	Blood-vessel-rich tissue behind the retina, needed for nourishment of the eye
Optic nerve	Nerve in back of the eye; carries visual impulse from the retina to the brain
Optic disk	Connects the optic nerve to the retina

The eyeball is moved by six small muscles which are controlled by nerves. All parts of the eye work together in order for the eye to operate properly. When light hits the eyeball, the light rays are bent by the cornea and lens to sharpen the image. The object becomes focused. The light passes through the vitreous body and places an image of the object on the retina. The retina then sends this visual image via the optic nerve to the brain, where it is interpreted.

Normal visual acuity is measured as 20/20. This is an arbitrary designation based on the ability to read a line of letters or symbols of a given size from a distance of twenty feet. If your vision is less than 20/200, it would mean that you would not be able to read even the largest letter on the chart from a distance of twenty feet. If this condition were not correctable, you would be considered legally blind. Legal blindness is also defined as having peripheral vision that is less than 20 degrees. Average peripheral vision (the ability to see to the side) is about 180 degrees. This means that an average person can see a half circle from the side of his left eye to the side of his right eye.

Diabetes is a leading cause of blindness in adults. The longer a person has diabetes, the greater the chances of developing eye complications. Eye changes due to diabetes occur in 80 percent of patients who have had diabetes for twenty years. These eye changes are usually of a mild form, but 3–10 percent of diabetic persons develop severe eye disease. These statistics were obtained prior to the recent intensive efforts at diabetes control.

Diabetes may damage vision by causing diabetic retinopathy. This refers to abnormal changes in the blood vessels of the retina and will be discussed later. Other complications of the eye caused by diabetes include blurred vision, glaucoma and cataracts. The latter two complications are seen not only in people with diabetes but occur in the general population as well.

Blurring of Vision

Blurred vision has no relationship to the serious eye complication of retinopathy. Rather, the blurred image comes as a reaction of the eyeball to changes in diabetes control. When diabetes is out of control, you lose fluids through polyuria. This fluid loss occurs in the eyeball as well. Because the eyeball is hollow, changes in its shape can occur with loss of fluid. When diabetes control is resumed, fluid returns to body areas, including the eyeball. Edema, or swelling of the lens, may occur. The lens cannot focus properly because of these changes. Often, eyeglasses are not prescribed for three to four weeks following the diagnosis of diabetes or following poor diabetes control, because the lens of the eye is not focusing properly. As control improves, the eyes should focus normally. This blurring of vision does not lead to blindness.

Glaucoma

Glaucoma is another complication that is seen in those with diabetes, but it also occurs commonly in non-diabetic patients. Glaucoma refers to increased pressure in the eye which may cause damage to the optic nerve. The damage results in visual impairment. Glaucoma is a major cause of blindness. It usually occurs in patients over 40 years of age. If detected early, the most common form of the disease may be controlled with drugs. In other cases, surgery may be necessary. Some patients have no symptoms initially. Later, symptoms of glaucoma include reduced vision, eye pain, bright flashes or rings of light. Glaucoma is detected through the use of a tonometer. This instrument measures eyeball pressure. Your ophthalmologist (a doctor who specializes in the care of eyes) will test for glaucoma during an eye exam. Early detection of glaucoma is essential so that medication such as eye drops can be prescribed or surgery can be performed.

Cataracts

Cataracts associated with diabetes are a leading cause of blindness in the United States. A cataract is a clouding of the lens of the eye. The clouding interferes with the passage of light to the retina. The first sign of a cataract developing is gradual, painless blurring of vision. Cataracts can usually be successfully removed by surgery and vision can be restored. There are four main types of cataracts. One is called "senile" and is a common form associated with aging. "Congenital" cataracts occur at birth. "Traumatic" cataracts develop following an injury to the eye. "Secondary" cataracts result from another disease, such as diabetes. Cataracts may develop from diabetes because of a buildup of by-products from the breakdown of glucose, in this case sorbitol. This type of cataract can be treated surgically. Because the lens of the eye is removed, its function must be taken over by spectacles, a contact lens or a permanent artificial lens that is implanted in the eye.

Diabetic Retinopathy

Diabetic retinopathy is the most frequent eye complication of diabetes. Currently, about 80 percent of all those having diabetes for over twenty years will show signs of this disease. Yet only a small percentage will develop serious problems that threaten vision.

Remember that the retina receives visual images. As a result of microangiopathy, the blood vessels that nourish the retina leak. The blood vessels may develop weak areas that balloon out or become narrowed or blocked. The retina may then become starved for oxygen as its blood supply is lost. These changes are characteristic of "background" retinopathy. The development of bulges on the walls of blood vessels (microaneurysms), fluid leaks (exudates) or blood leaks (hemorrhages) do not usually have any effect on vision. However, blurring of vision may occur if the macula is affected.

In the advanced state of diabetic retinopathy, called proliferative retinopathy, new, abnormal blood vessels are formed within the retina. The formation of new vessels (neovascularization) is a response to lack of oxygen supply to the retina. These new vessels are fragile, with thin walls. They easily break and leak blood into the vitreous humor. A vitreous hemorrhage can cause temporary or permanent loss of vision. Neovascularization may also cause scar tissue formation. When the scar tissue shrinks, it pulls the retina away from its wall, resulting in retinal detachment. Retinal detachment, if untreated, will lead to blindness.

All of these complications, including proliferative retinopathy, vitreous hemorrhage and retinal detachment, can be assessed and treated by new methods available today. Eye problems can be detected early by regular visits to your ophthalmologist.

Diagnosis of Retinopathy

The diagnosis of background retinopathy can be made by your doctor, using a special instrument called an ophthalmoscope. This lighted instrument allows him to obtain a magnified view of the retina when looking through your dilated pupil. Fluorescein dye angiography will confirm the diagnosis of proliferative retinopathy. Here, a dye is injected into your arm and carried through the bloodstream to the retina. By means of a special rapid-action camera, photographs of the retina can be taken. The doctor then can see the actual flow of dye through the blood vessels. He can better evaluate retinal circulation in your eye as he looks for the presence of neovascularization or leaky vessels.

Diabetic retinopathy frequently produces no symptoms. If you see floating objects or cobwebs in front of your eyes, notify your doctor. Although these may not mean you actually have retinopathy, you should be examined. Because diabetic eye disease may at first produce no symptoms, visit an ophthalmologist at least once per year. He or she will detect problems before you have symptoms.

Treatment of Retinopathy

Today there are specific treatments available to protect you against serious complications of retinopathy. Photocoagulation (laser therapy) is used to reduce the risk of blindness. A laser is a device that produces a beam of light that is used to seal off leaking vessels. ("Laser" is an acronym for Light Amplification by Stimulated Emission of Radiation.) Heat from the laser beam is used to seal many small areas of retinal tissue. This destroys new blood vessels, discourages the growth of future blood vessels and prevents loss of vision.

Laser therapy has become a commonly used treatment that is simple and relatively pain-free. It can usually be done on an outpatient basis, without the use of pain medication. Three types of laser therapy are used. The Ruby laser delivers intense red radiation and is useful when multiple hemorrhages are present. The Argon laser is a green laser that has great accuracy and can pinpoint smaller areas of damage. The Zenon arc is a white laser beam that produces a more widespread and deeper therapy; it cannot be localized and therefore is not used frequently.

Vitrectomy is another new treatment for diabetic eye disease. Prior to this development, little could be done if there was a large hemorrhage into the vitreous humor. The clear fluid of the vitreous would be colored with blood, and light could not be transmitted, resulting in blindness. Vitrectomy consists of removing tissue and blood from the vitreous of the eye and replacing it with clear fluid. Many people who have undergone vitrectomy have had partial or total sight returned to them.

Prevention of Eye Disease

You play an essential role in preventing eye disease. Prevention includes striving for normoglycemia, obtaining care from an ophthalmologist and becoming aware of the risk factors that will aggravate the occurrence of diabetic retinopathy. Your eyes may look and feel fine. However, without an examination performed by an ophthalmologist, using specialized instruments, early problems will not be detected. Eye exams are not painful. They are not time-consuming or threatening. They *are* necessary for your health. Although the philosophy of this book has been devoted to your role in diabetes self-management, it is important to note that you cannot discover eye complications without the assistance of an ophthalmologist.

Another part of prevention of diabetic retinopathy is increasing your awareness of risk factors that will aggravate the course of diabetic retinopathy. These include cigarette smoking and hypertension. Cigarette smoking, as a result of its narrowing effect on blood vessels, may worsen diabetic retinopathy. It causes less blood and consequently less oxygen to flow through the blood vessels. Cessation of cigarette smoking is necessary for many aspects of diabetes self-management. Uncontrolled hypertension may also aggravate diabetic retinopathy through its damaging effect on the blood vessels of the eye.

Continued Research in Diabetic Retinopathy

There have been exciting new developments in research directed at diabetic retinopathy. The National Eye Institute has been responsible for sponsoring several different studies that have been invaluable in providing recommendations for detection and treatment of diabetic retinopathy.

The National Eye Institute sponsored the Diabetic Retinopathy Study (DRS) begun in 1971. This study involved more than 1,700 patients, enrolled in fifteen medical centers, for the exclusive study of eye disease. It showed that photocoagulation reduces visual loss by 60 percent in advanced stages of diabetic retinopathy. Presently, the National Eye Institute is supporting a new clinical trial called the Early Treatment Diabetic Retinopathy Study (ETDRS). This study is designed to determine whether photocoagulation should be used earlier in the course of eye disease to slow its progress and reduce the risk of blindness. This study is also testing whether daily doses of aspirin may affect the progression of diabetic retinopathy by slowing its progress.

The National Eye Institute also supports the Diabetic Retinopathy Vitrectomy Study (DRVS). This involves patients in fifteen medical centers. The study is designed to determine whether it is better to perform vitrectomy immediately following the occurrence of a hemorrhage or to continue, as is currently done, to wait one year for the blood to clear on its own. It will also determine whether vitrectomy reduces visual loss in people with severe proliferative retinopathy who have not had a vitreous hemorrhage.

In conclusion, the most helpful and positive developments are the use of photocoagulation and vitrectomy to treat diabetic retinopathy. The many studies that are in progress involving large numbers of patients will provide valuable information concerning diabetic eye disease. If you are interested in further information on the detection and treatment of eye disease, write to the Office of Scientific Reporting, National Eye Institute, Bethesda, MD 20205. The National Eye Institute is a component of the National Institutes of Health, U.S. Department of Health and Human Services. Other facilities that will give you needed information concerning diabetes and eye disease are listed in the "More Useful Information" section under "Community Resources."

DIABETES AND YOUR KIDNEYS

The kidneys are part of the urinary system, which is described in detail in the "More Useful Information" section under "How Your Body Works." They are bean-shaped organs which lie at the back of the abdominal cavity. Their major function is to purify the blood. Blood enters the kidney through the renal artery. The kidney contains important working units called nephrons. These units do the actual filtering of the blood.

The nephrons are able to filter the blood by means of a complex circulation pathway. There are glomerular capillaries within each of the nephrons which are responsible for the exchange of fluids and particles. As blood passes into the nephron, it is filtered of impurities. Some substances are reabsorbed from the urine back into the bloodstream. Water, electrolytes, protein, glucose and other substances may be reabsorbed and passed back into the blood through the renal vein. Waste products are excreted (passed from the body) in the form of urine. Urine is formed in the Bowman's capsule of the kidney and then passed to the bladder to be finally excreted from the body. Besides acting as a filter, the kidney regulates the amount of fluid and salt present in the body.

Diabetic Nephropathy

Complications affecting the kidney are referred to as diabetic nephropathy. People who are at risk for developing diabetic nephropathy are those who have become diabetic before the age of 40 and are insulin-dependent. As many as half of all insulin-dependent diabetics were estimated to develop diabetic nephropathy prior to today's intervention of strict blood glucose control. For this reason, you must learn about kidney disease and the newer advances in treatment of diabetic nephropathy. Kidney disease can occur from medical problems other than diabetes. Kidney stones and inflammation of the kidneys (nephritis) are unrelated to diabetes and cause serious kidney complications. The first approach to kidney disease is to determine if the problem is correctable. Examples of correctable disorders are urinary-tract obstruction or infection. The doctor will perform certain tests to see if diabetes is the cause of your kidney disease.

Diabetic nephropathy develops because of changes in the filtering function of the kidney due to diabetes. These changes occur slowly and usually do not appear until after the disease has been present for about ten years. Then, a condition known as glomerulosclerosis may develop. This damage to the glomeruli (special blood vessels that allow for filtering) occurs as the walls of these small blood vessels (basement membrane) thicken. The filtering system of the kidney becomes less efficient. Substances such as protein leak into the urine instead of being kept in the blood. When protein is lost in the urine, blood proteins, particularly albumin, may be lowered. Albumin holds water within the blood vessels throughout the body. Without enough albumin, water leaves blood vessels and goes into tissues. Excessive water in the tissues is called edema, and may be a sign of damaged kidneys. (There are other causes of edema besides kidney damage.) Decreased albumin, large amounts of protein in the urine and edema are signs of kidney damage. Progressive, irreversible damage to the kidneys is called chronic renal failure.

Chronic renal failure usually progresses slowly. Because the kidney has a great deal of reserve function, symptoms are usually not noticed until about 90 percent of kidney function is lost. When the filtering ability of the kidney decreases to about 25 percent of normal, renal insufficiency occurs. Laboratory tests such as the creatinine and blood urea nitrogen (BUN) are used to estimate kidney function. A creatinine clearance test is a precise test to analyze both urine and blood and helps your doctor estimate the remaining percentage of kidney function. When the filtering capacity of the kidney falls to less than 5–10 percent of normal, uremia or end-stage renal disease has occurred. Fatigue, anemia, nausea and high blood pressure may develop. Treatment is necessary and will be discussed later.

Kidney disease is managed conservatively until approximately 90 percent of kidney function is lost. You would be asked to stop smoking and your blood pressure would be strictly controlled. Your goal would be to attain the best possible diabetes control. These measures may all help to slow the progress of kidney disease. During this time you should be under the care of a nephrologist (a doctor who specializes in diseases of the kidney). He will try to balance your intake of food, fluid and electrolytes with your kidneys' remaining ability to excrete these properly.

The nutritionist becomes an important resource for the diabetic person with kidney disease. Your diet may now be different from what you were previously eating. Some diabetes self-management routines may be changed as well. As kidney disease progresses, the renal threshold increases and causes inaccurate urine test results. Less urine will be excreted, so less is available to test. Blood glucose monitoring is the best alternative for testing during this time. Frequent hypoglycemic episodes are more common as the requirement for insulin decreases. This is due to the kidneys' failing ability to break down and excrete insulin. Instead, insulin remains in the bloodstream for a long period of time.

During this time, it is essential that you and your family develop a special relationship with your doctor. You should be able to discuss the development of renal failure openly and receive information. Dr. Eli Friedman, who specializes in diabetic nephropathy, describes the need for a "life plan" for diabetics with nephropathy. Often, when patients develop renal failure from diabetes, they have been poorly educated, managed and controlled. They have not received the proper information to prevent the development of kidney disease. A life plan for diabetics with kidney disease includes intensive diabetic control, close consultation with a nephrologist and an ophthalmologist as well as a coordination of diabetes care, rehabilitation counseling and increased education about diabetes. The development of a life plan for subsequent therapy may help the diabetic person face this difficult adjustment.

You cannot live without working kidneys or a substitute for them. Today, there are three major treatments of chronic renal failure. The therapy chosen depends on the individual situation. Treatment of chronic renal failure involves the use of hemodialysis, peritoneal dialysis or transplantation.

Treatment of Kidney Disease

Hemodialysis refers to cleansing of the blood of harmful waste products. Twenty percent of all hemodialysis patients in the United States have diabetes. During hemodialysis, the patient is attached to a machine which acts as a substitute for the kidneys. Blood passes through the plastic artificial kidney machine, is cleansed of waste products and returns to the body. Hemodialysis is the most widely used treatment for kidney failure. The federal government pays for the treatment of kidney failure and is now encouraging the use of home dialysis. Home dialysis is less expensive and more comfortable. Patients stay in their own homes and are given their own dialysis treatments without having to travel to a center two or three times a week. The success of rehabilitation of a dialysis patient depends on the individual's physical status and emotional adjustment to the loss of kidney function. Family support, as always, is important in this adjustment.

Peritoneal Dialysis

Peritoneal dialysis involves the insertion of a cleansing fluid into the peritoneum (a membrane in the abdomen covering the internal organs). This membrane can easily absorb fluid that will help transfer waste products out of the body. A small plastic catheter is inserted into the abdomen through a minor surgical procedure. A cleansing fluid (dialysate) is poured into the abdominal cavity through this catheter. The fluid stays in place in the abdomen for a specific amount of time. This peritoneal membrane is supplied with blood vessels, so wastes from the blood can flow out from the peritoneal membrane. After a short time, the dialysate with the absorbed wastes can be drained out of the body. This procedure is referred to as CAPD (continuous ambulatory peritoneal dialysis).

The procedure can be performed by the patient at home or at work several times a day. Fluid drains into the abdomen when the individual hangs the dialysate container above his head. Fluid drains out when the container is placed below his abdomen. In some cases, insulin may be added to the solution and glucose control achieved along with the dialysis. One must be meticulous in handling the peritoneal dialysis equipment to avoid infection. An important feature in the success of peritoneal dialysis is the individual's commitment to participate actively in the treatment.

Transplantation

Another option in the treatment of kidney disease is surgical transplantation of a kidney. Two out of every three diabetic kidney recipients have been shown to have functioning kidneys at least three years after surgery if they received a transplant from a living, related donor. One-half of the recipients will continue to have a functioning kidney for at least three years if the transplant comes from someone who has recently died and is unrelated. The failure rate is high but must be looked at in terms of past statistics. Approximately fifteen years ago, there was little to no chance for successful kidney transplants for diabetics. Kidney transplantation can also stabilize visual problems for at least three years in the majority of recipients. Patients receiving kidneys are able to return to work and family responsibilities without the pressure and time commitments of dialysis. This is the most positive aspect of transplantation.

There are the usual problems inherent in organ transplantation, including tissue rejection. During the rejection process, the body realizes that the transplanted kidney is a foreign organ and makes efforts to reject it. Various drugs are used to prevent rejection. It is difficult to obtain suitable kidney donors. It is better if the donated kidney comes from a relative. The general public needs more education on the importance of organ donation.

The choice among the various options for the treatment of diabetic kidney disease may seem confusing to you. It is a choice that must be discussed fully with your doctor and your family. The people who advocate transplantation do so because they feel it offers more complete rehabilitation. For younger patients who have family members willing to donate a well-matched kidney, transplantation may be the best option.

Kidney failure results in the need for treatment using dialysis or transplantation. Very often, patients may have diabetic nephropathy and not develop end-stage renal disease (kidney failure). They will continue to function without the need for dialysis. In fact, they may need little if any treatment for their kidney disease. Both transplantation and the improvement of dialysis devices are the subjects of intense research.

Your Self-Management

You have a role in the detection and prevention of diabetic nephropathy. One area that we have already mentioned is your participation in a health management program to ensure good diabetic control. A second area is keeping close contact with your doctor, making appointments for regular checkups and obtaining laboratory tests to determine kidney function, at least annually or more often. If you have hypertension, it is in your best interest to keep it controlled. If you smoke cigarettes, you should quit immediately. Another aspect of self-management for people who have had insulin-dependent diabetes for many years is testing urine protein at home. Because the appearance of large amounts of protein in the urine is an early sign of diabetic nephropathy, some patients are choosing to use a simple dipstick test at home to check their urine. This could be done once every three months. However, do not be alarmed if trace amounts of protein are present in your urine. This can be related to many things, including normal breakdown of body cells, and does not mean you have diabetic nephropathy.

DIABETES AND YOUR NERVOUS SYSTEM

Diabetic Neuropathy

Diabetes is associated with a variety of complications in the nervous system. The nervous system, along with the endocrine system, coordinates all activities of the body. The nervous system receives messages from the body's external and internal environment. It also carries messages from one part of the body to another. These messages are in the form of electrical impulses which are carried through nerves. The specialized cells of the nervous system are called neurons. The nervous system can be divided into three parts: the central, peripheral and autonomic systems. These are reviewed in the "More Useful Information" section under "How Your Body Works." Diabetes can interfere with these communications and can break down the transmission of nervous impulses from one area to another. This is called diabetic neuropathy. In the majority of cases, the neuropathy is slight and does not produce serious symptoms. Although diabetic neuropathy affects men and women equally, it is not common among young people with diabetes. It is related to the duration of diabetes.

Diabetic neuropathy is believed to result from excess sorbitol and/or reduced myoinositol in nerves. Both of these abnormalities in metabolism result from hyperglycemia. Glucose is able to enter nerve cells even in the absence of insulin. Therefore, in poorly controlled diabetes (with high blood glucose and low insulin levels) an excess amount of glucose enters nerve cells. Some excess glucose is metabolized to sorbitol (a sugar alcohol). Accumulation of sorbitol leads to damage of the nerve cell. A similar process may occur in the lens of the eye, resulting in the formation of diabetic cataract. Myoinositol is necessary for proper functioning of nerves. It is excreted in the urine in large amounts in uncontrolled diabetes. Reduced levels in nervous tissue may contribute to diabetic neuropathy.

Lowering blood glucose corrects both these abnormalities. Although there is much that remains to be discovered about neuropathy, it is clear that it results from hyperglycemia. Diabetic neuropathy is preventable by maintaining a normal blood glucose. In its early stages the symptoms of neuropathy may be improved by normalization of blood glucose. There are four major kinds of neuropathy and these will now be described.

Distal Symmetrical Polyneuropathy

This is the most common type of peripheral neuropathy. If you think of the "periphery" of your body as your feet, lower legs, toes, hands and fingertips, you will be able to understand the name peripheral neuropathy. Two symptoms of peripheral neuropathy are pain and paresthesia. Paresthesia refers to tingling sensations. Tingling is often associated with a loss of sensation to touch. It can be differentiated from the common "pins and needles" that all people experience by the amount of time that symptoms persist. It usually lasts for more than twenty minutes. Numbness, often without pain, is present. When pain occurs it is sometimes severe, usually coming when you are at rest and often occurring only at night. This type of pain, in the lower extremities, is also characteristic of neuropathy. Difficulty with balance may also occur.

How is peripheral neuropathy diagnosed? Your doctor will ask you questions to gain an accurate history of possible peripheral neuropathy. He will also test the nervous responses of various parts of the body. These tests usually include sticking the skin of the bottom of the foot and ankle with a pin to determine sensitivity to pain. Touching with a tuft of cotton determines feeling. Hot and cold sensitivity and the response to the vibrations of a tuning fork are evaluated. The doctor also taps the knee and ankle with a reflex hammer to see whether or not you respond with normal reflexes.

Many cases of painful neuropathy improve after a period of three to six months. Often, when someone is experiencing painful peripheral neuropathy, he may become depressed, have a poor appetite and lose weight. Peripheral neuropathy often improves with normalization of blood glucose levels. Certain medications may also be useful in controlling symptoms.

We have spoken of the feet and lower legs, but the hands and fingertips can also be affected by peripheral neuropathy. If the ability to feel painful sensations is not present, the diabetic person with neuropathy may burn himself when cooking. All items that are potentially harmful to the feet and lower legs, hands and fingertips, such as heating pads and hot-water bottles, should be avoided. Proper foot care is essential and is described in Chapter 20.

There are other kinds of peripheral neuropathy. One of them, called Charcot's joint, involves deterioration of the joints of the foot or the ankle. Without sensation in the foot and ankle, the bones of the joint may move in an abnormal way without producing any painful reaction. Continued walking on this joint would cause gradual destruction. A foot that has developed Charcot's joint appears shortened and widened. The arch of the foot is flattened. Today, various orthopedic appliances, such as a walking cast, are available to correct the condition and make it easier to walk normally. This condition is relatively uncommon.

Foot drop is another condition seen in diabetic peripheral neuropathy. As a result of damage to motor nerves, the foot cannot be raised upward. An ankle and foot brace can help keep the foot in a normal position until recovery is complete.

A neuropathic foot ulcer may result from peripheral neuropathy. This ulcer develops on the bottom of the foot at a site of pressure. Yet, due to a lack of sensation, the pressure isn't felt. If the feet are not examined on a daily basis, the injury may become extensive. Some ulcers develop because the blood supply is insufficient to keep the area healthy. The neuropathic ulcer usually has an appropriate blood supply but it is difficult to treat. Because the ulcer has developed due to pressure, part of the treatment involves relieving the pressure. There are special shoes which can be worn to relieve pressure on the foot. If the ulcer becomes infected, antibiotics are prescribed. At times, surgery is necessary.

These types of neuropathies can be frightening, but they can often be controlled by maintaining normal blood glucose levels. Seeing your doctor regularly and taking medication to reduce discomfort will also help. Practicing good foot hygiene and staying slim so that excess weight will not be a burden on your feet and lower legs are valuable self-management tips.

Autonomic Neuropathy

Autonomic neuropathy involves nerves which function without your conscious control. It may be helpful to think of this as "automatic" neuropathy. It affects internal organs which usually act automatically. These nerves supply the gastrointestinal tract, bladder, genital organs and the small blood vessels and sweat glands of the skin.

Loss of the normal sweating response may occur with neuropathy, especially in the lower extremities. Some people then have increased sweating in their upper extremities. Diabetic neuropathy may also affect the urinary bladder. Nerve damage may prevent the bladder from emptying properly. This is known as bladder atony. Sometimes more than a quart of urine can be retained in the bladder. Normally, the nerves of the inner walls of the bladder would be stimulated and would communicate the need to urinate when the bladder is full. However, when neuropathy is present, the feeling of pressure of a full bladder may be lost. Recurrent urinary tract infections may result from paralysis of the bladder. If you notice that your lower abdomen is bloated, and that you have not been urinating regularly, bring this to the attention of your doctor. The treatment available for this condition involves medications which stimulate the bladder to empty. Antibiotics can also be helpful if infection is present.

The gastrointestinal system may also be affected by diabetic neuropathy. A condition known as diabetic diarrhea may result from diabetes' effect on the nerves that control the small intestine. This diarrhea may occur sporadically in between normal bowel habits and periods of constipation. It often occurs at night. At times, there is a lack of control of the bowel, which may cause embarrassment. Although diabetic diarrhea may be severe, it does not usually affect general health. Antibiotics and antidiarrheal medications are used to treat diabetic diarrhea.

Another form of autonomic neuropathy that affects the GI tract is called delayed gastric emptying. There is a loss of tone in the muscles of the stomach, resulting in a delay in emptying of the stomach. There is a lack of consistency in the time it takes food to enter the small intestine. Patients with this disorder may have to seek detailed dietary advice. Drugs are available that stimulate the emptying of the stomach.

Autonomic neuropathy also has an effect on the cardiovascular system. A condition known as orthostatic hypotension may result. As you stand up, blood usually rushes to the feet. Blood vessels constrict to prevent blood pressure from dropping. If the nerves that control these blood vessels become damaged, the blood vessels may not prevent blood from settling toward the feet. Less blood then becomes available for the brain, causing dizziness. You may have experienced this if you got up too quickly from a lying to a standing position. This can be prevented by changing positions slowly. The use of pressure stockings and certain medications may improve this condition.

Because of neuropathic changes in the cardiovascular system, diabetic persons may have a "silent" myocardial infarction. A silent myocardial infarction refers to a heart attack without the important warning symptom of chest pain. Chest pain is communicated as a nervous impulse, and if the impulse is lacking, heart attack may occur silently. Know the other warning signs of a heart attack, including nausea, vomiting, perspiration, anxiety and extreme weakness.

Another form of autonomic neuropathy that is commonly seen is a decrease in sexual function. This will be further discussed in Chapter 19.

Diabetic Amyotrophy

Proximal motor neuropathy occurs in the thigh muscles. It is also called amyotrophy. The overlying skin may become sensitive and painful. The muscle of the thigh shrinks because its nerve supply is damaged. Often, people experiencing this condition lose weight, become fatigued and are unable to climb stairs or walk rapidly. This condition is rare and recovery usually occurs within two years.

Cranial Mononeuropathy

Symptoms of this form of neuropathy include double vision, eyelid droop and pain surrounding the eye. This is caused by damage to the cranial nerves that control the eye. The symptoms develop rapidly and usually clear completely within three to four months. Patients with cranial neuropathy may need pain medication and may also have to wear an eye patch in order to gain visual comfort while the condition persists.

As you can see, most neuropathies can be treated. For this reason, it is most important that you become aware of various symptoms of neuropathy and bring them to the attention of your doctor. A doctor specializing in treatment of neurological disorders is called a neurologist.

Retinopathy, nephropathy and neuropathy are known as a triopathy of diabetes complications. They are results of the metabolic abnormalities that occur in diabetes and therefore can be avoided by good control. The statistics quoted in this chapter for the likelihood of development of diabetic triopathy are based on patients who have not been optimally educated or controlled. Again, promotion of health and avoidance of illness are the goals of this book. You must develop the self-control necessary to prevent complications in the future. For those who have already developed complications, there have been remarkable advances in treatment in recent years. The treatment of diabetic retinopathy through laser therapy is an example of these major advances.

19

Sexuality, Pregnancy and Family Planning

SEXUALITY AND DIABETES

In recent years there has been an increasing amount of public interest in sexuality. Motion picture films, television shows and best-selling books have all dealt with this topic. People are realizing that they have a right to receive accurate and complete information about their sexual concerns. You, as a diabetic person or as a family member of someone with diabetes, need to know the effect diabetes has on sexuality.

What is sexuality? Sexuality does not refer to sexual intercourse alone. Sexuality is a part of human nature and is involved in human relationships. Sexuality has to do with our sense of ourselves as a man or a woman, our feelings of intimacy and enjoyment of sensuality, our individual and unique fantasies, the things which "turn us on" or "turn us off." Sexuality is a part of a person's natural desire for closeness with others.

Any medical condition that interferes with sexual and reproductive functions threatens human sexuality. For over a hundred years, diabetes has been known to have an effect on male sexual functioning. In this chapter, we will look at sexual problems of both male and female diabetic persons. The communications and adjustments necessary for the diabetic person experiencing sexual difficulties will also be discussed.

Much information about human sexual response was gained through the work of Masters and Johnson in the 1960s. The human sexual response varies from person to person and can be divided into four stages. The excitement stage begins when an individual responds to sexual stimulation. In the plateau stage, physical responses to sexual tension heighten. The orgasmic stage is one of intense pleasure with climax of sexual tension. During the resolution stage, there is a return to the unstimulated state.

What happens to a man physically during sexual intercourse? For a man, sexual functioning includes arousal, erection and orgasm with ejaculation. Penile erection occurs as a reflex. Nerves are stimulated which result in expansion of the penile arteries. The blood flow to the corpora cavernosa (spaces inside of the penis) then increases. Blood is retained and helps to expand and congest veins so that an erection (tumescence) occurs. This nervous stimulus must be present in order to have an erection. The male reproductive system is further explained in the "More Useful Information" section under "How Your Body Works."

Male Sexual Dysfunction

Erectile dysfunction or erectile impotence is the inability to get and keep an erection of sufficient firmness to sustain sexual intercourse. Diabetes can affect the ability to get and maintain an erection. If an impairment in the nervous system interrupts or prevents the proper nervous stimulation, the penile arteries will not dilate and the penis will not become erect. In diabetic autonomic neuropathy, certain pelvic nerves may be damaged, resulting in impotence. This type of sexual difficulty occurs in approximately half of all men who have had diabetes for many years. In diabetes, this problem is termed erectile impotence rather than sexual impotence because the difficulty is with the process of getting and keeping an erection alone. Other aspects of sexual function such as libido (sex drive) and ejaculation may remain unaffected by diabetes.

Erectile impotence in diabetic men is also associated with damaged nerve fibers (neuropathy). Diminished blood flow due to atherosclerosis is another complicating factor in the development of impotence. Thus impairment of either the nervous system or the circulatory system may lead to sexual problems. When diabetes has either effect on male sexual functioning, a slow progressive impotence may develop. Impaired erections (difficulty in getting or maintaining full erections) may occur for six months to two years or more before total erectile impotence occurs.

Impotence can also be linked to blood glucose control. Males may have transient (temporary) impotence when diabetes is out of control. Complete impotence that has developed in a well-controlled diabetic male may be a permanent condition, but should be evaluated by a health professional who is expert in assessing whether the loss of erection is based on other physical or psychological causes.

Other causes of impotence include use of certain drugs (particularly some antihypertensive medications), other endocrine diseases and certain types of operations. Impotence may also occur due to testosterone deficiency. A blood test for the hormone testosterone is important in determining if there is an endocrine basis for impotence. Testosterone levels in diabetic males with or without impotence are usually normal. It has not been helpful to give injections of testosterone to improve impotence in these cases. In fact, testosterone may only further stimulate the libido and not improve the erectile process, worsening the entire situation.

All men may, at one time in their lives, experience difficulty in sexual functioning. Thus it is important to differentiate whether the impotence in a diabetic male is due to diabetic neuropathy or other causes. If you see your doctor for help with the problem of erectile impotence, he may ask you specific questions to try to determine if the cause of impotence is psychological. Psychological causes of impotence can occur in all men, with or without diabetes. Often the psychological adjustment to a chronic illness such as diabetes can interfere with sexual relationships.

Psychological impotence may be selective in the sense that it may be present with one partner but not with another, or at times of stress, anger or depression and not at other times. Your doctor might ask you if impotence occurs during all sexual encounters with all sexual partners, if relevant. Nocturnal erections and emissions usually occur when psychological impotence is present. Your doctor may ask you if you still are having morning erections (on waking up) or if you notice you have an erection when your bladder is full as you arise in the morning. He may ask you whether you still have the ability to have an erection when you masturbate. Erection at any of these times would probably indicate a psychological cause of impotence. A history of the onset of impotence helps to differentiate whether it is from a psychological or a physical cause. Psychological impotence may occur suddenly, whereas diabetic neuropathy may cause a gradual potency problem. The testicles may lose sensitivity as well.

When diabetic neuropathic impotence is suspected, tests can be performed to confirm the diagnosis. One of these tests is known as NTP (nocturnal tumescence of the penis). Everyone, during sleep, experiences regularly occurring periods of rapid vertical and horizontal eye movements. These are known as REMs. Usually, three or four periods of REM sleep occur during an average night. During this time spontaneous erections in men also occur. Normally, there are erections during REM sleep in men of all ages as well as in men who complain of impotence without evidence of organic disease. In order to evaluate this, a man is usually referred to a Sleep Disorders Clinic. There, a gauge is placed on the base of the penis. This monitors and documents periods of penile tumescence (the engorgement of the penis with blood) while he is asleep. There is no nocturnal penile tumescence when impotence is due to diabetic neuropathy. Diminished blood flow due to atherosclerosis may also result in a blood supply that is not adequate for erection.

What is available for a man who is experiencing erectile impotence due to diabetes? First, the degree of control of the diabetes must be assessed. When diabetes is out of control, weakness and malnutrition may occur. When diabetes is controlled and health restored, normal potency may again be achieved. Sometimes, episodes of impotence are due to hypoglycemia. If hypoglycemia is a problem, especially early in the morning, two or three Life Saver candies prior to sexual intercourse have been reported to make a difference. If diabetic autonomic neuropathy is present, there is no specific therapy for erectile impotence at this time. Mechanical devices, such as the penile prosthesis, have been devised and may be beneficial for certain patients.

Surgical implantation of penile prosthetic devices have been used to treat erectile impotence. There are two types of penile prostheses. For certain patients, the Small-Carrion prosthesis can be implanted surgically. With this device, two implants made of silicone rubber, acrylic or polyethylene are inserted and a permanent erection is maintained. These implants are rigid enough to prevent the penis from buckling during intercourse. The erection can be held at the stomach when jockey-type briefs are worn and will not be detected through clothes. This procedure is considered simple and is well tolerated by most patients. The major disadvantage to this treatment is the presence of a permanent semi-erection.

Another prosthesis available for use is inflatable and allows the erection to be controlled. Scott-Bradley-Timm developed this in 1973 and many men have now successfully used this prosthesis. The device consists of a pump, fluid storage area and inflatable cylinders which are surgically implanted. The erection is triggered by the pump in the scrotal sac. When the pump is pushed, fluid is pumped into the hollow implants in the penis and an erection results. When the pump mechanism is again pushed, the fluid is returned to the reservoir and the penis loses the erection. This procedure is more expensive and complex. However, an advantage of this device is that it is undetectable.

Another sexual dysfunction that occurs in diabetic men is retrograde ejaculation. The internal sphincter connecting the urethra to the bladder may relax due to autonomic diabetic neuropathy. When this occurs, seminal fluid containing sperm will flow back into the bladder during ejaculation, not out of the urethra. Men experiencing this associated sexual difficulty are not impotent. They are aware of having orgasm but no ejaculate is passed. This is a cause of sterility. If you are having symptoms of retrograde ejaculation, it is important that you bring this to your doctor's attention. Certain medications may be used to treat this condition. If the problem persists and infertility is a result, sperm may be extracted mechanically from the urine and used for artificial insemination. This condition is found in 1–2 percent of diabetic men.

Male and female sexual functioning are alike in physiology. The glans or head of the penis is similar to the clitoris. The skin of the shaft of the penis is similar in sensitivity to that of the labia minora and the skin of the scrotum of the male is similar to the labia majora in the female. Nerve pathways are alike in that the spinal centers controlling sex organ reflexes are present in both males and females. During female sexual response there is local blood vessel congestion. This vasocongestion resembles the male erection process. During sexual arousal, the labia and the tissues of the lower third of the vagina become swollen with blood, and lubrication of the vagina occurs. Orgasm is characterized by a series of rapid contractions of the uterus and vagina. The nervous system stimulates the lubrication necessary for the female during sexual intercourse, and the spinal reflex center stimulates the female orgasmic response. The female reproductive system is further explained in the ''More Useful Information'' section.

Female Sexual Dysfunction

Because of the similarity in the physiological processes of sexual function in males and females and because both sexes experience diabetic neuropathy equally, it is surprising that there isn't more known about sexual difficulties in diabetic women. It is more difficult to document the effect of diabetes on female sexuality. Although impotence is a well-recognized complication of diabetes in men, there is no such clear-cut effect in the female population.

In one study of sexual functioning, a group of 125 diabetic women were compared with an age-matched group of 100 non-diabetic women. Total absence of orgasm was reported by 35 percent of the diabetic women and only 6 percent of the control group. These diabetic women stated that they had gradually developed orgasmic problems after the onset of diabetes. In another, similar study, 100 diabetic women were interviewed. Over half of these women had demonstrated neuropathy. Approximately 80 percent of the diabetic women reported that they still had orgasms. This figure is comparable to the non-diabetic population. There was also no difference in sexual desire or the ability to achieve orgasm between those diabetic women who had and those who did not have evidence of neuropathy.

You can see the conflicts between these two studies. Does diabetes lead to reduction or loss of orgasm in females? This is a topic that has not yet been fully explored. It is more difficult to obtain direct clinical evidence of orgasm in a female. Only recently have clinical testing devices been developed to assess sexual aspects of the female diabetic. These include a vaginal photoplethysmograph. This instrument measures vaginal blood flow during sleep and is similar to the NPTs that were previously described for men.

Another associated problem seen with the diabetic female is dyspareunia (painful sexual intercourse). Painful sexual intercourse may be due to many factors, such as emotions, lack of lubrication or vaginitis. Vaginitis is a common condition seen in diabetic women. Monilial vaginitis occurs when fungus overgrows in the presence of high blood and urine glucose. Pain, burning and swelling of the genitalia will make intercourse difficult, if not impossible. There is usually a vaginal discharge. This form of vaginitis may be treated by Mycostatin vaginal suppositories and good diabetic control.

Intercourse may also be painful if the vagina is not lubricated sufficiently for the penis to enter. If sexual arousal does not occur, lubricating fluids are not released into the vagina and sexual intercourse will be difficult. Menopausal women may find vaginal dryness a problem. Lubricating cream such as K-Y Jelly (not Vaseline) and certain medications are available to improve vaginal lubrication. Increased sexual stimulation prior to intercourse will also increase lubrication. If you are experiencing this problem, your condition should be fully evaluated. Do not hesitate to speak with your diabetes specialist, family doctor, gynecologist or nurse regarding sexual problems.

Other parameters of your health will also be assessed. If your diabetes is not controlled, your sexual response may not be at a high level. Achievement of blood glucose control is necessary in order to improve your sexual response.

Knowing that diabetes can be associated with sexual problems may help you communicate freely with members of the health-care team regarding your sexual problems. But because sex is such a personal aspect of your life, everything else concerning diabetes may be discussed with the exception of sexual problems. If you are not asked about possible sexual difficulties, do not hesitate to volunteer such information. It is equally essential that you communicate with your partner about problems that are present. It is important to discuss the feelings that these problems cause.

Sexual counseling may be helpful for many individuals. If nothing else, it may correct misinformation. Sexual functioning does not have to be associated only with having intercourse with an erection and ejaculation for a male and an orgasm for a female. Intimacy can be achieved by a variety of sensual acts including massage, caressing and kissing of many different parts of the body. Warmth, intimacy and physical gratification are possible without sexual intercourse. Disturbances in the area of sexual function and adjustment may hurt your own self-image. It is important that you do not allow negative feelings to distort your view of yourself, to define yourself as a "failure."

It is not an easy task to discuss sexual problems, even with a professional. If you do have a problem, make an appointment with your doctor and speak frankly about this subject. Be prepared to answer some of the following questions: Have you lost the desire for sex? Do you have pain during intercourse? Are you unable to reach orgasm? Females should be prepared for a pelvic exam in which the doctor will look for infections in the vagina or possible problems with pelvic organs. Blood may be drawn to decide whether hormonal disorders are a problem. Both men and women should be prepared to give a diabetes history. How long has diabetes been present? Is your blood glucose controlled? Are there other signs of diabetic neuropathic complications?

Your doctor may also ask about your feelings. Are you angry, fearful, depressed about your sexual performance? Are you constantly watching your own self during sex, afraid that you will not have an orgasm or erection? Your doctor may also ask about other medications that you may be taking, such as tranquilizers or blood-pressure pills, and whether you are consuming too much alcohol, all of which can interfere with sexual intercourse.

Your doctor may advise you regarding open communication with your partner. If you are upset about your present sexual communication, this distress may be relieved by open conversations. You may need a change in the timing of some of your diabetes self-management routines in order to facilitate sexual functioning. If you are testing your blood, monitoring your urine or giving an insulin injection immediately before sexual intercourse, you may be feeling anxious, rushed or distracted. Talk about these feelings with your partner, as well as your doctor.

Often, with something as complicated and emotional as sexual expression, the partners cannot handle the problem alone. You probably have received help with other aspects of diabetes self-management, such as learning home blood testing and insulin administration. Do not hesitate to ask for help in the professional realm of sex counseling. A positive, fulfilled sex life should not be denied to a person who has diabetes.

Remember, too, that your doctor or diabetes health team may not be adequately prepared to offer you the sexual counseling that you need. Instead, you may need to seek out the expertise of a sex therapist. Counseling can help you learn how to deal with both physical and emotional aspects of impotence. Better communication may evolve between you and your partner. Investigate the credentials of the sex therapist that you choose. Often, large medical centers have a human sexuality program where you may seek help. By contacting your local medical center's Obstetrics-Gynecology, Psychiatry or Endocrinology Department, you may be able to find a listing of such centers. The American Association of Sex Educators, Counselors and Therapists, too, will provide you with information. Refer to the "Community Resources" section at the end of this book for the address.

Sexuality is part of man's natural desire for closeness with others. Any problem that interferes with sexual function is a threat to human sexuality. Sexual difficulties may be the result of psychological or physiological problems. To differentiate between the two, your doctor will evaluate you thoroughly. Diabetic autonomic neuropathy may damage pelvic nerves and cause erectile impotence. Atherosclerosis, certain medications, some endocrine diseases and poor blood glucose control can also cause impotence in men. Sexual problems in women may be the result of neuropathy, painful sexual intercourse or poor diabetes control. Treatment of sexual dysfunction may take many paths. Men may be candidates for a penile prosthesis. All are advised to maintain good diabetes control. You are also encouraged to communicate openly with the health-care team. If your doctor doesn't ask you, you may have to start the discussion yourself. Communication with your partner is also essential. Finally, you may need the expertise of a sex therapist to help you learn to deal with the physical and emotional aspects of impotence.

Part of one's sexuality involves entering various developmental stages of life. For a woman, pregnancy is an important psychological, developmental and physical stage. The next part of this chapter will discuss pregnancy and family planning.

PREGNANCY AND DIABETES

Planning for a family is a most exciting and fulfilling time of life. For the woman with diabetes it may become a time of anticipation, emotional upheaval and concern. You may have many additional questions regarding yourself and the soon-to-be-born baby. It is essential for you to understand the relationship between pregnancy and diabetes.

Prior to the discovery of insulin, women with diabetes rarely became pregnant. Those that were able to become pregnant often faced a poor outcome. In the beginning of the twentieth century, the infant death rate was extremely high. However, as the years progressed, the twentieth century has become a remarkable time for pregnant women with diabetes. Refinements in diabetes management for mothers and infants have led to a 95 percent chance for a successful outcome.

Physicians now realize the great importance of rigid control of blood glucose. Several research studies have shown that those women with fasting plasma glucose levels of 60–90 mg./dl. and postprandial blood glucoses of 120 mg./dl. experienced a lower incidence of infant death. The results have been quite different in women maintaining a blood glucose of 200 mg./dl. throughout pregnancy. There seems to be no doubt that blood glucose control positively affects the outcome of the pregnancy.

Presently, 1 in 200 pregnancies occur in diabetic females. Another 5 in 200 will develop diabetes during pregnancy (gestational diabetes). Prior to 1960, the fetal death rate was as high as 30 percent. Now, it is only 5 percent. Although the death rate has declined, there are still significant congenital problems.

We will now describe physiological changes occurring in diabetes and pregnancy, methods of testing for control during pregnancy, as well as tests needed prior to the time of delivery. Changes in insulin regimen and self-management practices during pregnancy will also be discussed.

It is important for you to understand that having a normal blood glucose value and a normal hemoglobin A_{1C} prior to and at conception are important to the outcome of your pregnancy. Diabetes in good control prior to conception may prevent congenital malformations. Malformations occur before the eighth week of pregnancy, often long before you know you are pregnant. Ideally your diabetes should be well controlled, with your hemoglobin A_{1C} in a normal range at the time of conception. Your pregnancy should be planned.

Many physical changes occur during pregnancy. If a woman is prone to the development of diabetes, diabetes may become apparent during pregnancy. This is called gestational diabetes. Also, women who already have diabetes may find their control more difficult. Women who were successfully controlled in the past by diet therapy alone may find they need to use insulin during pregnancy. Insulin-dependent mothers-to-bé will require changes in insulin dosage as the pregnancy progresses. Your blood glucose must be strictly controlled throughout pregnancy. Your capillary blood should be frequently monitored. Your fasting blood glucose should remain between 60 and 100 mg./dl. Your blood glucose should rise no higher than 120 mg./dl. after meals.

White's Classification

In 1948, Dr. Priscilla White devised the White's classification for pregnant diabetics. This is a useful tool in predicting the outcome of diabetic pregnancies.

It classifies diabetic pregnancies according to the duration and severity of diabetes. It helps to individualize medical and obstetric care. Duration and severity of diabetes mellitus is indicated by the presence or absence of vascular complications. According to the classification, the incidence of infant (fetal) death increases in proportion to the severity of diabetes. The classification follows.

Class A: Blood glucose control is maintained by diet alone.
Class B: Onset of disease is age 20 or older and duration less than 10 years.
Class C: Onset of disease is age 10 to 19 and duration is 10 to 19 years.
Class D: Onset is less than age 10 or duration 20 years or more or evidence of vascular disease.
Class F: Diabetic nephropathy present
Class R: Malignant proliferative retinopathy
Class T: Pregnancy after renal transplantation
Class G: Multiple obstetric failures
Class H: Cardiomyopathy

Changes in Diabetes Control During Pregnancy

FIRST TRIMESTER

The first trimester refers to the first three months of pregnancy. Many women experience more insulin reactions during early pregnancy. This occurs for many reasons. If you have morning sickness with nausea and vomiting, your food intake will not match your daily insulin dose. Also, the maternal blood glucose is transferred to the fetus. In addition, your body may become unusually sensitive to insulin. Insulin reactions may come on very quickly, often without warning. Several steps can be taken to combat this. Your insulin dose may have to be decreased during these first few weeks. You may need smaller, more frequent meals. Some women have 3 meals plus 3 snacks daily. The basic rules of hypoglycemia should always be followed. These include wearing identification and carrying a simple carbohydrate on your person.

SECOND TRIMESTER

The second trimester refers to the middle three months of pregnancy. At this time, contrainsulin hormones start to be produced by the placenta. These hormones include human placental lactogen, estrogen and progesterone. In addition, maternal cortisol levels increase tremendously. Both of these factors play a role in increasing blood glucose levels. Now, the mother has to be aware of the possibility of ketoacidosis as insulin requirements rise. Starvation ketosis, too, may also develop if your caloric intake is not adequate. Ketosis must be prevented because ketones may be harmful to the development of the fetus. This can be determined if your blood glucose is normal but you are spilling acetone in your urine. It means that your body fats are being used for fuel.

THIRD TRIMESTER

The third trimester refers to the final three months of pregnancy. Now, your insulin needs may be 50 percent or greater than during your pre-pregnancy days. You may be taking a split, mixed-dose, or multiple injections. The contrainsulin hormones are secreted in extremely large amounts. In addition, insulinase, an enzyme that helps break down insulin, is also made by the placenta, adding to the difficulty in controlling your blood glucose. Throughout this third trimester as well as the entire pregnancy, proper timing of meals and medication and frequent blood testing are essential.

Pregnancy as a Developmental Stage

A psychological adjustment is necessary for all women when they learn that they are pregnant. Pregnancy can be viewed as a normal part of development. The diagnosis of diabetes can assume crisis proportions for some women. It necessitates a reordering of priorities, as well as adjusting roles and relationships within the family and society. The pregnant woman must also cope with physical and emotional changes.

If you have had diabetes for a long time, you may have had many experiences with hospital care, some of which might not have been favorable. Become educated and prepared for changes that will occur so you can avoid frustration and resistance when changes occur in your management. Previous education concerning diabetes self-management must be reinforced. Many new skills must be learned in order for you to deal successfully with both your pregnancy and diabetes.

Gestational Diabetes

Gestational diabetes is hyperglycemia which is recognized for the first time during pregnancy. The blood glucose usually reverts to normal during the postpartum period or after birth. However, one-third of gestational diabetic mothers will develop diabetes within an 8-year period of time.

Women will be tested for gestational diabetes when a mother-to-be has glycosuria on more than one occasion, is overweight or has a strong family history of diabetes. The mother will also be tested, if in the past she gave birth to an infant weighing more than 10 pounds, had a past history of unexplained stillbirths, neonatal deaths or congenital anomalies.

Testing for gestational diabetes is done through the use of an oral glucose tolerance test. This means that after drinking a sugar beverage the blood results should be no higher than the following:

| | *Blood glucose* |
Time	*mg./dl.*
Fasting	90
1 hour	170
2 hours	145
3 hours	125

If two or more values are met or exceeded, the test is considered abnormal. One to 2 percent of all pregnancies result in the development of gestational diabetes. However, if you are already at risk for developing diabetes during pregnancy, the best advice is to control your weight and intake of simple carbohydrates. Do not allow yourself to gain more weight than the recommended 25 pounds. Sometimes women are able to control their weight perfectly, but because of the stress of pregnancy, the blood glucose continues to rise. Therefore, these women have to start taking insulin, usually for the duration of pregnancy. If you have gestational diabetes, make sure you return to your ideal body weight after the baby is born and remain at that weight. Have blood tests taken regularly so that a reemergence of diabetes is not overlooked.

Management of Diabetes During Pregnancy

As your pregnancy continues, many diabetes self-management practices will be followed. Basic self-management does not change. You will still need to identify hypoglycemia and differentiate it from diabetic ketoacidosis. You must wear identification at all times stating that you have diabetes, and carry a simple-acting carbohydrate to combat hypoglycemia. You will still need to maintain preventive foot-care practices but you will need to learn new aspects of diabetes self-management.

If you have been in good control and under the care of a doctor on a regular basis, this will continue during your pregnancy. Yet it is necessary to see your doctor more regularly and receive the best prenatal care that you can. There may be some changes and differences in your labor and delivery and your baby's progress after birth. The need for your use of high-risk centers for diabetic women, the use of the team approach for diabetes maternal and child care, as well as the use of intensive care nurseries, may all be new to you.

During your pregnancy you may see an obstetrician, an endocrinologist and a perinatologist. A perinatologist is a doctor who specializes in care of women undergoing high-risk pregnancies. These doctors will assist you in the care of your pregnancy, your diabetes and any special complications that arise during this time. You may see a nurse that specializes in obstetrical care, as well as a nurse that specializes in the care of your diabetes. You will see a nutritionist since dietary intervention is an important aspect of proper pregnancy care. Be prepared for an early hospitalization, a variety of tests prior to labor and delivery, and a short separation from your infant after birth.

Your insulin dose and schedule may change. The dose may increase to double the usual amount as the pregnancy progresses. You will almost certainly take multiple injections of insulin. This does not mean that your diabetes has worsened, but rather that the insulin will work more effectively for you and the baby. Some women are using insulin pumps for the duration of the pregnancy. This technique has also been successful in maintaining normal blood glucose values. See the chapter on Insulin for more information.

During pregnancy, home blood glucose monitoring becomes essential in assessing and maintaining maternal blood glucose control. Many women are doing this 6–8 times per day. Your blood glucose control is the single most important factor in the outcome of your pregnancy. Good control is directly related to giving birth to a healthy baby and can only be established through a monitoring program. You will be testing your blood at home using blood glucose test strips, preferably in conjunction with a meter. We would strongly recommend the purchase of a blood glucose meter at this time. When you are self-monitoring, your fasting blood glucose test should be no higher than 100 mg./dl. with values never exceeding 150 mg./dl. The hemoglobin A_{1C} or glycosolated hemoglobin is an excellent reflection of blood glucose control and will be checked several times. It should stay within normal limits.

Nutrition During Pregnancy

Diet has always been the cornerstone of diabetes control but it assumes a particularly important role during pregnancy. Dietary goals include meeting the nutritional needs of the mother and the developing fetus, as well as maintaining maternal blood glucose within normal physiological limits. The pregnant woman requires approximately 300 extra calories per day. Your meal plan may be divided into 3 meals and 3 snacks. Consistency in the timing of meals as well as the nutrient composition is essential. Frequent feedings may be helpful if you experience morning sickness, or take multiple injections of insulin. Your intake of protein, vitamins and minerals will be increased. Other nutrition recommendations during pregnancy are similar to women not pregnant. This means your meal plan should include complex carbohydrates and polyunsaturated fats rather than saturated fats. If you are obese, pregnancy is not a time to lose weight. Your total weight gain should be about 22 to 27 pounds. Your nutritionist can assist you in readjusting your caloric intake.

Effects of Diabetes on the Mother-to-be

Diabetes will affect the mother-to-be's chances of having a successful pregnancy. Good maternal blood glucose control can prevent many complications. Diabetic pregnant women have a higher incidence of pre-eclampsia (characterized by high blood pressure, water retention and protein in the urine) especially if vascular complications are present. There is an increased incidence of Caesarean section. This often occurs due to the excessive size of the baby. Polyhydramnios, which refers to excess amniotic fluid, often occurs. Pregnant diabetic women may have more urinary and vaginal tract infections, and more spontaneous abortions (miscarriage).

Effect of Diabetes on the Fetus

Much research has indicated the incidence of stillbirths and congenital defects to occur in relation to poor control or diabetic ketoacidosis. In women whose pregnancy is classified as D to R, stillbirths may be a result of placental insufficiency due to vascular complications. This means the placenta may not function properly in transferring nutrients to the fetus.

An increased risk of illness to the baby is certainly due to prematurity. Respiratory distress syndrome (RDS) is directly related to prematurity. The infant's lungs have not fully developed. This may be due to the excess fetal insulin secreted in response to the excess maternal glucose. Tests are available to assess the fetus' pulmonary maturity. Congenital anomalies may also occur as in any birth. Again, it is important to stress that early intervention is necessary so that blood glucose levels before the pregnancy are well within the normal limits.

Some conditions, while not fatal, are serious and may affect the infant delivered to a diabetic mother. One of these is called macrosomia. This is excessive size for gestational age. Babies of diabetic mothers have often been described as looking as though they had stuffed themselves at a 9-month feast. The chubby appearance occurs because maternal blood glucose is easily transmitted to the fetus causing an increase in fetal insulin production. Since one role of insulin is to deposit fat, this excess insulin causes an increased deposition of fat, glycogen and protein, resulting in a baby that is heavier and larger than normal. In women with vascular complications and diabetes of long duration, macrosomia is not seen as often. Another condition that may occur to the infant is neonatal hypoglycemia. Fetal insulin levels are increased and will remain so after the delivery, yet the maternal blood glucose is no longer present. This excess insulin will cause hypoglycemia. Infants are given glucose intravenously, to prevent this.

Hyperbilirubinemia is often observed. He or she will have to be observed for jaundice and possibly receive blood transfusions. Jaundice is a yellowness of the skin. It is due to excess bilirubin in the blood. Bilirubin is the yellow color in bile, a product of the liver. This problem can be easily controlled within the hospital setting. Hypocalcemia or low blood calcium may also occur in conjunction with hypoglycemia.

Tests Prior to Labor and Delivery

You will be asked to undergo several tests prior to the delivery of your baby. Various types of monitoring will be done to evaluate the status of the baby and yourself. *Ultrasonography* measures fetal growth rate. You may have this done several times during your pregnancy. Sound waves are utilized to ascertain the size of the baby's head, the location of the placenta and the amount of the amniotic fluid present. To help determine the most appropriate time for delivery, the *Estriol* test will measure the well-being of the baby. Estriol is a hormone produced by the fetus and the maternal placenta. It can be measured after week 30 in the mother's blood and urine. Consecutive readings are compared and a significant decrease in average values indicates fetal distress. *Non-stress testing* measures the fetal heart rate in response to spontaneous movement. The acceleration of fetal heart rate with movement shows a relatively healthy fetus. An unresponsive heart rate may signify fetal distress. *Oxytocin stress testing* measures the ability of the fetus to withstand the stress of labor when uterine contractions are induced chemically. It aids in monitoring the fetal heart-rate response pattern. The *L:S Ratio* (lecithin-sphingomyelin) test measures fetal lung maturity via amniocentesis; it will determine the amount of surfactant present in the lungs. Surfactant aids in the maturation process of the baby's lungs. A ratio of 2:1, L:S, indicates the baby's lungs have matured. The appropriate ratio will decrease the likelihood of the respiratory distress syndrome being present when the baby is born. There has been some controversy in the use of the L:S ratio as the sole indicator of lung maturity. This is because diabetes may cause a delay in fetal lung maturity and RDS may still occur, despite the ratio. Therefore, some physicians will also test for the presence of another substance called phosphatidylglycerol. It seems that RDS rarely occurs with a phosphatidylglycerol value of 3 percent or more, regardless of the L:S ratio.

These tests are time-consuming and may be fatiguing to the mother-to-be. They will not be as frightening if you anticipate and understand them. All tests must be interpreted in relation to the others to determine the accurate time for delivery. During the test you will be supported by your physician and labor- and delivery-room nurses. Do not hesitate to ask questions. Remember you are giving birth to the infant and you must be fully informed on all matters.

Besides the tests that have already been described that relate to the baby, keep in mind that you will be tested throughout your pregnancy in regard to your diabetes. Your general health and well-being is important to sustain the pregnancy. You will want to avoid all complications related to diabetes. For this reason your eyes will be checked frequently for detection of diabetic retinopathy. You will also have blood tests that will determine kidney function and your blood pressure will be closely monitored to identify hypertension. You will have to be in close contact with both your physician for your diabetes and physician for care of your pregnancy during this time, as well as the rest of the diabetes team.

Labor and Delivery

Management of your delivery may include giving a small amount of your pregnancy dose of intermediate insulin in the morning and then monitoring blood glucose values closely to see the need for further insulin. I.V. insulin may be constantly infused while blood glucose levels are monitored throughout labor and delivery, although recent studies have demonstrated that most women need very little insulin during labor and delivery. I.V. glucose may be given to meet energy needs as labor and delivery progresses.

At the delivery, the neonatologist will be present to care for the infant. Your baby may need I.V. fluids (glucose) or oxygen. Your insulin requirements will drastically be reduced; you may need less insulin for a short amount of time than you did pre-pregnancy.

Breast-feeding

You may have questions about what will follow after the labor and delivery. Will you be able to breast-feed? Mothers who have diabetes may breast-feed their infants. Insulin should be taken rather than oral agents in order to control diabetes. Oral agents would be passed into the breast milk and would lower the infant's blood glucose; this does not occur with insulin. Your insulin requirements may be less while you are breast-feeding. Your diet must include an extra 500 calories above your pre-pregnancy diet. This will make up for the energy expended by milk production. Drink adequate fluids to compensate for the significant fluid losses that occur with each nursing session. Consult your physician prior to weaning the baby so appropriate insulin and dietary alterations can be made. Episodes of hypoglycemia may occur during or shortly after breast-feeding. Drinking an 8-ounce glass of milk, containing 12 grams of carbohydrate, before nursing, may help prevent this. Continue to test your blood glucose several times per day.

Contraception and Family Planning

It is important to add a note about contraception. For the woman who has diabetes, contraception is especially important. A successful pregnancy is one that is well planned and one where your diabetes is in good control. Try to talk freely with your doctor about your diabetes control before beginning a family. Obtain special counseling regarding the use of birth control devices. Oral contraceptives have been found to affect diabetes control, causing an increase in insulin requirements. Their use would be discouraged during breast-feeding, since they pass into the breast milk. The intrauterine device is still controversial in its use. It may increase the risk of infection and may not be the method of choice for you. Breast-feeding is not a method of contraception. This is an "old wives' tale." Conception can occur during this time. If you are breast-feeding you still need a method of birth control. The diaphragm may be an appropriate contraceptive device but it must be used properly and used each time you have sexual intercourse.

A healthy pregnancy with a successful outcome is a very real possibility for the woman with diabetes. Preplanning for a family, excellent prenatal care, as well as close contact with your doctor are all essential. The key to the success of the pregnancy is control of maternal blood glucose. Many women welcome the challenge of diabetes self-management and pregnancy. Frequent blood glucose monitoring, multiple injections of insulin and increased contact with the health-care team are essential aspects of proper diabetic pregnancy care.

20

Foot-Care Principles

Preventive foot care is an essential component of diabetes self-management. Your risk of developing foot problems can be greatly reduced by following principles of foot hygiene and preventive foot care. Far too many foot injuries and complications occur because the diabetic person is not educated about the importance of caring for the feet. In this aspect of diabetes self-management, the responsibility lies primarily with you as opposed to your doctor. For example, recognizing eye complications depends on your health-care provider. You cannot look into your own eyes, at the retina, to discover diabetes' effects. Yet, without tools or instruments, you can easily observe and even prevent foot complications.

The danger of possible foot problems cannot be overestimated. In the United States, 50 to 70 percent of all amputations not due to injuries occur in people with diabetes. Also, after one amputation, over 50 percent of patients have a second amputation within one to five years. These statistics are presented not to frighten you but to make you aware of how inattention to foot care can lead to serious complications. Three factors may be at work to produce foot damage: peripheral vascular disease, neuropathy and infection.

Peripheral vascular disease (PVD) is a diabetic complication and refers to an inadequate blood supply to the extremities due to blocked arteries. Blocked blood vessels may occur as part of the general process known as atherosclerosis. Peripheral neuropathy may also result in decreased sensation in the foot. The feet become more vulnerable to cuts or scrapes that may go unnoticed because of an absence of feeling. A person with poorly controlled diabetes may have

TABLE 22
VICIOUS CYCLE OF FOOT INJURIES

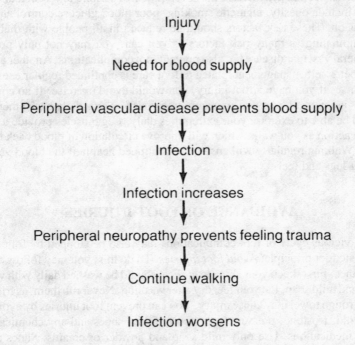

Injury

↓

Need for blood supply

↓

Peripheral vascular disease prevents blood supply

↓

Infection

↓

Infection increases

↓

Peripheral neuropathy prevents feeling trauma

↓

Continue walking

↓

Infection worsens

difficulty resisting and combating infection. Infection may result from even a minor trauma (injury) to the foot.

These three factors which result in damage to the feet can create a vicious cycle. A small trauma to the foot can result in an infection. In order to combat infection, the area demands more blood supply. If the blood supply is reduced by peripheral vascular disease, the infection will spread. Because of a lack of feeling in the foot, you may not be aware of the infection or trauma. You may continue to walk, causing more trauma. The condition will worsen, the infection will increase and blood supply will again be inadequate to fight off the infection. The vicious cycle will continue. This cycle may lead to permanent damage of the foot. (See Table 22.)

RISK FACTORS WORSEN FOOT COMPLICATIONS

The vicious cycle of foot complications can be stopped by attacking the conditions that lead to foot damage. One of the major risks is peripheral vascular disease. If peripheral vascular disease progresses to the point where blood supply to an extremity is totally decreased, tissues die and amputation may be necessary. Certain risk factors will increase the development of peripheral vascular disease. These include obesity, cigarette smoking, poor blood glucose control and hypertension. These risk factors should be reduced in all people with diabetes. By eliminating as many risk factors as you can, you may not only prevent peripheral vascular disease but also prevent foot complications. Another aspect of diabetes self-management related to foot care is continued regular exercise. Of course, if you have a foot injury, you would avoid exercise. If no complications are present, and you are examining your feet on a daily basis, then you should be able to exercise your extremities daily. Leg muscles provide a massaging action as you walk, which will improve circulation of blood back to the heart. Walking regularly will ensure the continued health of the blood vessels in your legs and feet.

AVOIDANCE OF FOOT INJURIES

The vicious cycle of foot complications may also be stopped by following one basic foot principle: *Avoid foot injuries*. To do this, you may follow a few guidelines. First, keep your skin clean. Feet should be washed daily with warm water and mild soap. Pat your feet dry after washing. Never rub them, as friction from a rough towel may cause injury. You can prevent foot injuries by avoiding heat, cold, frostbite, pressure from poorly fitting shoes and any chemicals or strong medications. Use only mild soap and powder or creams. Shoes are a necessity and should be worn, even at home and at the beach, to prevent foot injury. Secondly, a podiatrist (a specialist in foot care) should be consulted for properly fitting shoes. If you have recurring foot problems, customized therapeutic shoes may be the answer. If your podiatrist prescribes special shoes, it is essential that you wear them. A third preventive factor is nail care. Avoid cutting your own nails whenever possible. Filing nails is preferable to cutting them. If the nails are too thick to be comfortably filed, they should be trimmed by a podiatrist. Finally, if you are unable to see a podiatrist to cut your nails, soften your nails by soaking them in warm water for about ten minutes before cutting them. Clean gently around the nails with a soft brush. Do not rush the procedure. Use a good light and cut your nails slowly, following the natural line of the nail. Do not dig into the corners and do not attempt to cut your nails too short.

Preventive foot care involves following the guidelines listed below for proper care of your feet. Always wear shoes or slippers, whether at home, at the beach or in your backyard. Never go barefoot. Always wear shoes that fit properly. Wear boots for only short periods of time. When you purchase a new pair of shoes, break them in slowly and carefully.

Avoid foot soaks. Although soaking the feet for long periods of time may seem comfortable, it is damaging. Feet should be washed with a mild soap and patted dry with a soft towel. Use powder and lotion appropriately. Don't keep your feet too moist or too dry. Emollients are needed to keep the skin soft and free from dryness. Emollients include lanolin, vegetable oils, mineral oils and Vaseline. Simple baby powders can be used to combat perspiration of the feet. Avoid plastic shoes, nylon hose, rubber or artificial materials that will cause your feet to perspire. Cotton socks will absorb moisture, not trap it.

Never apply heat of any kind to the feet. Use lukewarm water when bathing. Avoid hot-water bottles and heating pads, to prevent accidental burns. If peripheral neuropathy is present, you will not feel a burn when you apply heat to the feet. Keep your feet warm by wearing socks.

Consult your doctor if any foot injuries arise. Any pain, redness or swelling should be brought to your doctor's attention. Pain in your calves during exercise should also be reported to your doctor. It may indicate inadequate circulation. Avoid any type of "bathroom surgery." Bathroom surgery refers to your use of corn-remover remedies, scraping calluses off with metal tools or using razor blades. If you feel a special treatment is needed, it is your responsibility to contact a health-care team member. In this case, arrange a visit to the podiatrist. Avoid using strong, burning or colored medications on the feet. This is important for two reasons. Harsh medications may burn the feet. Secondly, colored medications will cover up a developing infection and prevent you from noticing it.

Many people, who have no foot problems and do not have diabetic neuropathy, find this emphasis on foot care difficult to understand. It may be safer for you to assume that sensation is poor in your feet. In this way you can engage in preventive care to avoid foot injuries. You will also learn good habits that will last you a lifetime.

Be aware of habits that interfere with circulation to your feet. One common habit is crossing the legs at the knee. The popliteal artery lies behind your kneecap. If you cross your right leg over your left leg, you block that artery in the right leg and decrease circulation toward your feet. Although old habits are hard to break, avoid crossing your legs. Women should avoid tight pantyhose, panty girdles, garters and knee socks. Examine your legs after taking off undergarments. Are there lines or indentations where knee socks or a girdle has been? These garments may be too tight and decrease your circulation. With men, high knee socks may result in the same problem.

DAILY SELF-INSPECTION

Even if you follow principles of foot care, foot problems can develop. The only way you can discover an injury is by daily self-inspection of your feet. In no way does this replace the role of the podiatrist in foot-care management.

Rather, it helps you discover a foot problem and alerts you to contact the podiatrist. Checking your feet can easily be incorporated into your daily hygiene after a bath or shower. It can also be a separate activity prior to retiring at night. It should take an average of two minutes to examine both feet; that's two minutes of prevention.

How do you examine your feet? When you are inspecting and assessing the condition of your feet, ask yourself the following questions:

1. Are my toenails filed (straight across, not diagonal at the corners)?
2. Are my feet clean? (How about the soles?)
3. Does the color of my feet look O.K. (not too pale, not too red)? Use a light if necessary. If you are overweight and cannot see your feet, use a mirror to help examine your feet. Ask someone to help you if necessary.
4. Does my skin look dry? Is it wet with perspiration? (Hopefully, neither will occur if you are using lotion and powder correctly.)
5. Is there any swelling? (Elevate those feet whenever you can!)
6. Is the skin broken anywhere? (Check the soles again.)
7. Do I have any numbness or tingling in my feet?
8. Do I have any painful areas?
9. Are my feet still sensitive to changes in temperature? (Can I feel the cold bathroom tile when I come out of the shower?)
10. Are my shoes sturdy and in good condition? (You need good support.)
11. Are my shoes made of leather? (Your feet need to "breathe.")
12. Do my shoes fit me well? (Any pressure points will lead to irritations.)
13. Am I wearing socks or stockings that are loose enough? (You need to keep that circulation moving.)

An inspection can be completed as easily as completing the questions above. Be aware of the importance of looking at your feet and shoes on a daily basis. If problems arise, know the team member to contact, your podiatrist. Remember, the podiatrist is specially trained not only to provide you with foot care but also to educate you in the proper care of your feet. Use him to learn about proper care of your feet. Review these situations that call for notifying your podiatrist.

NOTIFY YOUR PODIATRIST IF THE FOLLOWING OCCUR:

1. Cuts or scrapes that do not heal
2. Redness or swelling spreading along the foot
3. Ingrown, infected toenails
4. Trauma to the foot
5. Discoloration of the foot
6. Loss of sensation in the foot
7. Any pain, redness or swelling of the foot

Like all persons with diabetes, you must take special care of your feet because you have a higher risk of developing peripheral vascular disease, peripheral neuropathy and infection. Several risk factors causing peripheral vascular disease can be controlled. These include obesity, cigarette smoking, blood glucose and blood pressure. Prevent injury to your feet by keeping them clean and avoid exposing them to heat or cold. Wear well-fitting shoes and avoid any type of bathroom surgery. Inspect your feet on a daily basis to make sure they are free from injury. Finally, see your podiatrist as needed.

21
Vacation and Travel Tips

Travel can be viewed as a challenge to your self-management program. Some say that diabetes is a problem that is always present and one can never vacation away from the disease. This is true, but vacationing does not have to be viewed negatively. You will be able to vacation with diabetes successfully if you incorporate a few basic principles of diabetes management into your vacation plans. This chapter will be divided into three sections, outlining plans you must make before you leave, travel considerations while en route and potential problem solving after you arrive at your destination.

BEFORE YOU LEAVE

Think through your travel plans and determine how diabetes may affect them. Deal with problems prior to leaving home. Consulting a guidebook to foreign countries may help you to anticipate new situations. An important first step in advance planning is to see your doctor. Ask him how you should adjust your medication and testing techniques while you are away. Also, ask for a letter describing your diabetes treatment and for a prescription for insulin and syringes. By discussing with your doctor potential problems that could arise, you can prevent them from developing.

Immunizations

Your doctor may suggest that you receive certain immunizations if you are traveling to foreign countries. This can be done at least three to four weeks before your departure. Immunizations may cause some physical discomfort, and the reaction may upset your blood glucose control. If you have questions regarding whether immunizations are necessary, write for "Immunization Information for International Travel," available from the Superintendent of Documents, U.S. Government Printing Office, Washington, DC 20402.

Individual Medical History and Prescriptions

Prepare a written medical history as part of your advance planning. You should always know your medical history, whether or not you are vacationing. Your medical history can be written down and carried with you on vacation. This would include medical conditions that you have, allergies and your use of medications. The medical history is an important document and should be stored safely, with your prescriptions. Taking along prescriptions will eliminate any problems if your medicine or supplies are lost.

Supplies

How do you prepare for your daily diabetes routine when you are away? A key to any preparation is obtaining extra supplies. Take along extra insulin, syringes, alcohol swabs, oral hypoglycemics and urine- or blood-testing equipment. A good rule is to take twice as much as you would normally need.

In order to calculate how much insulin you need for your travels, you must know the amount of units that you take per day. Divide the total amount of insulin in the bottle by your daily dose in order to see how many days the insulin bottle will last. Then double this number and take along the appropriate extra supply of insulin. In case you run out or lose your insulin while you are away, you can obtain insulin all over the world. Foreign labels may have to be deciphered. In the "More Useful Information" section, under "Travel Tips," you will find a list of insulin availability throughout the world. The use of Regular insulin during illness may be necessary when you are away. Take Regular insulin with you in order to be prepared for an emergency. Remember to bring twice the amount you need of your oral hypoglycemics.

Plan to bring extra urine-testing supplies with you. Most people find that while traveling they prefer to use a strip or stick method, such as Tes-Tape, Diastix, Ketodiastix or Ketostix. Clinitest tablets can also be obtained in foil-wrapped packages. These make travel easy. Continue to monitor your blood glucose in foreign countries. Both the Ames Company and Bio-Dynamics manufacture portable home blood glucose monitoring equipment.

Emergency Resources

Before you leave home, you should be aware of the resources that are available for emergency help. It may make you feel more comfortable about traveling when you realize that diabetes is an international disease. The International Diabetes Federation is located at 10 Queen Anne Street, London, W1M OBD, England. Telephone: London 01-637-3644. By writing to the IDF you can obtain information about foreign insulins as well as a list of English-speaking diabetologists. It will also provide you with a list of international diabetes associations. International travelers may obtain a doctor through Intermedic, 777 Third Avenue, New York, NY 10017. Membership in Intermedic entitles you to a copy of a directory of participating doctors in over 200 foreign cities. The American embassy or consulate in the country where you are traveling can also help provide you with necessary information about medical resources. Your hotel, tour guide or travel agent will help you in obtaining the address and telephone number of the American embassy.

If you are traveling in the United States, your local affiliate of the American Diabetes Association will give you the telephone number and address of affiliates and chapters located in various areas of the country. You may also write to the American Diabetes Association, 2 Park Avenue, New York, NY 10016, for help in this matter.

A list of emergency phrases in foreign languages that deal with diabetes is helpful. Refer to the "More Useful Information" section, under "Travel Tips," for a listing of emergency phrases such as "I have diabetes," "Please get me a doctor" and "Sugar or orange juice, please." These are translated into French, Spanish, German and Italian. Words such as "Coca-Cola" are international in their use. If you are experiencing hypoglycemia, you can easily ask for this. Think of this book as a resource, too. Take it with you when you travel so that you may refer to specific topics.

In summary, before you leave, you will want to speak with your doctor, plan in advance for the materials and extra supplies that you need and know the resources that are available to you when you travel. See the travel checklist which follows.

TRAVEL CHECKLIST

1. Insulin
2. Syringes
3. Oral drugs
4. Urine-testing equipment
5. Alcohol swabs

6. Extra snacks
7. Prescription for insulin and syringes
8. Antidiarrheal or stomach medication
9. Good walking shoes
10. Instant glucose
11. Regular insulin
12. Identification tag
13. Extra pair of glasses
14. Glucagon
15. Self-monitoring equipment

Travel by Car

When traveling by car, keep extra snacks with you to avoid hypoglycemia, because you may be geographically separated from food. Be prepared for the possibility of your car breaking down. Try to maintain a time schedule for eating meals and snacks. If you are driving, it is important that you avoid hypoglycemia by eating at regular mealtimes, avoiding fatigue and keeping carbohydrates in the car. These can include graham crackers, sugar packets, fruit or fruit juices. The amount of food you take depends on how long you will be traveling. If you are driving, and attempting to meet a deadline, this may be a source of stress. Try to have rest periods, with stops every one or two hours. At this time, get out of the car and walk around to improve circulation. Try to avoid the stress of meeting a travel deadline when vacationing by car.

Do not keep insulin or any medication in the glove compartment, in the trunk or on the dashboard where it will be exposed to high temperatures. Store the insulin in the interior of the car. Expensive travel kits are not necessary. Any well-supported small travel case that you have at home can be used to safely store your insulin supply, syringes and alcohol swabs. Insulin does not have to be refrigerated, but it should not be exposed to undesirable temperatures.

Travel by Plane

When traveling by airplane, there are certain details that must be preplanned. You may request a diabetic meal beforehand. You may wish to inform the flight attendant that you have diabetes. This may help you later if you need any special assistance, such as treatment for hypoglycemia. Carry your own snack in case of a delayed flight or mealtime. This is an example of being in control of your disease and reducing any stress that may be associated with traveling. You then do not have to depend on anyone else to make your travel time pleasant. In an airplane, if you need to give yourself an injection, inject only half as much air in the bottle as you do normally. Cabin air pressure is lower than ground air pressure, and not as much pressure is needed inside the bottle to draw out insulin.

Insulin should not be stored in the baggage compartment of an airplane. First, there is the risk of having luggage lost. Second, luggage areas are kept at near-freezing temperatures. Insulin should not be frozen. So travel with your insulin supplies stored with you in a carry-on case. In fact, keep all medication with you.

Changing Time Zones

If you are traveling by air and changing time zones, you may need to adjust your insulin dosage. Discuss insulin adjustments necessary for travel with your doctor. When traveling from west to east the day becomes shorter. Travel from east to west causes the day to become longer. Flying north and south does not interfere with time zones as drastically. For example, a trip from New York to Paris will shorten the day by six hours. A trip from Paris to New York will lengthen the day by six hours. Large insulin doses such as those above 20 units may overlap if you are traveling from west to east and adjustments must be made. A good rule to follow is to lower the insulin dose on the day you arrive at your destination by the portion of the day lost. For example, if you go from New York to London, you may arrive after a night flight at 10 A.M., when it would be 4 A.M. at home. You have shortened your day by six hours. You are losing 25 percent of the day while en route to the east. Therefore, you would take 25 percent less of your normal insulin dosage on the day that you arrive. For example, 25 percent of 40 units is 10 units; 40 units minus 10 units is 30 units. You would take 30 units that day. This applies to NPH and Lente insulin. When dealing with Regular insulin, if your blood glucose results are normal, you may be able to eliminate the Regular insulin entirely. Check this with your doctor.

If you are flying west, you are adding extra hours and may need an extra dose of Regular insulin upon arrival. You may determine whether you need additional insulin by self-monitoring and following your doctor's advice. Many doctors prefer to have their patients test their blood while en route and supplement accordingly with small amounts of Regular insulin. If you take oral hypoglycemics, you are less likely to have problems with overlap. If you are taking oral hypoglycemics twice daily and traveling to the east, it may be possible for you to skip the first dose of your medication when you arrive.

Travel by Bus or Train

When traveling by bus or train, be prepared for the same delays that may occur with other forms of transportation. A delay in public transportation may cause you to have hypoglycemia. Stand up and walk frequently while on a long bus or train trip to improve your circulation. Here, too, travel with your insulin supply stored with you. If you are traveling to places where the temperature will be well above 70° F., use insulated bags to keep your insulin cool.

Travel by Boat

It is not necessary to arrange for special meals in advance when taking a cruise. The vast amount of food served on a cruise may be a temptation to anyone on a restricted diet, but many of the foods that are presented would be available in a diabetic meal plan. Choices must be made according to what you are able to integrate into your meal plan. Portion control techniques are a most important strategy in order not to gain weight. On a cruise you may suffer seasickness. Ask your doctor for a prescription for Bonine, Dramamine, Marezine or Transderm-V. These medications may prevent you from experiencing constant nausea and vomiting.

Continue Testing

If travel to your destination takes more than three to four hours, testing must be incorporated into your travel schedule. Sticks or strips for urine testing may be convenient. You may make a quick trip to the bathroom on an airplane and pass a test stick under a stream of urine. If you have become adept at blood glucose monitoring, the fingerstick procedure can be done in seconds. If you must take an insulin injection while you are traveling and are concerned about drawing up the insulin from the vial while in a moving vehicle, you may fill your syringe prior to travel. You should not prefill your syringe for any longer than a twenty-four-hour period.

No matter how you are traveling (car, bus, airplane or cruise), the basic principles remain the same. Preplan, take adequate supplies of equipment with you and prevent hypoglycemia by carrying extra snacks. In these ways, you can easily incorporate diabetes into your travel plans.

AFTER YOU ARRIVE

When you have arrived at your destination, you will probably want to see as much as you can in a short period of time. Avoid overexertion. If strenuous exercise is planned, rearrange your diabetes routine by decreasing your insulin dosage or increasing your food intake prior to exercise. Protect yourself against exhaustion while sightseeing by taking adequate rests. If it has taken you a long time to reach your destination, the first twenty-four hours may be better spent resting and "catching up" than in overactivity.

"Don't Drink the Water"

This has become a standard joke in certain places such as Mexico, Central and South America, Asia and Africa. The joke will not seem funny if you are one of the unfortunate individuals who contract "turista" or "Montezuma's revenge" (prolonged diarrhea). Ask your doctor about the advisability of taking medication to prevent traveler's diarrhea. Avoid water and ice cubes, milk products, ice cream, cheeses and cream sauces. Be wary of any vegetables and fruits that you do not peel. If turista does strike, you may feel nauseous and vomit or have diarrhea, which will interfere with nutritional requirements of diabetes. Have your doctor prescribe medications such as Kaopectate and Lomotil. Follow sick-day rules and drink tea, clear soups, or eat bland foods such as rice. Make sure that you eat and drink sweetened foods and liquids to ensure that you are taking in enough carbohydrates. These include bottled Coke or ginger ale. Continue to take your insulin as prescribed. See the following nutrition tips for the tropics.

NUTRITION TIPS FOR TRAVEL TO THE TROPICS

1. Avoid fresh milk.
2. Avoid untreated water and ice.
3. Avoid raw freshwater crabs or clams.
4. Avoid rich or creamy sauces.
5. Avoid unpeelable fruits and uncooked vegetables and lettuce.
6. Avoid raw or undercooked freshwater fish and rare meat.

Dietary Concerns

Another important aspect of travel is the cultural differences in dining times. In many European and Latin American countries, dinner does not begin until 9 or 10 P.M. You do not have to miss the experience of dining late while traveling. Instead, refer to Chapter 14 for specific guidelines. Another dietary concern during a vacation is the use of alcohol. Many people say that they drink alcohol only during a festive occasion such as a vacation. If you do not usually drink alcohol in other settings, be careful to limit yourself to only one drink, particularly if you are not eating at the same time. Remember the hypoglycemic effect of alcohol. Avoid sweetened tropical drinks. Their potency is often disguised by their sweet taste. Instead, choose a white wine spritzer or a tall scotch and water.

Importance of Diet

While on vacation, it is important to maintain your weight and not go far off your diet. Set a goal of maintaining your weight rather than losing weight at vacation time. It may help to review your Exchange System prior to leaving home. Ask questions in restaurants about food preparation. Use portion control and behavior modification techniques in an effort to maintain your weight. You may not know how *arroz con pollo* fits in on an Exchange List, but you should be able to tell the difference between an average and a large portion. While on vacation, do not skip meals. When traveling, many people follow a modified American plan, with breakfast and dinner included, at their hotel. This may lead to skipping lunch. If you take insulin, it is important that you eat your meals consistently and strive for the same timing and nutrient composition of foods that you follow at home.

You may find that U-100 insulin is not always available when you are traveling in foreign countries. Many foreign insulins are available in U-40 and U-80 concentrations. The number of units that you need to control your blood glucose does not change when a change in concentration is made. If you need 40 units of U-100 insulin daily, you will need 40 units of U-80 or U-40 insulin. The only thing that will change is the amount of fluid. This means that the syringe you use to draw up the insulin must correspond to the concentration of insulin that you're using. For example, if you have to switch to U-40 insulin, make sure you obtain U-40 syringes so that you will draw up your dose accurately. Remember, the 1 cc. of the syringe you're using must contain the same number of units as the 1 cc. of the insulin you are using.

Foot and Skin Care

Proper foot care is essential during vacation times. As part of your preplanning, you should have broken in your shoes properly and provided for an extra pair of walking shoes to take with you. Do not overdo walking when you first begin your vacation or you may develop blisters or a foot ulcer. These will cause physical harm as well as prevent you from enjoying the rest of your vacation. If you do develop a blister, do not break it. Unbroken skin helps to protect you from developing an infection. Do not walk without shoes, even on the beach. Follow foot-care principles on vacation as you would at home.

It is also important to protect your skin. Avoid getting a sunburn. Think of your skin as the most important protective organ of your body. Sunburn may also lead to dehydration, which may affect your blood glucose control. Use a sunscreen containing PABA (paramino benzoic acid). This will prevent burning from the rays of the sun, particularly when it is used properly and reapplied after swimming. Limit your exposure to the sun so that you will tan gradually.

Prepare for vacation by preplanning for situations before you leave, while en route and after you arrive. Before you leave, ask your doctor about medication adjustments and obtain prescriptions for medication. Get necessary immunizations and extra supplies for self-monitoring. While en route, store your insulin with you, learn how to adjust insulin when traveling to different time zones and preplan your meals for transportation delays. After you arrive at your destination, avoid overexertion and prevent foot problems. Try to stick to your meal plan and preplan to prevent hypoglycemia. Bon voyage and stay healthy!

22

Research

F. G. Banting and C. H. Best, in 1921, were able to recover insulin from the pancreas on a budget that only paid for the dogs used in their experiments. By contrast, the questions that must now be answered concerning diabetes require space-age technology (and consequently space-age funding). Although pharmaceutical firms and private foundations (including the ADA and JDF) contribute funds, the bulk of funding for diabetes research comes from the federal government, through the National Institutes of Health (NIH). This federal agency conducts research in its own facilities (intramural) and awards grants to investigators throughout the United States (extramural). The commitment and wealth of the United States government has made us the world leader in biomedical research. The extent of federal funding may be appreciated by the fact that in 1979 the National Institute of Arthritis, Diabetes and Digestive and Kidney Diseases (NIADDKD) had $100 million allocated to research related to diabetes.

Federal funding is legislated by Congress and is therefore subject to public influence. While the NIADDKD has a budget of $100 million, the budget of the National Cancer Institute approaches $1 billion. It is vital for diabetic individuals to be politically active to influence legislators to provide funding for diabetes research. The current level of funding resulted from such pressure, which led to the passage of the National Diabetes Mellitus Research and Education Act of 1974. This act resulted in an expanded and coordinated national diabetes research effort. There are two committees (the Trans-NIH Diabetes Mellitus Coordinating Committee and the Diabetes Mellitus Inter-Agency Coordinating Committee) that are responsible for coordination of diabetes research. The Trans-NIH DMCC coordinates research in diabetes for the NIH. The DMCC is responsible for coordination of diabetes research within the federal government. The scope of its responsibility is shown below. In this chapter, the major areas of federal support will be summarized to provide an overview of current diabetes research.

The Diabetes Mellitus Coordinating Committee (DMCC) is responsible for coordinating diabetes research. The following government departments are involved with the DMCC:

Health Care Financing Administration
Food and Drug Administration
National Institute of General Medical Sciences
Social Security Administration
Center for Disease Control
Division of Research Resources
National Center for Health Statistics
National Center for Health Services Research
National Eye Institute
National Institute of Child Health and Human Development
National Institute of Allergy and Infectious Diseases
National Heart, Lung and Blood Institute
National Naval Medical Center
Health Resources and Services Administration
Veterans Administration
National Institute of Dental Research
National Institute of Mental Health
U.S. Department of Agriculture
National Institute of Neurological and Communicative
    Disorders and Stroke
National Institute on Aging
National Institute of Environmental Health Science

Before discussing the particulars of this coordinated attack on diabetes, the distinction should be made between basic and clinical research. Basic biological research involves the investigation of the anatomy, physiology and biochemistry of living things, frequently at the cellular level. Clinical research involves the investigation of a disease process or its treatment in human subjects. It is often difficult for the uninformed to understand why research should be supported on the cellular level. For example, why study receptors on the cell membrane? The answer is simple. Clinical research is the application of basic research findings to human subjects. Without basic research, there would be no advances in relevant applied clinical research. It was basic research that identified the lack of insulin from the pancreas as the cause of diabetes. Without this knowledge, insulin could not have been extracted and used to save the lives of insulin-dependent diabetic patients. A more recent example is the basic cellular research on recombinant DNA (genetic engineering). These basic studies led to technological advances that have resulted in the production of human insulin.

The next part of this chapter will review some of the research goals and/or accomplishments of various units of the DMCC. It is important to remember that each unit has various functions and responsibilities for many different diseases. Therefore, only those functions that are related to diabetes will be described here.

The National Institute of Child Health and Human Development is carrying on research on the prevention of diabetes. It is investigating gestational diabetes, infant mortality and congenital defects and the risk factors for the development of diabetes in infancy. It is also studying the genetic and immunological aspects of diabetes in childhood. Investigations are under way to study metabolic fuels and how they affect fetal development. Fetal lung maturation in diabetic pregnancy is under study to determine why infants of diabetic mothers have a higher incidence of RDS (respiratory distress syndrome).

The National Institute of Dental Research is investigating dental complications and diabetes. Specific areas of investigation include periodontal disease in children and the relationship of periodontal disease to the immune system. This institute studies the increased susceptibility to and the microbiology of periodontal disease in diabetics, and the greater frequency of cleft palate in the children of diabetic mothers. Peripheral orofacial (pertaining to the mouth) neuropathies, such as loss of salivation, taste and smell, are also under study.

The National Eye Institute is studying the cause and treatment of diabetes-induced eye problems. The institute is examining factors influencing blood flow and edema of the retina, as well as risk factors for microangiopathy. It is also investigating basement membrane thickening and the metabolic pathways for sugar alcohols. This institute supported studies that demonstrated the usefulness of photocoagulation for retinopathy.

The National Heart, Lung and Blood Institute supports studies on diabetes and the heart and blood vessels. It is probing accelerated plaque formation in diabetes and the contribution of diabetes to congestive heart failure. It is also examining the interrelationship between obesity, diabetes and hypertension.

The National Institute of Arthritis, Diabetes and Digestive and Kidney Diseases plans, develops and implements comprehensive national diabetes programs. It has supported research on the structure and function of pancreatic hormones and enzymes and the genetic nature of diabetes. It is also supporting a variety of lines of investigation that have successful islet cell transplants as a long-term goal.

Alternative delivery routes for insulin are under study. Appropriate computer programs for insulin pumps and refinement of the present pumps to make them safer, more effective and more reliable are under investigation. The Division of Research Resources is also involved in the area of islet cell transplants. It is also developing clinical studies of diet and exercise regimens for the Type II diabetic person.

The National Institute of General Medical Sciences supports studies on the effect of drugs on carbohydrate metabolism and the release of pancreatic hormones. The interaction of hypoglycemic drugs with other drugs is also under study. It is interested in the development of new oral medications for diabetes.

The Alcohol Abuse and Mental Health Administration acts to decrease psychosocial and behavioral problems associated with diabetes. It is examining individual and family coping patterns, adaptation to the diagnosis of diabetes in children and various types of stress on diabetic individuals. In addition, it is probing the effect of acute and chronic alcohol intake on the pancreas and various phases of glucose metabolism in rats. The psychological and endocrinological aspects of diabetes in those with and without sexual difficulties are also under study.

The National Institute of Neurological and Communicative Disorders and Stroke fosters and coordinates research into the cause, prevention, diagnosis and treatment of neurological and communicative disorders. This institute is studying diabetic neuropathy. The effect of the nervous system on the pancreas and the role of the central nervous system in regulating nutrient balance are also being studied.

Overall future plans for diabetes research as outlined by the DMCC include:

Improving insulin delivery services to improve glucose control
Transplanting pancreatic islet cells
Obtaining new knowledge of the causes of insulin-dependent and non-insulin-dependent diabetes
Learning more about how insulin regulates glucose metabolism
Learning more about the secretion, action and regulation of hormones
Learning more about nutrition
Learning more about the prevention and treatment of obesity

LIKELY ADVANCES FOR THE FUTURE

Major advances in basic research are unpredictable. They often result from a stroke of genius or just plain luck. However, the application of basic findings to clinical uses involves technological development and is more predictable.

Although it is difficult to be precise concerning how long it will be before these applications are available, the following will attempt to predict the future of diabetes research.

Human insulin is now being mass-produced, using recombinant DNA technology. This will provide an endless supply of insulin. It is likely that human insulin will reduce or eliminate the problems of insulin allergy and lipodystrophy and may decrease immunological insulin resistance.

Improved methods of insulin delivery will become available. The devices used will be miniaturized and safe; closed-loop delivery systems will be developed. Unfortunately, even the closed-loop system does not perfectly simulate normal insulin secretion. This is why islet cell transplants are desirable. A major problem with the transplants involves the drugs that must be used to suppress the immune system so that the islets will not be rejected by the body. Containers for the islet cells will be developed that permit insulin to be secreted but do not allow the larger molecules (antibodies) that damage the islets to enter.

Several advances in drug therapy may be anticipated. There is evidence that sulfonylureas lower blood glucose in part by an effect on insulin receptors; other drugs will be developed that increase the number of receptors or the affinity for insulin. Aldose reductase inhibitors will be available. These inhibitors prevent the accumulation of sugar alcohols in the tissues of the eyes and nerves and may reduce the incidence of diabetic microangiopathy. Further understanding of the accelerated atherosclerosis that occurs in diabetes should answer the question whether it is beneficial to take drugs such as aspirin which inhibit thromboxane release by platelets. Thromboxanes may cause abnormal clumping in platelets, an early step in the formation of an atherosclerotic plaque. Second-generation sulfonylureas will be marketed.

Other advances may not be forthcoming in the next decade but are possible by the end of this century. The virus or viruses responsible for Type I diabetes may be identified and a vaccine may be developed to prevent insulin-dependent diabetes. In 1982, the amazing feat was accomplished of chemically analyzing the human gene that produces insulin. The gene was found to be biochemically abnormal in patients with diabetes. Genetic engineering may in the future provide the means for gene transplantation to eliminate the susceptibility to either Type I or Type II diabetes. Thus it is possible to foresee the prevention and elimination of diabetes mellitus. The time frame for these developments, however, is certainly in excess of ten years and may be much longer.

As an informed person, you should begin to critically evaluate research findings. The media will present you with a variety of research findings in every area of diabetes. Be aware of misleading press releases and misleading claims of cures for diabetes. It is in the nature of the media to try to attract readers or viewers; reporting may be fragmentary, inaccurate and sensational. The great interest of the public in "medical breakthroughs" has resulted in media coverage of scientific meetings and arrangements for delivery of medical journals to the press prior to their arrival at your doctor's office. It is likely that you will read a synopsis of an article from the prestigious *New England Journal of Medicine* in the New York *Times* before your doctor has received his copy of the *Journal*! You may become aware of the names of people who are presently doing *credible* research in the area of diabetes. You can find these names when you read magazines such as *Diabetes Forecast,* a publication of the American Diabetes Association. This magazine will provide you with accurate information.

When you begin to analyze material presented in newspapers, on TV or radio or in magazines, you must also observe whether the number of persons studied is substantial. Conclusions based on just a few patients may not be valid. Make sure the research methods do not seem outlandish. Knowing the institution where the research was done is sometimes helpful in deciding whether an article is credible. Look at the authors and institutions conducting the research and where the research was published. Is it published in a worthwhile medical journal or is it a small filler in a newspaper column? This is all part of critically evaluating medical literature, as well as not believing everything you read just because it is in print. In addition, you should also ask the opinion of your doctor or your local ADA affiliate before you accept the latest "breakthrough." Never change your diabetes self-management program on the basis of information derived from the media without consulting your doctor or health-care team member.

Insulin was discovered over half a century ago; the hope for advances in the treatment and eventual prevention and cure of diabetes has never been brighter. Nonetheless, it is important that your expectations remain realistic and that you learn how to obtain accurate information. Subscribe to *Diabetes Forecast*. Discuss media reports with your doctor. Support research by fund raising for your diabetes affiliate and by influencing your congressmen to support diabetes research.

23

Health Resources and Your

Personal Health

This chapter will review a variety of diverse information regarding your health care. You are part of a comprehensive health-care system. The purpose of this chapter is to increase your awareness of health-care delivery and the health-care team.

PHILOSOPHY OF SELF-CARE

Self-care has been described as the process by which a lay person functions on his own behalf to engage in activities to promote health. This usually involves health maintenance, disease prevention, self-treatment and participation in the use of professional services. It involves a decision-making process as choices of treatment options are made. Self-care builds confidence in your own ability to handle health-related problems. Through it, your relationship with the health-care system will change.

WHAT IS THE HEALTH-CARE DELIVERY SYSTEM?

The health-care delivery system is made up of health-care professionals and organizations that are providers of care. In the past, the health-care delivery system focused primarily on illness. The system has recently become more health-oriented at the same time that it tries to meet the special needs of the ill. The professionals making up the health-care team are a group of people working together for a common purpose. Each member of the team works to provide quality care for you, the consumer. Each individual member has a specific role. You are the central player in the health-care team. Patient-centered care is a new concept. In the past, due to demands of institutions, individual patients' needs were sometimes sacrificed. Now, such concepts as primary nursing (the assignment of the same nurse to the same patient for the duration of his hospital stay) and patient education have changed that. You are able to collaborate with the health-care professional in determining your health goals.

WHO MAKES UP THE TEAM?

You will meet a variety of people in the health-care system if you are hospitalized. The health-care team is composed of physicians, dentists, nurses, nutritionists, physicians' assistants, pharmacists, social workers, podiatrists, laboratory technicians and other trained individuals.

THE PHYSICIAN

A physician (doctor) has a medical degree and oversees your health-care program. He or she has been trained in the diagnosis and treatment of illness. A physician's education begins with receiving a bachelor's degree. He then attends medical school for four years. Before graduation from medical school he will serve as an extern. An externship or clinical clerkship is a time period when a medical student receives training in a hospital. Upon completion of medical school, the student receives his medical degree (M.D.). He then becomes an intern. An intern is a doctor who practices medicine under the supervision of hospital staff for a year after graduation from medical school. This is done to gain experience and to meet specific requirements for state licensure. This is also called the first postgraduate year or PGY-1. During this year, the intern may take his licensing exam. This license means that a specific agency of the state government has granted permission to practice medicine within the jurisdiction of that state. With today's expansion of technical knowledge, it is unusual for a physician to enter a practice after completion of only one postgraduate year. The intern may continue as a resident and enter his second and third postgraduate years, participating in patient care under the supervision of practitioners in clinical areas. A residency may last from three to seven years, depending on the chosen specialty.

A licensed physician may also meet specific requirements to become board-certified in his specialty or subspecialty. A specialist is a physician who limits practice to certain diseases, to the diseases of a specific organ or to a certain type of therapy. Each specialty, with its required training, is listed below. Each specialty has a specific board certification that a physician may acquire. A specialty board grants recognition to the physician after predetermined qualifications have been met and an examination has been passed. Board certification is not licensure. A physician may practice a specialty even if he is not board-certified.

MEDICAL SPECIALTIES

Allergist/Immunologist Must have 3 years of training in internal medicine or pediatrics plus 2 years of training in allergy/immunology to diagnose and treat allergies and diseases of the immune system

Anesthesiologist Must have 4 years of training to render patients insensible to pain during surgery

Colon-Rectal Surgeon Must have 4 years of general surgery and additional training of no less than 1 year in colon-rectal surgery

Dermatologist Must have 2 to 4 years of training to treat diseases of the skin

Family Practitioner Must have 1–3 years of training to provide comprehensive health maintenance and medical care to the entire family

Internist Must have 3 years of training to give comprehensive care to adults

Neurologist Must complete 1 year of approved training, then another 3 years to diagnose and treat diseases of the brain and nervous system

Neurosurgeon Must have 1 year of training in general surgery and an additional 5 years of specialized training to perform surgery on the brain and nervous system

Nuclear Medicine Specialist Must have 2 or more years of preparatory residency training and an additional 2 years in nuclear medicine to provide diagnostic, therapeutic and investigational uses of radionuclides

Obstetrician/Gynecologist Must have 3 years of training to diagnose and treat diseases of the female, including treatment during pregnancy

Ophthalmologist Must have 3 years of training to diagnose and treat diseases of the eyes

Orthopedic Surgeon Must have 5 years of training to perform surgery on the locomotion structures of the body, especially the skeleton, joints, muscles and fascia

Otolaryngologist Must have 5 years of training to treat diseases of the ear and upper and lower respiratory tract

Pathologist Must have 3 years of training to study tissues removed during surgery or autopsy

Pediatrician Must have 3 years of training to diagnose and treat diseases in children

Physical Medicine and Rehabilitation Specialist Must have 3 years of training to provide care in the clinical and diagnostic use of physical procedures and aspects of medical rehabilitation

Plastic Surgeon Must have 3 years of general surgery, then 2 years of extra training to provide functional and aesthetic treatment for congenital (from birth) or acquired defects

Preventive Medicine Specialist Must have 3 years of training to provide care in the prevention of the occurrence of mental and physical illness

Psychiatrist Must complete 1 year of approved training and then another 3 years to diagnose, treat and prevent mental illness

Radiologist Must have 4 years of training to use radioactive substances and X rays in the diagnosis and treatment of diseases

Surgeon, General Must have at least 5 years of surgical training to deal with manual and operative procedures to correct problems and repair injuries

Thoracic Surgeon Must complete the requirements of the American Board of Surgery and 2 additional years to treat disorders of the lungs, esophagus, diaphragm and cardiovascular system

Urologist Must have 5 years of training to diagnose and treat diseases of the urogenital tract in men and the urinary tract in women

A subspecialist has completed one to three years of additional training in a particular subspecialty. In the area of internal medicine there are nine subspecialties. Two years of subspecialty training is undertaken after completion of a three-year residency in internal medicine. Thus, the subspecialist who cares for you is an internist with further specialized training. See the following list of internal medicine subspecialties. As a person with diabetes, you should also know that the ophthalmologist can subspecialize in diseases of the retina and the cornea.

INTERNAL MEDICINE SUBSPECIALTIES

Cardiology (diseases of the cardiovascular system)
Endocrinology-metabolism (diseases of the endocrine glands) (diabetes)
Gastroenterology (diseases of the gastrointestinal tract)
Hematology (diseases of the blood)
Infectious disease (communicable diseases)
Medical oncology (cancer-related diseases)
Nephrology (diseases of the kidney)
Pulmonary disease (diseases of the lung)
Rheumatology (diseases of the bones and joints)

Once in practice, the physician may become a fellow of his particular specialty organization. This may be indicated by initials after the physician's name. For example, he may be a Fellow of the American College of Surgeons (F.A.C.S.)

or a Fellow of the American College of Physicians (F.A.C.P.). Fellows are members of a college or honor society dedicated to improving the state of the art in their specialty. They have been recognized by their peers. You may also see the initials P.C. after a physician's name. This means "professional corporation." It is a legal phrase indicating how the physician conducts his business affairs and has nothing to do with the physician's qualifications.

A doctor of osteopathic medicine (D.O.) is a health-care professional whose academic training is similar to that of a medical doctor with additional emphasis on the manipulation of bones. Educational requirements include a bachelor's degree and four years in an osteopathic school. He may enter an osteopathic or an American Medical Association-approved residency that is usually three years in duration. Upon completion of osteopathic school, the D.O. is eligible to take a state licensing exam.

THE DENTIST

Aside from the general dentist, there are specialties within dentistry. These include the following:

	EXTRA TRAINING
Public health dentist	
Prevents and controls dental diseases and promotes dental health through organized community efforts	1 year
Endodontist	
Diagnoses and treats oral conditions that arise as a result of problems of the dental pulp	2 years
Oral pathologist	
Studies the nature of the diseases affecting the oral and adjacent regions	3 years
Oral and maxillofacial surgeon	
Diagnoses and surgically treats diseases, injuries and defects of the oral and maxillofacial region	3–4 years
Orthodontist	
Supervises and corrects the growing and mature dental structures	2 years
Pedodontist	
Practices and teaches comprehensive, preventive and therapeutic oral health care of children from birth through adolescence	2 years

Periodontist
Diagnoses and treats diseases of the supporting and surrounding tissues
of the teeth   2 years

Prosthodontist
Restores and maintains oral functions by the restoration of natural teeth
and replacement of missing teeth   2–3 years

THE NURSE

Nursing is the diagnosis and treatment of human responses to actual or potential health problems. The nurse is responsible for the care of individuals in cooperation with other health personnel. Nurses may be found working in hospitals, clinics, communities and industrial areas. Nurses must gather relevant information on patients' needs and then plan and implement appropriate nursing care. Nurses can be educated in various ways. They can attend a nursing school affiliated with a hospital or enroll in an associate degree college program or a four-year baccalaureate program. At the completion of these programs, graduate nurses are eligible to take the state licensing exam to receive their registered nurse (R.N.) titles. They may also continue education by earning a master's and a doctoral degree in nursing. Nurses may then specialize in one area, such as teaching, administrative or clinical practice or research.

THE NUTRITIONIST

The registered dietitian or nutritionist is educated to provide nutritional care to individuals or groups. He or she is involved in helping people to select and obtain food for health or during illness. The registered dietitian initiates dietary interventions to improve patients' nutritional status and consults with hospital staff regarding problems affecting patients' food intake. She assesses the nutritional status of patients and may formulate menus for therapeutic diets. The nutritionist has completed an undergraduate program in home economics or nutrition. Graduates of dietetic programs may also apply for a dietetic internship. The nutritionist is encouraged to become a member of the American Dietetic Association and must successfully complete the examination for professional registration. Nutritionists may go on for advanced education and receive a master's or a Ph.D. degree in nutrition.

THE PHYSICIAN'S ASSISTANT

The physician's assistant (P.A.) provides patient services under the direct supervision of a physician. The assistant may take patients' histories, perform complete physical exams and counsel patients and their families. Educational requirements usually include two years of undergraduate studies in the areas of science and the humanities and one year of full-time patient-care experience. The P.A. program lasts an additional two years, after which the student becomes certified and receives a bachelor's degree in physician's assisting.

THE PHARMACIST

The registered pharmacist (R.Ph.) compounds and dispenses drugs, advises you on medication and provides information on drug interactions. They often keep patient records on file. The pharmacist receives a bachelor of science degree in a five-year pharmacy program. He or she completes 1,000 hours of an internship and must pass a licensing exam to receive the title of registered pharmacist. Pharmacists may also further their education by receiving a master's degree in pharmacy, pharmacy administration, clinical pharmacy or pharmacology, or a doctorate in pharmacology.

THE SOCIAL WORKER

Social workers perform social service and patient counseling functions. They also assist patients in obtaining community resources. They initially receive a bachelor of science degree in social work. The social worker may receive a master's degree in social work (M.S.W.) and then become eligible to take the state licensing exam to receive the title of certified social worker. A social worker may also become a member of the Academy of Certified Social Workers (A.C.S.W.). This is awarded by the Association of Social Workers.

THE PODIATRIST

A podiatrist (D.P.M.) specializes in the care of your feet and advises you about proper-fitting footwear. A podiatrist must have a bachelor's degree and complete a four-year podiatry program. He may then enter an internship program and pass a licensing exam to become a licensed doctor of podiatric medicine.

THE LABORATORY TECHNICIAN

The laboratory technician performs routine tests in a medical setting for use in the diagnoses of disease. He or she usually completes four years of college to obtain a degree in medical technology. In addition, he or she completes a year of internship, after which he or she is eligible for the registry exam with the American Society of Clinical Pathologists.

ANCILLARY PERSONNEL AND VOLUNTEERS

Nurse's aides and orderlies are ancillary personnel who help in patient care. They work under the supervision of a registered nurse. Volunteers in the hospital setting are usually distinguished by uniforms. They perform many useful tasks, such as reading to patients, transporting patients from unit to unit and delivering mail and flowers. If you are hospitalized, look at the name tag of each person who enters your room. The name tag will identify the hospital employee by name and description. If you cannot read the name tag, or the person is not wearing it, be assertive and ask for the person's name and position.

WHERE CAN YOU RECEIVE HEALTH CARE?

There are various kinds of hospitals, offering different types of services. Any hospital you choose should be accredited by the Joint Committee on Accreditation for Hospitals (JCAH). The purpose of this organization is to establish standards for hospital services.

Health care may be obtained in a primary-care center such as a physician's office or clinic. Primary care refers to a first contact, including diagnosis and treatment, psychological support, patient education and general health maintenance. This is known as ambulatory care or outpatient care. Hospitals can be considered secondary- or tertiary-care centers, although they may also provide primary care. A secondary-care hospital is usually a community hospital. Your doctor has access to practice in such a hospital. Tertiary-care hospitals provide an advanced level of treatment, such as kidney dialysis, open-heart surgery and high-risk maternal care.

Hospitals may treat acute, chronic or specific diseases. One type of hospital is known as a voluntary, non-profit or community hospital. A teaching hospital is usually affiliated with a medical school. Modern advances in medical techniques are frequently developed in teaching hospitals. These hospitals aid in the education of medical students, interns and residents. Teaching hospitals offer an intellectual atmosphere with the continuous presence of hospital-based doctors (interns and residents). A public hospital is a tax-supported facility serving the community. It can be a city, county or military VA hospital. There is usually a permanent full-time staff of physicians in all medical areas. The quality of care you receive depends on the overall quality of the institution.

TYPES OF MEDICAL PRACTICES

Physicians may enter into different practice arrangements. Solo practice refers to a physician in private practice without partners. Group specialty practice is a group of physicians of the same specialty working together. These may include, as examples, two obstetricians or five pediatricians in a group. It is helpful for some doctors to practice in a group, as there can be frequent professional exchanges. They can share responsibilities such as night and weekend calls as well as office expenses. Multi-specialty groups are also available. These include doctors of several specialties, such as family practice, obstetrics/gynecology, pediatrics and internal medicine. Here you do not have to be referred to an outside center for care unless you require advanced care. Doctors may also practice within a health maintenance organization (HMO). HMOs combine health insurance and health-care delivery. The HMO provides care for a fixed premium which is paid monthly (often by a person's employer). Prepayment for all-inclusive health care within an HMO differs from the more traditional fee-for-service arrangement, wherein a doctor charges a patient for each specific type of care each time it is rendered.

HOW TO CHOOSE YOUR DOCTOR

When selecting a doctor, review the American Medical Directory or the Directory of Medical Specialties. You can find these research books in the library. They will tell you the education and qualifications of board-certified physicians. Compile a list of the names and specialties of the doctors you may want to visit. Check each doctor's hospital association and the medical school from which he graduated. Determine where he completed his internship and residency. Your doctor should also be one with whom you can establish a good rapport and who is easily accessible.

REACHING YOUR DOCTOR BY PHONE

You will, on occasion, have to reach your doctor by telephone. You will have to get your message across to the person answering the phone. This person may be the office manager or receptionist. She is responsible for screening phone calls in a way that protects the doctor from unnecessary interruptions. The doctor may give the receptionist certain guidelines for screening calls or the receptionist may make her own decisions as to which patient message is urgent. If you cannot speak to the doctor at the time of your call, leave a clear and concise message. Explain your problem in an assertive manner. Tell the receptionist that the doctor has told you to call for this particular reason. Make sure you know exactly when the doctor will return your call.

If you must reach your doctor after office hours, maintain the same assertive attitude with the answering service. If your phone call is urgent, make sure that the service understands and is able to reach your doctor as soon as possible. Always ask how long it will be until the doctor returns your call. Have your list of questions ready for the doctor, and if you do not receive a return call within a reasonable time, phone again. Remember, when you leave a message, you may be speaking to an answering service or a receptionist who is not necessarily trained in patient needs. They should not speak in a curt or impatient manner. However, they may not have adequate sensitivity to patients, so the responsibility of getting your message answered lies in your own communication skills.

THE PHYSICAL EXAMINATION AND ITS IMPORTANCE

The Initial Exam

You will be seeing your doctor often to receive care for diabetes. Part of this care will involve the physical examination. The initial office visit may cause much anxiety. You may be concerned about your weight, blood glucose or degree of control in relation to complications. You may feel intimidated in a crowded waiting room. Your doctor and his office staff may seem rushed. In order to get mentally prepared for this experience, make a list of questions you want to ask so you remember to ask each one. Take your time and make sure you understand each answer. Do not worry about taking up too much of the doctor's time. If you are taking too long, your doctor will probably tell you that he cannot answer everything in one day. Having a friend or relative with you during the office visit is helpful. Often people become so anxious they miss some statements. A friend can be an objective listener.

The taking of your history, which precedes the physical exam, is organized in a specific way to allow your doctor to learn about your past and present health.

Be prepared to give a concise, organized description of your past health. Avoid irrelevant details which will prolong the history taking. The doctor will want to know about the main problem that led you to make an appointment to see him. This is known as the chief complaint. You can think of the chief complaint as the title of a story. It is used to establish the priorities for the rest of the examination process. You will then be asked for a history of your present illness. This is telling the story of the chief complaint. Again, be organized, and use short sentences. The doctor will ask questions to clarify your situation. You can provide historical information such as medication, X rays or lab test results. He will inquire about your medical history, such as background information about your health, hospitalizations, surgeries, allergies and medications. He will ask about your family history and illnesses that your parents, grandparents, siblings and children might have had. He will take a social history, which includes your occupation, use of alcohol, tobacco and other drugs, as well as your exercise program and recreational pursuits. The history will end with a review of systems. At this point, the doctor will ask specific questions related to different body systems. Examples of such questions would be the following: do you have headaches, nosebleeds, blurred vision, difficulty swallowing, chest pains, difficulty breathing, stomachaches, constipation, sexual problems, difficulty passing urine, leg cramps?

During the physical examination, the doctor will examine the various parts of your body that he has just questioned you about. He will use a standard type of physical assessment which includes inspection, palpation, percussion and auscultation. Inspection is the visual examination of the body without the use of instruments. Palpation is the examination of a part of the body by means of touch. Light pressure is used to feel the size of organs and the quality of skin. Percussion is striking an area with the fingers. The sound produced helps to detect enlarged organs or collections of fluid. Auscultation is examination by listening, with the aid of a stethoscope, to sounds arising from various organs (usually the heart, lungs and abdomen).

The doctor will also measure vital signs that will help him assess your overall cardiac and respiratory function. Your blood pressure and pulse will be measured. Your temperature, if needed, will be taken. Your rate of respiration (the number of times you breathe per minute) will also be determined. In order to monitor your diabetes, the doctor will carefully examine specific body parts. For example, he may perform an eye exam even though you visit an ophthalmologist. He may examine your feet, inspecting your toenails. The doctor may also perform a neurological exam using various tools to test your reflexes and your response to various sensations on your extremities.

Several laboratory tests may also be performed. A complete blood count (CBC), hemoglobin and hematocrit are helpful in indicating the presence of infection and anemia. A lipid (fat) profile includes cholesterol, triglycerides, HDL, VLDL and LDL. A urinalysis will be performed to detect the presence of protein, sugar, acetone, bacteria or blood and to determine the pH of the urine. All men over 40 should have a rectal exam and their stool examined for occult (hidden) blood. Additional automated blood tests may be performed which can indicate problems with various organ systems. However, diseases are not usually diagnosed on the basis of one blood value. The history, physical exam, blood work and other special tests are combined so that the doctor may see the total picture. Blood tests that may indicate a problem with the biliary tract (the gallbladder and bile ducts) include bilirubin, alkaline phosphatase and albumin. Abnormal serum levels of creatinine, urea nitrogen and albumin may signal kidney disease. Abnormal levels of electrolytes such as potassium, chloride and sodium may indicate water and mineral imbalance.

Your doctor may request that you have blood work done while fasting. This means that you will not have any food or beverage for a specific number of hours prior to the blood work. In addition, you would not take any medication for diabetes prior to the test. However, on the morning of the laboratory test you would be able to take all other medications with a small amount of water. Remember, if you take medication for diabetes, bring it with you along with food to eat after your blood specimen is drawn.

Much of the time of the visit will be spent on the history, physical exam and laboratory work. You may also need time to speak with your doctor about matters of importance to you. Yet all this as well as the physical exam may not be done in one day. If your doctor is unable to spend as much time with you as you need, you may have to make another appointment to speak with him.

You may also need to speak with your doctor again if you have received some upsetting information that you need a few days to think over. You may have so many questions to be answered pertaining to your situation that you become overwhelmed. Your best action is to return for another office visit with a clear mind. This allows for improved communication between you and your doctor. Make sure you are able to express your feelings to him. Tell him you are upset or confused about the information. Remember that your doctor is not a mind reader and may not be able to detect your feelings by facial expressions.

You may need to undergo special tests to diagnose other medical problems. At this time also you may have to follow special test diets. For example, this is the case if you must undergo a barium enema. You should expect that there will be some disruption in your pattern of control. Your insulin dose and food intake may change. Your goal should be to avoid hypoglycemia and marked hyperglycemia. Always try to schedule your tests early in the morning. If you had to undergo any test that required you to fast, you would not take your insulin in the morning of the test, nor would you eat. You would still need to take insulin later in the day, but the amount would vary according to your doctor's instructions.

The Follow-up Exam

Each year you should receive a complete physical exam just like your initial exam. However, to help evaluate your diabetes, you should see your doctor for interval exams. These may be necessary on a monthly basis or may be performed only every three or four months. The frequency of the visits depends on how stable your diabetes is, the type of diabetes you have and the presence or absence of complications.

THE PATIENT'S BILL OF RIGHTS

Today's emphasis on the patients' participation as consumers of health care led to the development of the Patient's Bill of Rights. Patients should not be ignorant and passive about their health care. Health-care providers should not be on pedestals but should be educators and partners in decision making. The patient-provider relationship should be changed from one of total patient dependence on the professional to interdependence in the health-care decision-making process. This requires different responses from both the patient and the health-care provider. The Patient's Bill of Rights can be applied to the hospital setting. If you have a chronic illness, you may be exposed to hospitals more often and it is important that you are aware of the Bill of Rights. The Bill of Rights was prepared by the American Hospital Association (and is reprinted below with permission of the AHA, copyright 1972). The patient has the right to:

1. Considerate and respectful care.
2. Upon request, the name of the physician responsible for coordinating his care.
3. The name and function of any person providing health-care services to the patient.
4. Obtain from the physician complete, current information concerning the diagnosis, treatment and prognosis in terms the patient can be reasonably expected to understand. When it is not medically advisable to give such information to the patient, the information should be made available to an appropriate person on his behalf.

5. Receive from his physician information necessary to give informed consent prior to the start of any procedure, or treatment or both, which, except for those emergency situations not requiring an informed consent, shall include as a minimum the specific procedure, or treatment or both, the medically significant risks involved and the probable duration of incapacitation, if any. The patient shall be advised of medically significant alternatives for care or treatment, if any.

6. Refuse treatment to the extent permitted by law and to be informed of the medical consequences of his action.

7. Privacy to the extent consistent with providing adequate medical care to the patient. This shall not preclude discreet discussion of a patient's case or examination of a patient by appropriate care personnel.

8. Privacy and confidentiality of all records pertaining to the patient's treatment except as otherwise provided by law or third party payment contract (payment by an insurance carrier).

9. A response by the hospital, in a reasonable manner, to the patient's request for services customarily rendered by the hospital consistent with the patient's treatment.

10. Be informed by his physician or delegate of the physician of the patient's continuing health-care requirements following discharge and that before transferring the patient to another facility the hospital first informs the patient of the need for such a transfer.

11. The identity, upon request, of other health-care and educational institutions that the hospital has authorized to participate in his treatment.

12. Refuse to participate in research and that human experimentation affecting care or treatment shall be performed only with his informed effective consent.

13. Examine and receive an explanation of his bill regardless of sources of payment.

14. Know the hospital rules and regulations that apply to his conduct as a patient.

15. Treatment without discrimination as to race, color, religion, sex, national origin or source of payment.

The Patient's Bill of Rights is an educational resource for a person who is hospitalized. You should not lose any human rights by being hospitalized. You can maintain your rights by asking questions of your health-care provider. Have a list of questions written down so you will remember to ask each one. Obtain as much information as you need. Have all your treatment alternatives described to you. Provide your doctor with feedback when you are dissatisfied or pleased and, finally, search out self-help groups to be sure that you are receiving current information regarding your particular concern. Often, because of the stress of hospitalization, patients revert to a type of behavior which is passive and helpless ("the sick role"). Assertive behavior is essential to your well-being at all times, but particularly during hospitalization. More tips on how to be assertive with health-care providers will now be discussed.

THE ASSERTIVE CONSUMER

Assertiveness, assertive behavior, assertiveness training—what is it and why is it important? Assertiveness is behavior that is healthy and constructive. To be assertive is to communicate in a direct, forthright manner. When you are aggressive, you tend to dominate or project overtones of hostility in your communication. Aggressive behavior involves communicating at the expense of others. You ignore the rights of others in an attempt to dominate. Aggressive behavior reflects anger. Your overlying expression of hostility may be communicated more than the essence of what you originally wanted to communicate. When you are passive, you avoid all kinds of communication. Passive behavior avoids unpleasant or risky situations and allows others to take control. You usually will not get your message across and may end up angry and resentful with yourself. Both methods of communication are ineffective.

In this section, role-playing situations are described to show you the difference between assertive, aggressive and passive behavior. Hopefully, you will begin to change aggressive and passive behaviors to become assertive. You are a consumer. Therefore, you must assert yourself in your role as the most important member of the health-care team.

Assertive behavior includes the expression of feelings and ideas in a clear manner. It is standing up for your own rights, but in a way that doesn't interfere with the rights of others. This is honest and direct communication.

First you must identify what feelings you wish to express, express them and get feedback from your actions. By using assertiveness in simple situations, you can learn to assert yourself in your social, family and professional life and as a health-care consumer.

Before learning assertive behavior you must analyze your present behavior. How do you handle conflict? How does your family handle conflict? How do you feel when you speak up in a crowd? Is your voice loud, angry or harsh? Review the following examples of assertive, passive and aggressive behavior.

You've been waiting in a doctor's reception area for over a half hour. A person who has just come into the reception area is taken directly into the doctor's inner office. The doctor's secretary looks at you and says, "You will be taken in shortly." Which of the following is your response?

1. You smile at the secretary sweetly.
2. You frown and remain seated.
3. You stand up and yell at the secretary, "How dare you take another person in before me! I have been waiting here a half hour! How dare you! Get me the doctor immediately!"
4. You say, "I was here before the person who has just gone in. Is there a reason why I am waiting such a long time to see the doctor?"

The assertive answer would be number four. You are telling the truth and communicating directly that you have been waiting a long time. You are also bringing attention to the fact that someone else has just gone into the office. You are asking a direct question: "Is there a reason?" Remember that perhaps there *is* a reason. Perhaps the patient who has just been ushered into the inner office has an emergency. You will be able to receive an answer from the secretary. This will cause a reduction in your own stress. Smiling will not be interpreted by the secretary as any kind of dissatisfaction on your part due to the long wait. You will not have communicated any discomfort to her. The second answer is still demonstrating a passive kind of behavior. Although you may be unhappy with the situation, you have not spoken up and have not asked for the reason why you have been waiting. The secretary has no way to interpret what your frown means. The third reaction is aggressive action; its hostile overtones would probably offend the secretary. You may not receive any answer as to why you have been waiting. You may just be kept waiting.

The health-care system may be confusing. Health-care institutions have their own rules and regulations and terms. All these factors lead to your discomfort when asking questions of health-care professionals. If you assume, from the beginning, that the health-care professional is busy and may not have time for you, you are starting with a self-defeating attitude. You will not obtain the information you need. One technique used when speaking with health-care professionals is to identify your feelings about the situation. A statement to health-care professionals such as "I feel uncomfortable taking your time to ask such questions," or "I know how busy you are, but I do have questions," will accomplish this. You can also use the "broken record" technique when speaking with health-care professionals. If the health-care professional gives you unclear information and then ends the conversation, you can ask the question over again. Although this may seem odd, and you may feel foolish repeating the same questions, this "broken record" allows you extra time to gather thoughts. It emphasizes to the health-care professional your need for further clarification of information.

Remember that these are all things you can do as part of self-directive behavior (behavior that you initiate). Often, patients think that health-care professionals should be aware of their needs, so they feel they do not have to use assertive techniques to communicate. You cannot expect all health-care professionals to always be attuned to your needs. In a fragmented, busy health-care system, this is not realistic. With the use of assertive techniques, you will be able to communicate effectively with all health-care professionals. However, assertive techniques may not help you in the emergency room. Various aspects of the emergency room will now be discussed.

THE USE AND MISUSE OF THE EMERGENCY ROOM

The emergency medical care system has been misused in the past due to a breakdown in communication between patients and doctors as well as a lack of physician availability. Often, if people cannot get in touch with their doctors, or do not have primary-care physicians, they use the emergency room (ER) for primary care. This can lead to dangerous overcrowding. You should visit the ER only in an acute (sudden onset) situation. People are attended to in the ER according to their time of arrival and their need. The ER personnel decide who must be seen first. The more severely ill must be attended to before anyone else. It is not only dangerous but costly to have people crowd into the ER. The ER should not be used as a substitute for a doctor's office. Yet if you do have to use an ER, you should be prepared with certain facts.

You can prepare for future emergencies by keeping a list of emergency phone numbers next to your telephone. The list would include the number of your doctor, the fire department, the closest hospital, your closest relative, the Poison Control Center and a private ambulance company. If you have a major illness or allergy, ask your doctor to help prepare you for a possible emergency by role-playing a situation. If there has been a poisoning, be prepared to bring the bottle of poison with you. Carry an identification card if you have a chronic illness or are taking medications.

Know the available emergency transport systems in your community. These include the volunteer fire department, the police and private ambulance companies. You should also know the quickest route by car to the closest emergency room. If you are going to the ER, you can assist the personnel by calling ahead and offering information about the emergency.

The environment in the emergency room may be crowded, busy and impersonal. When you enter the ER you may be asked to wait and it may be impossible to estimate how long it will be until you are seen. The clerical staff will ask you to complete forms. You must know your Social Security number and insurance carrier. You or your accompanying family member will be interviewed. You may meet doctors who will attend to your chief complaint but they may not perform a full examination. Nurses and other ER personnel, such as X-ray technicians, laboratory and medical technicians, will also assist you.

What Is an Emergency?

Major emergencies that require a visit to the ER include shortness of breath or difficulty in breathing or the sudden onset of severe pain in the chest, abdomen, head, back or neck. Be alert to emergencies such as large amounts of blood lost during vomiting or diarrhea, in the urine or from the vagina. Convulsions and unconsciousness, stupor, drowsiness or disorientation, especially if the person was previously alert, are reasons for a visit to the ER. An injury to the eye, burns and fractured bones warrant use of the ER. A skull or spine injury, a gunshot or knife wound or a severe cut should be treated in the ER. Poison ingestion, severe psychiatric problems and many snake and insect bites should also be treated in the ER.

Identification stating you have diabetes should always be worn. Tell family members or friends to call your doctor and/or take you to the ER if you experience deep, heavy breathing or if you are semi-comatose and unable to be aroused. Your knowledge of first-aid principles is important for you and your family. You can avail yourself of community resources such as the Red Cross programs and adult education programs to become knowledgeable in this area.

As a person with diabetes you are at risk for developing emergencies such as insulin reactions and diabetic ketoacidosis. Remember to make sure that you are using the ER appropriately. Learn the principles of first aid and be prepared for emergencies. Know how to get assistance fast. Oftentimes, after being brought to the ER you may be unable to leave because the doctor may determine that you need to be hospitalized. Emergency and elective hospital admissions will now be discussed.

HOSPITAL ADMISSIONS

Admission to a hospital is either emergency or elective. In an emergency situation, you may have gone to the emergency room for care. The doctor there may determine that you need further hospital care and should be admitted. If so, you will be held in the emergency area until you are stable enough to be transferred to a room. Sometimes a room is not available and you may remain in the ER until admission procedures are completed. Often, the members of your family will be asked to go to the admitting office and provide certain information. After the admission process is completed, your family will be able to see you once again, before you settle into your room.

The second type of admission is elective admission. This involves preplanning between you and the hospital. After the decision has been made that it is necessary for you to be hospitalized, your doctor's office staff will arrange for a date for admission to the hospital. After a date is set up for admission, you will usually receive communication from the hospital regarding preadmission testing, dates, times, finances, etc.

On the morning of admission you may be asked to fast and have certain testing done at the hospital. Recently, preadmission testing has become standard for surgical procedures. In this case, you would come to the hospital a few days before your admission and have your lab tests, EKG and chest X ray completed as an outpatient. On the day of admission you would be rapidly settled in your room.

If you are admitted electively, you may choose a private or a semiprivate room. Semiprivate rooms may have two or four people in them. Although you may request a certain type of room, this request may not always be granted, due to limited space. Insurance may not cover the cost of a private room. After arriving in your room, you will be oriented to your unit by nursing personnel. Such things as a call light to summon help, the use of bed side rails and the bathroom will be explained. Leave jewelry or large amounts of money at home. Only a limited number of clothing items should be kept with you. Many hospitals provide newly admitted patients with brochures explaining hospital procedures, visiting hours and religious consultations. If you have questions after being admitted, do not hesitate to ask them.

The next section will deal with common serious illnesses. They will be briefly discussed with emphasis on their detection and prevention.

HEALTH TIPS

Alcoholism

The National Institute of Mental Health defines alcoholism as ''an increasing need for alcohol in order to function.'' Many alcoholics can function without being intoxicated all the time. They have jobs and care for homes. This pattern can lead to denial of the existence of alcoholism. It is known that alcohol by itself is not enough to cause the disease; multiple factors are involved. There is frequently an unpleasant physical reaction to the withdrawal of alcohol, thus the treatment of alcoholism and the rehabilitation of the individual involve a detoxification process (withdrawal of alcohol). This is usually achieved with hospitalization for several days or weeks. Emotional support is also important. Many persons with alcoholism may have already lost the support of their friends and families. Therefore, a group such as Alcoholics Anonymous may be an important aid. These groups tend to focus on the peer-group process and a spiritual approach. For family members of an alcoholic, the group called Al-Anon is available. The addresses of these two groups are given in the "Community Resources" section at the end of this book.

Cancer

Receiving the diagnosis of cancer can be one of the most frightening experiences even though the outlook today is much better than it was forty years ago. Cancer will affect two out of every three families. Today, one out of every three cancer patients are alive five years after the initial diagnosis. Moreover, some cancers can now be cured. Cancer develops when a cell undergoes abnormal changes and a process of uncontrolled growth occurs. The cells grow in masses of tissues called tumors. The key to a favorable outcome is early detection and treatment. Beware of the following danger signs of cancer. These include:

Persistent hoarseness or cough for more than three weeks
Unexplained weight loss
A persistent sore
Change in bowel or bladder habits
Lumps or masses which appear where none was present
Increased size or change in color or appearance of any existing lumps, warts or birthmarks
Unexplained or abnormal bleeding

Tell your doctor immediately if you observe any danger signal.

BREAST EXAMINATION

Breast self-examination is the most important way to detect breast cancer. Regular breast self-examination is the best way of determining changes in breast tissue because you become familiar with your own breast tissue. All women after the age of 20 should perform a breast exam each month. In the premenopausal woman, this exam should be done 2 to 3 days after the end of the menstrual period. The postmenopausal woman should choose one day out of each month and consistently examine her breasts on that day. Most lumps are not cancerous. Some women have a normally lumpy type of breast tissue. This condition is known as benign fibrocystic breast disease.

To examine your breasts, first look in the mirror. Your arms should be at your side and then pulled over your head. What you are doing now is looking for a change in the size and shape of the breast. Next, lie flat on your back and examine one breast at a time. Examine the left breast first, using your right hand and pressing the tissue against the chest wall. Don't pinch the skin between your fingers. All breast tissue will feel a bit lumpy but remember that you are looking for changes in breast tissue. Move your hand around the breast in a circular fashion, working gradually from the outer edge to the nipple. Repeat with the right breast. Any lump detected should immediately be reported to your doctor. By examining your breasts regularly, valuable time will not be wasted before a lump is detected.

You may fit into a subclass of women who are at higher risk for breast cancer. This is the case if you are older than 50, have a mother or sister with a history of breast cancer or you have already had cancer in one breast. In this case, your doctor may also suggest mammography. This is a diagnostic tool, performed through X ray, to detect tumors before they can be felt.

PAP SMEAR

A Pap smear is a test performed by your gynecologist to detect the presence of cancer of the cervix. A speculum, a small instrument, is used to allow inspection of the vagina. After the speculum is placed, the cervix is examined and scraped with a spatula-type device to obtain a sample of cervical cells. This is examined under a microscope. Cells are classified according to certain characteristics. If your Pap smear appears abnormal, you may be asked to return for another test. This single test can detect 90 percent of all common types of cancer of the cervix. There is a good chance that an abnormal Pap smear will detect a cancer before it spreads. This test is usually done annually, although recent reports suggest that it may need to be performed only every three years. The American Cancer Society recommends that after two initial negative tests one year apart, you obtain a Pap test at least every three years. This includes women under 20 years of age if sexually active. Remember that this is a guideline, not a rule, and applies only to women without symptoms. Check with your own gynecologist for specific recommendations.

Tips on Surgery

Being told you need to have an operation is often a frightening experience. For the person with diabetes this will mean a temporary, yet total change in his self-management program. To be effective in the health-care system, you can follow a few rules prior to surgery. Begin by seeing your family doctor or internist. If your family doctor recommends that you visit a surgeon, determine if the surgeon is board-certified and a Fellow of the American College of Surgeons. Once the surgeon tells you surgery is required, it may be helpful to get a second opinion. After that is obtained, both your surgeon and your family doctor can discuss your situation with you and agree on the treatment. Your surgeon may treat you in the hospital or in his office, depending on the type of surgery being performed. You must make sure you understand all aspects of the surgery and/or alternatives. Ask to be informed of the risks, complications and benefits of the procedure. There is always risk present in any surgical procedure. If the benefits outweigh the risks, the procedure is undertaken. Seeking a second opinion is useful, especially if you will have to undergo surgery. The ultimate decision for surgery is yours. You must listen to the experts, know the risks, understand the treatments and then decide.

Facts About Over-the-Counter Medications

Over $10 million is spent each year on over-the-counter drugs. Drugs are available for many reasons: to wake up, to sleep, to lose weight, to gain weight, to reduce pain and anxiety levels. These drugs often treat symptoms but not the problem causing the symptoms. Simply because you are able to purchase medication over the counter does not mean the drug is safe. Drugs are chemicals used for specific purposes, but they also have unwanted side effects. All people do not need the same amount of medications and it is common for medications to be misused or used excessively. Use caution when taking any drug and avoid mixing drugs.

Often, people with diabetes may take several drugs at the same time. These may include prescription drugs for diabetes, hypertension or heart disease. A dangerous situation arises when you add over-the-counter analgesics (painkillers) or cough or cold remedies. Prescription drugs and over-the-counter medications may interact, causing a variety of health problems. When you speak to your doctor about medications, have your complete medical and drug history on hand. Be informed about your medications and know what they do, why they are prescribed, what their dangers are, how often and at what times you should take them.

Drugs are known by their chemical and brand names. The generic name for a drug is the term that describes the drug's chemical structure. The brand name is given by manufacturers and often is easier to remember. Always ask if the generic type of drug is available, since this type may be less expensive. Ask your doctor to prescribe generic drugs whenever appropriate. Check different pharmacies to compare prices of drugs. Many types of over-the-counter drugs are available for you. A list of a few and some notes of caution follow. *Analgesics* are mild pain relievers made of aspirin and/or acetaminophen. Often, caffeine may be included. *Cough remedies* are also available. Some of these cough medicines have large amounts of alcohol and sugars along with other ingredients. Be careful when using those medications with alcohol or antihistamines. This combination will usually cause drowsiness. There are a number of sugar-free cough syrups on the market. Several *eye washes* are available. These are often made of an ingredient such as ephedrine hydrochloride, which narrows tiny blood vessels of the eye, and an astringent such as zinc sulphate. Eye drops may mask symptoms of eye problems; avoid their use. Any difficulty with your eye should be reported immediately to your doctor. *Feminine hygiene sprays* are made of antiseptics, germicides and perfumes. They are deodorants. Feminine hygiene sprays can be irritating to the vaginal membrane and can disturb the pH of the vagina. Proper cleansing of the vaginal area makes their use unnecessary. *Sinus cold remedies* are frequently used to alleviate the congestion of colds. Decongestants, analgesics, stimulants and often ascorbic acid (vitamin C) may be added. In cold remedies, the antihistamine may cause drowsiness. The vitamin C may interfere with urine-testing results. In addition, the decongestants may elevate blood pressure levels in those with hypertension. *Sleep inducers* may contain an antihistamine as well as other components. Side effects of these medications may include blurred vision and dizziness. Their use is to be avoided. *Stomach aids* are frequently used for upset stomachs. Some stomach remedies contain aluminum hydroxide, which can cause constipation, as well as sodium bicarbonate, which can aggravate blood pressure levels.

A major part of health maintenance for diabetic persons involves applying hygiene principles. Proper hygienic care of the skin, hair, vagina, urinary tract and teeth will now be described.

HYGIENE PRINCIPLES OF DIABETES

What is hygiene? Hygeia was the ancient Greek goddess of health. Hygiene refers to the science of health and its preservation. Principles of hygiene can be applied to all systems of your body.

Skin

The skin is the protective covering of the body. When the skin is broken as a result of a cut or bruise, the body becomes vulnerable to infection. Skin can never be totally sterilized, but cleansing of the skin will reduce the amount of bacteria present. This will decrease your risk of infection if a cut or abrasion does occur.

Infections often occur in the areas where the skin rubs or touches other parts of the skin. This is seen in the groin, between the thighs, under the arms and the breasts. As skin areas touch one another, chafing may occur. This is known as intertrigo. It may be caused by friction or by excessive moisture, warmth or sweat. Obesity may cause the development of intertrigo. Not only is this condition a source of discomfort but it also may lead to the development of bacterial or fungal infections. If you are overweight, pay particular attention to cleaning and drying these areas of the skin. Infections may develop if these areas are not well cleaned.

Itching is known as pruritis and is commonly seen in diabetic persons. It may be generalized to all areas of the body and it may also be in specific areas such as the vagina. Strict personal hygiene and the use of moisturizing creams may help this condition. Your doctor may prescribe medication if the itching becomes severe.

Necrobiosis lipoidica diabeticorum is a rare skin condition associated with diabetes. It is found most frequently in insulin-dependent diabetic females. Here the skin becomes discolored, shiny and tight. The skin lesion usually appears on the lower legs and ankles. This is a harmless although disfiguring disorder for which no treatment is available at this time. All efforts are directed at preventing ulcers or infections from developing at this vulnerable spot. Another skin condition is known as diabetic dermopathy. Dermopathy refers to "shin spots," small brown spots which appear on the front of the legs. These spots do not cause pain or ulcers. They do seem to increase in appearance the longer you have diabetes and may result from trauma to the legs. Xanthoma diabeticorum involves skin lesions that result from uncontrolled diabetes. These lesions represent fat deposits in the skin and are a direct result of elevated blood lipids. They are orange-yellow plaques which may appear on the buttocks, forearms, elbows and knees. They usually disappear when diabetes is treated and controlled.

Avoid home remedies for any skin chafing or infection. Instead, bring these problems to the attention of your doctor or a dermatologist, a specialist in diseases of the skin. To prevent or alleviate these conditions you should take meticulous care of your skin and not allow skin to become too moist. Wear clothes that are made of natural fibers so that your skin can "breathe" easily through them. At times, when blood glucose is elevated, furuncles (boils) on the skin may appear. Diabetes control as well as proper hygiene can lessen this problem.

Hair

Hair is a protective covering for the body. It should be kept clean. In American society, ordinary social behavior dictates the removal of hair from certain areas of the body. Men may shave their faces on a daily basis. Women shave their legs and underarm areas. Your shaving equipment should be spotlessly clean. Always use a mild soap with lather or shaving cream in order to avoid cuts and proceed with smooth shaving.

FEMALE HYGIENE

Approximately one-half of the diabetic female population experiences vaginitis. Vaginitis is often caused by a fungus (yeast), *Candida albicans*. This fungus tends to grow more in the presence of elevated blood glucose. This is also known as a monilial infection and is characterized by a "cottage cheese" type of vaginal discharge.

If you develop symptoms of vaginitis such as itching, burning or vaginal discharge, see your doctor. Medication can be prescribed for this condition. The medication, either suppositories or creams, should be taken exactly as prescribed. You should avoid using home remedies such as harsh douches. Sometimes, because of the intimate nature of this problem, women hesitate to seek medical help. This is a mistake; it is essential to get proper treatment for vaginitis. Wearing cotton underwear will prevent moisture from being trapped in the vaginal area. Improving your diabetic control will reduce the occurrence of this type of infection. Careful personal hygiene will help avoid infections. This includes the following:

(a) use douches only on a doctor's advice, (b) wipe the perineal area (area between the vagina and rectum) from front to back only, to avoid contamination, and (c) clean the entire perineal area daily with soap and water.

Urinary Tract Infection

Diabetic females may be more prone to develop urinary tract infections than non-diabetic females. These infections may be caused by a transfer of bacteria from the vagina or rectum to the urethra. Poorly controlled diabetes may intensify a urinary tract infection. These infections must be recognized promptly, treated quickly and cured totally. Signs of a urinary tract infection include painful or burning urination, an urgent and frequent need to urinate, cloudy or bloody urine and fever or chills. If you have any of these symptoms, get medical help immediately. You will need antibiotics to kill the bacteria present in your urinary tract. Although your symptoms may disappear shortly after taking this medication, continue it so that the infection becomes totally cured. Follow the prescription exactly as your doctor has given it to you. It is essential that you practice careful personal hygiene to avoid infections.

DENTAL HYGIENE

Good dental hygiene is particularly important for the diabetic person. Uncontrolled diabetes may cause cavities, gum infections and tooth decay. Aside from the cosmetic importance of healthy teeth and gums, the mouth and the teeth are the gateway to your stomach. Since nutrition is so important in diabetes, you need to keep your mouth and teeth in good working order. In order to do this, learn about preventive dental care.

The adult has thirty-two teeth, which may last a lifetime if they receive proper care. The teeth are rooted into the jawbone. The crown of the tooth is the part of the tooth which can be seen. Plaque is a sticky film that develops on your teeth every day. Plaque can accumulate on the teeth if they are not cleaned thoroughly. Part of the plaque forms a hard deposit on the teeth known as calculus or tartar. If plaque and calculus build up, the gums may become inflamed. This inflammation is known as gingivitis. Gums may separate from the teeth and pockets of pus and bacteria may develop. This leads to the condition known as periodontitis or pyorrhea. The inflammation may spread to the jawbone.

Diabetes is so closely correlated with periodontal disease that some people find out for the first time that they have diabetes through a visit to the dentist. A classic warning sign of periodontal disease is the presence of bleeding gums. The single greatest cause of tooth loss in adults is gum disease. This may destroy the structures that support your teeth. Tell your dentist if you have bleeding gums.

How can you prevent dental problems? There are several ways available to you. These include proper diet, preventive care of the teeth and knowledge of symptoms of periodontal disease. Your teeth are designed to withstand much pressure each time you chew. In fact, chewing can be a useful exercise for healthy teeth and gums. Foods that require more chewing action help in preventing dental problems. These foods, usually rich in fiber, are part of a nutritious diet. They include cereals, breads, whole grains, raw fruits and vegetables. Simple carbohydrates such as candy and cake are not good for your teeth.

Another part of prevention is making your teeth resistant to decay through the use of fluoride. Fluoride prevents demineralization (the eating away of tooth enamel). Less tooth decay is found in adult populations that drink fluorinated water throughout their lives. You can check with your local health department to see if your water supply contains fluoride. Fluoride supplements are also available in drops, mouth rinses and tablets. A flouride toothpaste will give you extra protection against tooth decay.

Another aspect of dental care includes the proper brushing of teeth and the use of dental floss. Brushing your teeth after each meal or at least two times a day, upon arising and before retiring, will help. Teeth should also be cleaned professionally at least twice a year. Brush carefully, using a soft nylon brush with rounded ends. Brush your teeth in the area where your teeth meet your gums. Next, use short back-and-forth strokes to clean the outside surfaces of your teeth. Use an up-and-down motion to clean inside the front teeth. Finally, brush the edges of all teeth and the inside of your back teeth with back-and-forth strokes. Brush the upper surface of your tongue as well. Use dental floss to reach areas where a toothbrush cannot easily work. Remember, your teeth have four sides and flossing will help to remove bacteria. Using a sawing motion, guide the floss through tight places between the teeth. Use gentle motions as you floss up and down the sides of your teeth. Use a clean section of dental floss as you move from tooth to tooth. In order to check on how well you are cleaning your teeth, use disclosing agents. These contain vegetable coloring that can be applied to the teeth and gums. These stain the plaque that has not been removed and show you areas you have missed. Clean these areas more carefully in the future.

New advances have been made in the treatment of tooth and gum disease. One of these involves root canal therapy. A small opening is made in the tooth, exposing the root, and bacteria are cleaned away. Root canal therapy is viewed as painful by many individuals, but may be controlled with new pain-management techniques. A local anesthetic may be administered to make you comfortable. A tooth that otherwise might have been extracted may now be saved.

If you do need a tooth extraction or any type of oral surgery and you take insulin, certain adjustments in your insulin dose must be made. Remember, prevention is the key to successful self-management. If you were to take your normal dose of insulin and then have oral surgery, you would be unable to eat for many hours. You would run the risk of hypoglycemia. Always check with your doctor for advice during these special circumstances.

Begin a program of preventive tooth care by brushing your teeth on a regular basis, using dental floss and seeing your dentist at least once a year. Recognize that the dentist is an essential member of the health-care team. The dentist you see regularly may be well equipped to take care of many aspects of dental hygiene but will also refer you to specialists when necessary. The key to dental hygiene is prevention. Prevention is achieved with proper nutrition and daily attention to dental hygiene. Preventing dental problems will save you time, money and discomfort in the future.

CAREER PLANNING

Preparation for a lifetime career should occur before you enter the job market. Career planning and health insurance will now be discussed.

As an adult with diabetes you must carefully consider planning a career. There should be little reason for you not to enter the career of your choice. Follow your own interests in choosing a career. Become as highly educated and trained as possible. Use guidance and vocational counselors to discuss your ideas. School vacations or work experiences can be used to assess your interest in a specific career. Your general health and intellectual abilities are two considerations for career planning. Good control of diabetes is necessary for successful employment. Do all that you can to develop your intellectual skills. Remember, it will be important for you to maintain good general health.

The type of career you enter may depend on your type of diabetes. Persons taking insulin or an oral medication shouldn't work in positions where an accidental hypoglycemic event is dangerous. These jobs include driving commercial vehicles in interstate or foreign commerce, airplane piloting, working on scaffolding or with heavy machinery. Diabetic persons cannot enter the armed services. Positions such as registered nurse, policeman or fireman, which involve shift work, may make your self-management of diabetes more difficult due to the long and erratic hours of those professions. However, preplanning of meals, medication and daily routine can be achieved. If you are being treated with diet alone, there should be no job restrictions.

JOB DISCRIMINATION

It is illegal not to hire a person with diabetes on the basis of the disease alone. Title V of the Rehabilitation Act of 1973 states that all handicapped people should receive equal job opportunity and treatment. Also, programs and activities that receive federal assistance can't discriminate against the handicapped. In addition, employers must make reasonable accommodations for a person's condition. According to law, your ability to perform on the job must be fairly evaluated. You must be trained and promoted on the same basis as someone without diabetes. If you feel that you have been discriminated against in the work setting, you can write to the Handicapped Worker's Task Force, Department of Labor, 200 Constitution Avenue, N.W., Washington, DC 20210. You can also contact the Labor Department, the Human Rights Department or the governor's office in your state. Try to discuss any difficulties with your employer, when possible, before filing a complaint.

The Second Injury Law, in some states, gives companies protection in future compensation claims if they hire you. This encourages hiring people with a chronic illness. However, once you are hired, you should try to be an excellent worker. If you are poorly controlled, you are a poor role model for other people with diabetes as well as for future employers. It will help all persons with diabetes if you maintain good control and a good work record.

Persons with diabetes may be labeled "handicapped" in some parts of the country. You know your own physical limitations and the word "handicapped" may not specifically apply to you. Yet being labeled "handicapped" may be necessary to obtain certain benefits. To aid your plans for a career you should seek out government career counseling services. The government also offers financial assistance for job training. The Developmental Disabilities Program is a federal and state effort to help those with severe chronic mental or physical difficulties which developed during childhood. Services may include those that deal with a child's health, education, welfare and rehabilitation. Parents may want to contact their local Office of Vocational Rehabilitation. Remember, however, that uncomplicated diabetes is not considered disabling. Be honest with prospective employers about your diabetes. The American Diabetes Association states that persons with diabetes who are in good control can be excellent workers. You should be considered for a position on the basis of your qualifications. You should not be rejected for a position because you have diabetes.

Develop your educational skills. Obtain medical supervision. Stay well controlled, well motivated and well disciplined. Engage in proper job selection. Remember that the law does not permit discrimination based on diabetes alone. You are entitled to the same opportunities as a person without diabetes.

INSURANCE

The type and amount of insurance you purchase should be carefully thought out. The purpose of life insurance is to protect the family from financial disaster should the breadwinner die. Health insurance is also needed to protect against grave financial problems should a serious acute or chronic illness affect any member of the family. If you are not insured and then suffer a heart attack or other complications, you may find it difficult to obtain insurance. Make sure you obtain both life and health insurance.

Prior to 1940, life insurance was relatively unavailable for persons with diabetes. Today it is rare to be unable to obtain life insurance. Due to the improved life expectancy and better treatment for diabetes, more insurance companies have been prompted to provide insurance coverage. Insurance company requirements are stricter for obtaining health insurance. However, that, too, is available. You may be charged more for life or health insurance because you have diabetes. However, when obtaining life or health insurance, you will be evaluated on an individual basis. If you are in good control, you may not have to pay an extra premium. If you have a complication, you may pay extra. However, if you can correct the complication, the insurance company may reduce your premium. So if you are obese but lose weight and maintain the weight loss, your premium may be lowered. Remember, though, that once an insurance company "flags" you as having a complication, that fact enters a central file. So, at any time in the future, any insurance company you use will know you had a diabetes-related complication.

When you are applying for insurance, your doctor may be asked to document certain aspects of your control. These may include your weight, number of visits to him per year, evaluation of control, adherence to self-management activities and the presence of complications. You may be rejected if you haven't seen your doctor at least once in the past year. The insurance company may then want to do its own examination.

Other complications associated with diabetes will also affect your premium. These include obesity, hypertension, retinopathy and any stage of nephropathy. Your degree of control, as measured by the hemoglobin A_{1C}, may now be used by insurance companies. If a private company will not accept you on an individual basis because of your potential health problems, a group plan may be the best choice. A group plan makes you only a small part of the whole group, and it will be easier for you to be included. Membership in the American Diabetes Association and affiliates often includes eligibility for several group insurance plans.

HEALTH INSURANCE:
ACCIDENT AND SICKNESS POLICIES

Insurance can be tailored to your needs as well as your budget. Plans may be guaranteed renewable, which means that the policy provides coverage for a specific number of years during which time the premium cannot be increased. Plans may be non-cancelable, guaranteed renewable. This means the company cannot cancel your policy or change the premium. This is the most expensive type of policy, but may be beneficial for you later in life. Another policy is the optionally renewable policy. This means the option to renew or change the premium lies with the company. It may discontinue insurance whenever it wants. This type of coverage is the least expensive.

An individual or individual family plan is your choice if you cannot obtain a group plan. You can include your spouse and children under 19 years of age. Children over 19 who are unable to work due to a handicap may also be covered. Dependent children over 19 may be covered for an additional premium.

A group plan may be offered by an employer and may cover both employees and dependents. Premiums are generally lower than those with private insurance companies. You may be eligible regardless of any physical condition. A group plan may be formed with three or more people in an association. Your employer may pay for the entire plan or part of it. The coverage may or may not be adequate and you may have to pay some "out of pocket" fees. One benefit may be traded for a lesser benefit with each new policy year.

Blue Cross is an insurance carrier that covers hospital services such as room and board. In addition, it usually covers general nursing care as well as the cost of a sudden illness which requires a visit to the emergency room. It also covers presurgical testing and some home care which may be provided by nurses or health aides. Blue Cross pays physicians at a "going rate," or the usual fee in the area. Blue Shield usually covers surgery and medical costs as well. Check your policy to see if payment will be made for various elective procedures. Group Health Insurance or GHI covers medical costs such as office visits and some surgical expenses. It pays on a schedule of fees, per physician. Coverage by Major Medical may take over where other protection ends. Major Medical covers long hospital stays as well as extensive or multiple operations. There is usually a co-insurance clause included in the policy which states that you pay a certain percentage of the cost on your own. Private insurance companies vary in what they cover, and you should check specific items prior to purchasing the coverage. For example, office visits may not always be included and dental insurance may be under a separate policy.

MEDICARE AND MEDICAID

Medicare is available for those over 65 who are also eligible for Social Security. Disabled persons or those with chronic renal failure may also obtain Medicare. Others over 65 may purchase Medicare insurance. You should have two parts of Medicare insurance. Part A is free of charge and pays the cost of hospitals and skilled nursing homes, but does not cover doctor's bills. Part B can be paid for monthly. It covers doctor's bills, outpatient hospital services and other costs of various medical services and supplies. It does not cover a variety of medical costs, some of which include eyeglasses, hearing aids, dental bills and prescriptions.

Medicaid is assistance for low-income people. It is state-funded. Medicaid pays bills in whole or in part. You may be eligible for Medicaid if you are on welfare or are medically needy. Those eligible may include people younger than 65 but older than 21 who are blind or disabled with one or both parents dead or absent. Medicaid also provides for catastrophic illness where inpatient hospital costs would exceed 25 percent of your annual income. Medicaid may also cover inpatient nursing, outpatient nursing, outpatient clinic visits, laboratory fees, medications, eyeglasses, sickroom supplies and visits to a doctor, dentist, optometrist and podiatrist. Rules governing eligibility and payments for Medicare and Medicaid may change yearly depending on legislation. To determine current status check your local Social Security office.

You should know that some hospitals and doctors do not accept payment through insurance. They expect you to be responsible for paying your bills. Usually the insurance company will pay you the proper amount once you submit the proper form and your doctor's bill. Make sure you know in advance your doctor's procedures regarding this.

LIFE INSURANCE

Life insurance can be term or whole life. Term life insurance is usually less expensive and is purchased for a specific number of years: one, five, ten or twenty. Term insurance may be guaranteed annual renewable and convertible. This means it can be renewed when the term ends and converted from term to whole life at any time. Whole life insurance cannot be terminated by the company. It is more expensive, but you have coverage until death or retirement. Whole life insurance usually provides for a "cash-in value" whereby you can terminate your policy and receive cash value for your premium. The amount of cash you receive is usually less than what the total premium payments have been. However, as you get older, the amount of cash you receive is more than the payments. You can also receive a loan from your policy to use money. This money will then be deducted from your policy. You should never cash in your entire policy, since your coverage will be terminated.

Group life insurance is usually available from employers, who may pay part or all of the coverage. If you terminate your position, the insurance company is required by state law to offer you the option to convert, but only to the whole life form, not to a term policy. You can never be refused conversion once you have been covered under a group life insurance plan. Members of the American Diabetes Association may receive life insurance from John Hall and Associates, Inc. The address is given in the "Community Resources Directory" at the end of this book.

DISABILITY INSURANCE

Disability insurance helps replace income lost due to a disability. A disability is any illness or injury that prevents you from working. Excluded from this is elective surgery or any injury caused by your involvement in a criminal act. Most policies require patients to be partially or totally disabled before benefits are paid. Some policies have a waiting period before they take effect, but often payments may be received anywhere from 7 to 365 days. You can obtain disability insurance through your employer or, if self-employed, you may purchase it on your own.

COMMUNITY RESOURCES

Group community resources are helpful in your continued diabetes self-management. The library is an example of a community resource. The library carries many books on diabetes written by health professionals. It is useful to visit the library to review these books to keep up to date on information regarding diabetes. You will soon become an expert in judging the literature for yourself.

In 1940, the American Diabetes Association (ADA) was formed. Its members include over 3,500 doctors, research scientists, nurses, dietitians and educators. It is the leading voluntary health organization dealing with diabetes. Its main purpose is to teach people with diabetes how to live full and meaningful lives. To facilitate care for the patient, the ADA conducts professional seminars for health-care providers. The ADA is also responsible for educating the general public about the seriousness of diabetes and for helping the lay person to recognize the symptoms. Finally, the ADA is involved in funding numerous research endeavors. The ADA publishes three journals. *Diabetes* is a research journal specifically for health professionals. *Diabetes Care* is for professionals in clinical practice. *Diabetes Forecast* has bimonthly articles on nutrition, pregnancy, travel and many other topics of interest to the patient with diabetes. We strongly urge you to join the ADA and subscribe to *Diabetes Forecast*.

The Juvenile Diabetes Foundation was founded in 1970 by parents of diabetic children who believed that with research diabetes could be cured. The JDF is a voluntary health agency with chapters in many cities. Participants in the JDF may be parents or friends of those with diabetes. The JDF exists for fund raising for research to find a cure for diabetes.

Finally, diabetes clubs exist in many hospital settings across the country. They are organized by local American Diabetes Association affiliates, as well as by patients with diabetes. Diabetes clubs act as excellent support systems. They usually meet once a month for one to two hours. Guest speakers are professionals in the community who are invited to speak on a topic of interest to all patients. This formal presentation is followed by an informal discussion led by patients. You may contact your local ADA affiliate to learn how you can organize a diabetes club in your area.

This chapter has dealt with many aspects of your health. As a responsible self-manager it is necessary that you expand your knowledge from diabetes to general health and its maintenance. There are many health resources within the health-care delivery system. Professionals on the health-care team have extensive education in their specific areas. If you have diabetes, you will frequently have contact with many health-care providers, such as various doctors, a nurse, a nutritionist and a pharmacist. Choose your health-care professionals wisely, making sure they have appropriate credentials. Maintaining your personal health involves many factors. When you see a doctor for the first time, he will take a thorough history. A physical examination will be performed and certain laboratory tests will be ordered. You will need to see your doctor several times per year depending on your doctor's recommendation. The Patient's Bill of Rights has been developed to help increase your participation in your health care. The use of assertive behavior with health-care providers can help you express feelings and ideas in a clear manner. Assertive behavior can help you obtain the information you need regarding your health. At one time or another in your life, you may use an emergency room. Make sure you go during a true emergency. Be prepared for the environment in the ER. Prepare for an emergency at home by keeping essential phone numbers handy. Become familiar with some essential personal health tips. Avoid excessive alcohol use. If you are a woman, have a Pap smear as often as needed and perform breast self-examination monthly. Obtain a second opinion if you need surgery. Use over-the-counter medications as directed or with the advice of your doctor.

Engaging in proper hygienic practices is essential. Take care of your skin, keeping it clean and free from cuts. Diabetic females must take care to prevent vaginitis. If it develops, it must be treated properly. Urinary tract infections may also occur and require antibiotic therapy. Take care of your mouth and teeth because they are the gateway to your stomach. Brush your teeth thoroughly and floss daily. See your dentist regularly. Make daily hygiene practices part of self-management. Make sure you obtain adequate life and health insurance and plan for an interesting (as well as prosperous) career. Use your community resources, such as the American Diabetes Association and the Juvenile Diabetes Foundation, as often as needed.

More Useful Information

HOW YOUR BODY WORKS

In this section, the workings of the human body will be described. This information will act as a supplement to much of what you have already read.

The Structure of Living Things

The structure of living things may be classified into cells, tissues, organs and systems, in increasing order of complexity. Cells are the smallest units of living matter. Tissues are made up of the same types of cells. There are four main types of tissues: epithelial, connective, muscular and nervous tissues. Epithelial tissue is found throughout the body in such areas as the lining of the lungs, the skin and certain glands. Connective tissue is found in the walls of blood vessels, in the skin and in fat tissue. Muscular tissue includes skeletal muscle that is attached to bone. Smooth muscle tissue is located in the walls of organs such as the stomach. The action of smooth muscle cannot be consciously controlled (involuntary). Cardiac muscle is a specialized muscle tissue. The final type of tissue is nervous tissue. Nervous tissue carries messages among the body's organs.

Organs have specific functions and have their own blood and nerve supply. Organs may be made of several types of tissues in order to carry out their special functions. For example, the heart is an organ. Its function is to pump blood through the circulatory system. It has muscle tissue to pump blood, nervous tissue to stimulate the muscle to contract, connective tissue to separate its chambers and epithelial tissue to serve as a protective covering.

A system is a group of organs that perform similar functions or work together to perform one complex function. Prior to examining the various body systems, let's review the structure and function of cells. Cells are the basic units of all living matter. (See Figure 13.) Most cells can be seen only under a microscope. Your body is made up of trillions of cells. The cell is surrounded by a membrane

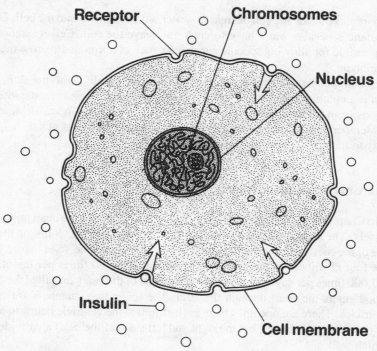

Figure 13. The cell and its functioning parts. Insulin enters the cell through the receptors.

which determines what will enter and exit from it. Cellular activity is directed by the nucleus. The nucleus lies in the center of the cell and contains chromosomes. Chromosomes are made up of thousands of genes. A human gene contains deoxyribonucleic acid (DNA), which contains material necessary for heredity. DNA tells the cell what to do. It gives a blueprint of what must be done to ribonucleic acid (RNA), which then does the actual work. Human genes for the production of insulin have been placed into bacteria. The bacteria are used to manufacture human insulin. Energy is necessary in order for the cell to work properly. The energy necessary for cell function comes from the breakdown of a high-energy compound known as adenosine triphosphate (ATP). This can be considered the power source of the cell.

A semipermeable cell membrane separates the inside of the cell from its liquid environment. It keeps an exact balance of liquid and other substances on either side of it. This balance is vital to life. If the concentration of particles (such as glucose) outside the cell increases, water moves out of the cell to balance this. This process is known as osmosis. The cells will then shrink. If the concentration of particles outside the cell decreases, water will then move into the cell. Other substances besides water have to enter and leave the cell. Cell receptors are responsible for allowing specific substances such as hormones to cross the cell membrane.

Certain body systems will now be described, beginning with the skin. The skin is a combination of waterproof, protective tissues. It protects the internal organs from infection, injury and dryness. It is a sensory organ. Pain, touch and temperature responses are felt through the skin. Its sweat glands help the body to maintain a normal temperature.

The Cardiovascular System

In Chapter 17 you learned about complications affecting the heart and blood vessels. The heart is a muscular organ about as large as a fist. It lies on the left side of the chest between the lungs and behind the breastbone. (See Figure 14a.) The four chambers of the heart beat continually 70–80 times per minute, or 100,000 times per day. The upper two chambers of the heart are called the atria. Blood enters the heart through the atria. The lower two chambers are called ventricles. There are openings from each atrium to the ventricle below to allow for the passage of blood, but the right and left sides of the heart are divided by a thick wall.

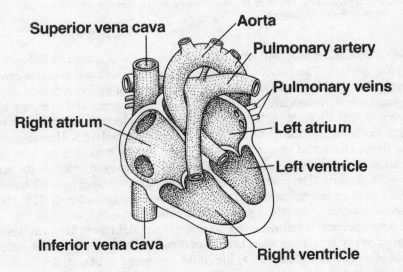

Superior vena cava

Aorta

Pulmonary artery

Pulmonary veins

Right atrium

Left atrium

Left ventricle

Inferior vena cava

Right ventricle

Figure 14a. A diagram of the heart

The movement of blood is controlled by the pumping action of the heart. The heart pumps five quarts of blood each minute. A natural pacemaker controls the pumping action. This pacemaker is made up of a small bundle of specialized cells that initiate electrical impulses. The impulses are influenced by the nervous system and hormones in the blood.

Both sides of the heart pump at the same time. Blood flows from the atria into the ventricles (diastole) while the valves open and then close to prevent backflow. When the ventricles contract (systole), blood is pumped out into the circulation.

Oxygen-poor blood is returned to the right atrium of the heart. It then passes into the right ventricle. The right ventricle pumps blood into the pulmonary artery, which takes it to the lungs. When the blood enters the lungs, it gives up carbon dioxide in exchange for oxygen. The oxygenated blood now travels back to the left atrium of the heart by way of the pulmonary veins. It enters the left ventricle, which pumps the oxygenated blood into the aorta. The blood passes from the aorta into smaller arteries and finally into the capillaries. The cells take up oxygen and nutrients from the capillaries in exchange for carbon dioxide and wastes. The wastes are then carried away as the blood now flows back from venules into larger veins until it reaches the heart. The process which began at the right atrium now begins again. Remember, too, the heart has its own blood supply, the coronary circulation. (See Figure 14b.)

The blood which is pumped through the body plays an essential part in the

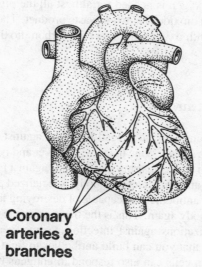

Coronary arteries & branches

Figure 14b. The heart has its own circulation.

functioning of your body. The fluid portion of the blood is known as plasma. The red blood cells are manufactured in the bone marrow and live for approximately 120 days. They contain hemoglobin, which carries oxygen to and carbon dioxide away from tissues. A decreased amount of red blood cells is called anemia. White blood cells are called leukocytes. They are formed in the bone marrow and lymphatic tissue. White blood cells help defend the body against infection and dispose of dead tissue. The white blood cells increase in number during infections. Blood also contains platelets, which help form blood clots.

You can now see how the heart works as a pump and how it uses the circulatory system to transport blood. Blood is also carried to the lungs, which are part of the respiratory system. This system will be described next.

The Respiratory System

The lungs lie on either side of the heart. (See Figure 15.) Air moves in and out of the lungs as they expand and contract. Normally, you take 14 to 20 breaths per minute, but breathing rate is affected by exercise, pain, general health and fitness. Breathing in will draw oxygen into the body while breathing out will expel carbon dioxide. Inside each lung are tiny air sacs called alveoli. It is here that the exchange of oxygen and carbon dioxide between the capillaries and the lungs takes place. Oxygen is needed for almost all the processes taking place in your body; carbon dioxide is a major waste product. The respiratory system supplies the blood with oxygen and rids it of carbon dioxide.

The Immune System

The immune system helps to defend the body against foreign substances. Lymphoid tissue, the spleen, bone marrow, the liver and lymph nodes are parts of this system, which is like an army that defends against foreign attack. When a foreign substance (antigen) enters the body, specialized proteins (antibodies) are produced. These antibodies are capable of destroying the foreign substance if it ever enters the body again. This is the basic principle of immunity. When you receive immunizations against infections, some weakened antigens are injected into you so that you can build antibodies to fight off certain diseases in the future. Certain cells can also respond to antigens by recognizing them as foreign and fighting and destroying them. This "cellular immunity" occurs in the rejection of transplanted organs.

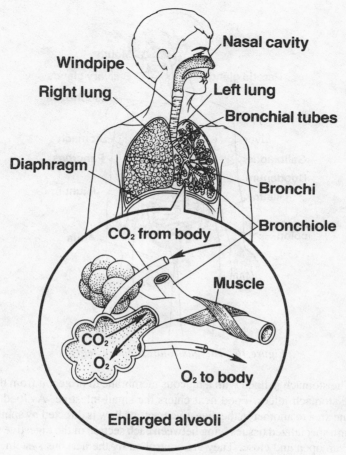

Figure 15. The respiratory system

The Gastrointestinal System (Digestive System)

Food contains important substances necessary for providing energy, building tissues and regulating body processes. In order for food to be used in this way, it must be digested and absorbed. The digestion of food into simple substances that can be absorbed into the circulation is the role of the gastrointestinal system.

Digestion begins as soon as food enters the mouth. Digestion is both a mechanical and a chemical process. After food is swallowed, it is moved through the gastrointestinal tract by involuntary muscle contractions called peristalsis. The stomach lies in the upper left area of the abdomen. An average meal will remain in the stomach for about three hours. During this time, stomach juices liquefy food so that it may easily pass into the small intestine. The stomach juices contain the enzyme pepsin, which breaks down proteins, and hydrochloric

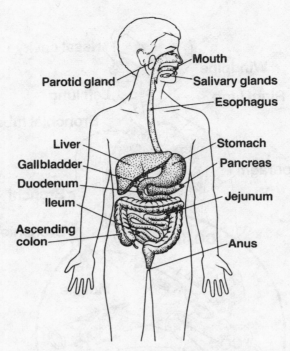

Figure 16. The gastrointestinal system

acid. The stomach is lined with a mucous membrane to protect it from the acid
and the stomach juices. Food next enters the small intestine. As food passes
from one area to another in the digestive tract, its flow is directed by sphincters.
These are specialized tissues lying between each section of the digestive system
which can open and close. They are controlled by the nervous system.

The small intestine is divided into three parts, the duodenum, the jejunum
and the ileum. Absorption is the process whereby digested food first enters the
cells in the lining of the small intestine and then enters the bloodstream. Absorption is dependent upon many factors, such as the presence of food in the
stomach prior to eating, the movement of food out of the stomach, the presence
of hormones and enzymes and the action of nerves. The remaining waste products continue to the large intestine, where water and salts (electrolytes) are
absorbed; they are then emptied from the gastrointestinal system.

Other important organs of the gastrointestinal system include the liver, the
gallbladder and the pancreas. (See Figure 16.) The liver has many important
functions, including the regulation of blood glucose. The liver also detoxifies
drugs and alcohol. It is capable of producing ketones (by-products of fat metabolism), blood proteins and bile (which goes to the gallbladder). The gallbladder stores and releases bile, which is necessary for the breakdown and
absorption of fats. The pancreas lies behind the stomach and has a commu-

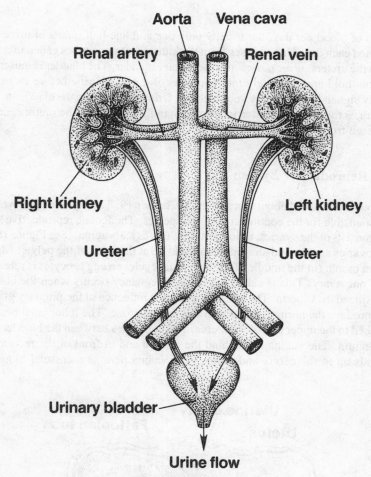

Aorta · Vena cava

Renal artery · Renal vein

Right kidney · Left kidney

Ureter · Ureter

Urinary bladder

Urine flow

Figure 17. The urinary system

nication (duct) to the small intestine. It weighs about a half pound. Important digestive enzymes made in the pancreas, such as trypsin, amylase and lipase, are released into the small intestine. Remember, the pancreas is also part of the endocrine system.

The Urinary System

The urinary system filters blood and eliminates waste products. (See Figure 17.) It also regulates water and salt (electrolyte) balance. This system is made up of the kidneys, ureters, urinary bladder and urethra. The kidneys are responsible for purifying the blood. A healthy kidney can purify over one hundred quarts of blood per day, but usually only one and one-half quarts of urine are excreted each day. Urine passes from the kidneys into two tubes called ureters. From the ureters, urine passes into the urinary bladder. The bladder is muscular and can hold approximately three-quarters of a pint of urine before its nerve supply signals you to empty your bladder. Urine passes from the bladder to the urethra, a tube that is shorter in women than in men. From the urethra, urine is passed from the body.

The Reproductive System

You have learned about this system in Chapter 19. The reproductive system is responsible for the continuation of the species. The female reproductive system consists of the ovaries, fallopian tubes, uterus and vagina. (See Figure 18a.) The ovaries are almond-shaped organs that lie at the sides of the pelvis. About once a month (in the middle of the menstrual cycle) an egg (oocyte) is released from one ovary. This is called ovulation. Pregnancy occurs when the oocyte is fertilized by a sperm. The ovaries, under the influence of the pituitary gland, also produce the hormones estrogen and progesterone. The fallopian tubes are attached to the upper part of the uterus. The uterus lies between the bladder and the rectum. The vagina lies behind the urethra and in front of the rectum. It extends up to the cervix and uterus. The vagina permits menstrual blood to

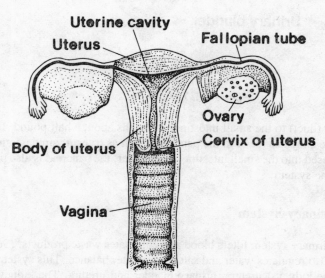

Figure 18a. The female reproductive system

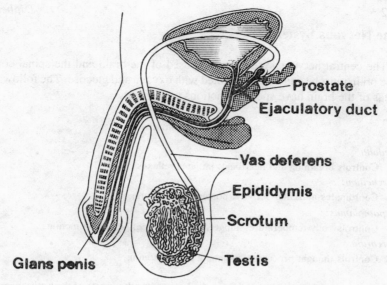

Prostate
Ejaculatory duct
Vas deferens
Epididymis
Scrotum
Glans penis
Testis

Figure 18b. The male reproductive system

escape from the uterus. It is the birth canal and receives the penis during intercourse. Menstruation usually begins between the ages of 10 and 14 but may not start until the age of 16 in some girls. Menopause usually occurs after the age of 45 and marks the end of the childbearing years. The ovaries no longer release oocytes and they secrete only small amounts of hormones. Menstruation stops at this time.

The male reproductive system includes the testes, epididymis, vas deferens, ejaculatory ducts and urethra. (See Figure 18b.) The scrotum, prostate gland and penis are other reproductive structures. The testes are located in the scrotum. It is here that sperm are produced. The hormone necessary for the development of male bodily characteristics, testosterone, is also produced here. The production of this hormone is under the control of the pituitary gland. As you can see, the role of the testes in the male is similar to the role of the ovaries in the female.

The epididymis is located at the upper part of the testis. Sperm mature in this area and enter the vas deferens. The vas deferens leads from the epididymis to the vicinity of the urinary bladder to form the ejaculatory ducts. The ejaculatory ducts empty into the urethra. The male urethra is located in the penis and has two functions. It carries sperm during ejaculation and it excretes urine. It secretes a substance which increases the movement of the sperm. The penis becomes congested with blood during sexual arousal, resulting in an erection. The circulatory, endocrine and nervous systems are all involved in producing a normal erection.

The Nervous System

The central nervous system is composed of the brain and the spinal cord. The brain must be constantly supplied with oxygen and glucose. The following areas of the brain have special functions to perform.

THE BRAIN AND ITS FUNCTIONS

Medulla:
Controls breathing and heartbeat; initiates reflexes
Cerebellum:
Coordinates muscular activity, posture, equilibrium
Hypothalamus:
Controls body temperature, hunger, water balance, pituitary functions
Cerebrum:
Controls thought processes, judgment and reasoning

Nerve impulses travel to and from the brain and other parts of the body through spinal nerves located in the spinal cord. (See Figure 19.) There are both motor and sensory nerves. Sensory nerves carry messages to the brain; motor nerves carry messages to muscles. There are twelve cranial nerves. They control such things as the sense of smell and taste as well as movement of the tongue and eyes and facial expression. A protective function of the nervous system (one that is often tested during a physical exam) concerns reflexes. In a reflex, a sensory message from the environment is carried to the central nervous system and an automatic motor response is carried to muscles to produce a reaction. This occurs without thinking. Pulling your hand away from a hot stove is an example of a reflex.

The autonomic nervous system controls processes which are not usually under conscious (voluntary) control. This system sends impulses to organs, glands and muscles. The routine regulation of heartbeat, of digestion and of blood pressure are examples of this system at work. The autonomic nervous system works through two divisions, the sympathetic and the parasympathetic. The sympathetic nervous system prepares the body for action in times of stress. The parasympathetic system works to slow the body's reactions and conserve energy.

The Endocrine System

The endocrine system acts in concert with the nervous system to control body processes. The endocrine system is composed of glands such as the hypothal-

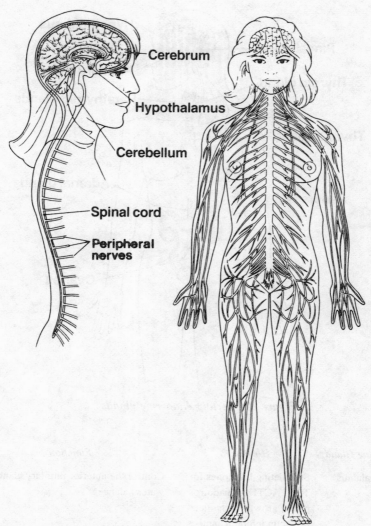

Figure 19. Your nervous system controls how you move your arms and legs as well as the workings of your internal organs.

amus, pituitary, pineal, thyroid, pancreas, parathyroid, thymus, adrenals (ovaries and testes). (See Figure 20.) Each of these is important in regulating the body's actions. Each gland releases specific hormones, which perform specific functions. The following is a partial listing of the endocrine glands and their hormones.

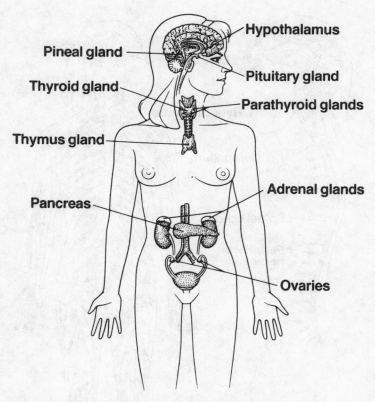

Figure 20. Certain endocrine glands

Endocrine Gland	Hormone	Function
Hypothalamus	Stimulating hormones for TSH, ACTH, gonadotrophins, growth hormone; prolactin inhibitor; antidiuretic hormone	Control the anterior pituitary gland and water balance
Pituitary	TSH (thyroid-stimulating hormone)	Stimulates activity of thyroid gland
	ACTH (adrenocorticotrophic hormone)	Stimulates activity of adrenal glands
	Gonadotrophic hormones	Stimulate sex glands Control ovulation

Endocrine Gland	Hormone	Function
	MSH (melanocyte-stimulating hormone)	Causes skin pigmentation
	Growth hormone	Stimulates growth of bone, muscle and organs
Pineal	Serotonin	Dilates and constricts blood vessels
	Melatonin	Decreases ovarian activity
Thyroid	Thyroxine (T_4), triiodo-thyronine (T_3)	Increase metabolism
	Calcitonin	Lowers blood calcium
Parathyroid	Parathyroid hormone	Increases blood calcium
Thymus	Thymosin	Fights off infection
Adrenals	Glucocorticoids	Help use glucose effectively
	Mineralocorticoids	Conserve salt balance
	Sex hormones	Stimulate reproductive organs
	Catecholamines (norepinephrine, epinephrine)	Respond to stress
Ovaries, Testes	Testosterone, estrogen, progesterone	Stimulate reproductive organs; secondary sexual characteristics

It is beyond the scope of this book to review the body systems in minute detail. However, we hope this information has improved your understanding of how your body works.

TYPES OF AVAILABLE INSULIN

	Product (Manufacturer)
Rapid-acting	Actrapid (Novo)
	Actrapid Human (Squibb-Novo)
	Semitard (Novo)
	Velosulin (Nordisk)
	Regular Iletin II (Lilly)
	Purified Regular (Squibb)
	Regular (Squibb)
	Semilente (Squibb)
	Regular Iletin I (Lilly)
	Humulin R (Lilly)

Intermediate-acting	Protaphane NPH (Novo)
	Monotard (Novo)
	Monotard Human (Squibb-Novo)
	Lentard (Novo)
	Insulatard NPH (Nordisk)
	Mixtard (Nordisk)
	NPH Iletin II (Lilly)
	Purified Isophane NPH (Squibb)
	Lente Iletin II (Lilly)
	Purified Lente (Squibb)
	Isophane NPH (Squibb)
	Lente (Squibb)
	NPH Iletin I (Lilly)
	Lente Iletin I (Lilly)
	Humulin N (Lilly)
Long-acting	Ultratard (Novo)
	PZI Iletin II (Lilly)
	Ultralente (Squibb)
	PZI (Squibb)
	Ultralente Iletin I (Lilly)
	PZI Iletin I (Lilly)

Reprinted with permission of Squibb-Novo, Inc., 1982.

FOREIGN PHRASES YOU SHOULD KNOW
BEFORE THE PLANE TAKES OFF

I am a diabetic

French: Je suis diabétique
          Juh swee *dee*-ah-bet-*eek*

Spanish: Yo soy diabetico
          Yo soy *dee*-ah-bet-*teek*-oh

German: Ich bin zuckerkrank
          Ick bin *zook*-er-krank

Italian: Io sono diabetico
          Ee-o so-no de-ah-*bet*-teek-oh

Please get me a doctor

French: Allez chercher un médecin, s'il vous plaît
              Ah-*lay* share-*shay* oon med-*sa(n)*, see voo play

Spanish: Haga me el favor de llamar al médico
              Ah-ga may el fa-*vor* day yah-mar ahl *med*-ee-co

German: Rufen Sie bitte einen Arzt
              Roof-en see *bit*-ah *eye*-nen *artst*

Italian: Per favore chiami un dottore
              Pair fah-*vor*-ray key-*ah*-me oon dot-*tor*-ray

Sugar or Coca-Cola, please*

French: Sucre ou Coca-Cola, s'il vous plaît
              Soo-cruh ooh Coca-Cola, see voo play

Spanish: Azúcar o uno vaso de Coca-Cola, por favor
              A-*zoo*-car o oo-no *va*-so day Coca-Cola, por fa-*vor*

German: Zucker oder Coca-Cola, bitte
              Zooker oder Coca-Cola, *bit*-ah

Italian: Zucchero o Coca-Cola, per favore
              Zooker-oh o Coca-Cola, *pair* fah-*vor*-ray

Orange juice

French: Jus d'orange
              Joo door-*ange*

Spanish: Vaso de jugo de naranja
              Va-so day *who*-go day nar-*ong*-ha

German: Orangensaft
              Or-*ong*-en-soft

Italian: Succo de arancia
              Sook-oh dee ah-*ron*-see-ah

Adapted with permission from *Vacation, Travel and Diabetes*, Becton Dickinson and Company.

---

* As you can see, Coca-Cola is an international word, so do not be afraid to say it if you are experiencing any signs of hypoglycemia. It will usually bring a quick response.

AVAILABILITY OF LILLY INSULINS OUTSIDE OF THE U.S.A.

COUNTRY	PROTAMINE ZINC INSULIN			REGULAR INSULIN			NPH INSULIN			LENTE INSULIN		
	M-140	M-180	M-110	M-240	M-280	M-210	M-340	M-380	M-310	M-440	M-480	M-410
Argentina	X	X	—	X	X	—	X	X	—	X	X	—
Bahrain	—	—	—	—	—	X	X	—	X	—	—	X
Barbados	—	—	X	—	—	X	—	—	—	—	—	—
Brazil	X	X	—	X	X	—	X	X	—	X	—	—
Canada	—	—	X	—	—	X	—	—	X	—	—	X
Colombia	—	—	—	X	X	—	X	X	—	X	X	—
Costa Rica	—	—	—	X	X	—	X	X	—	X	X	—
Dominican Rep.	—	—	—	X	X	—	X	X	—	X	X	—
El Salvador	—	—	—	X	X	—	X	X	—	X	X	—
Guatemala	—	—	—	X	X	—	X	—	—	X	X	—
Haiti	—	—	X	X	—	X	X	—	X	—	—	—
Honduras	—	—	—	X	X	—	X	X	—	X	X	—
Hong Kong	—	—	—	X	X	—	X	X	—	X	X	—
Israel	—	—	—	—	—	—	—	X	—	—	—	—
Italy	X	—	—	X	—	X	X	—	—	X	—	—
Jamaica	—	—	—	—	—	—	—	—	—	X	—	X
Japan	—	—	—	—	—	—	—	—	—	—	—	X
Malawi	X	X	—	X	X	X	X	—	—	—	—	—
Mexico	X	—	X	X	X	X	X	—	X	X	—	X
Neth. Antilles	—	—	—	X	X	—	—	—	—	X	—	—
Nicaragua	—	—	—	X	X	—	X	X	—	X	X	—
Panama	—	—	—	X	X	—	X	X	—	X	X	—
Peru	—	—	—	X	X	X	X	—	—	X	—	—
Puerto Rico	—	X	—	X	—	—	—	—	X	—	—	X
Switzerland	X	—	—	X	—	—	X	—	—	—	—	—
Thailand	—	—	—	X	—	—	X	X	—	—	—	—
Trinidad	—	—	—	—	—	—	X	—	X	—	—	—
Venezuela	X	X	—	X	X	—	X	X	—	X	X	—
Virgin Isl. (US)	—	—	—	—	—	X	—	—	X	—	—	—

X = Available, — = Unavailable

(Information made available by Eli Lilly and Company, 1982)

AVAILABILITY OF NORDISK INSULINS IN HIGHLY PURIFIED PORK QUALITY

COUNTRY	VELOSULIN			INSULATARD (NPH)			MIXTARD		
	40	80	100	40	80	100	40	80	100
Argentina	X	X	—	X	X	—	—	—	—
Australia	X	X	—	X	X	—	X	X	—
Austria	X	—	—	X	—	—	X	—	—
Belgium	X	—	—	X	—	—	X	—	—
Canada	—	—	X	—	—	X	—	—	X
Colombia	X	X	—	X	X	—	X	X	—
Costa Rica	X	X	—	X	X	—	—	—	—
Cyprus	X	—	—	X	—	—	X	—	—
Denmark	X	—	—	X	—	—	X	—	—
Ecuador	X	—	—	X	—	—	X	—	—
Egypt	X	—	—	X	—	—	X	—	—
Federal Republic of Germany	X	—	—	X	—	—	X	—	—
Finland	X	—	—	X	—	—	X	—	—
France	X	—	—	X	—	—	X	—	—
Greece	X	—	—	X	—	—	X	—	—
Iraq	X	—	—	X	—	—	—	—	—
Ireland	X	X	—	X	X	—	X	X	—
Israel	X	—	X	X	—	X	X	—	—
Japan	—	—	—	X	—	—	—	—	—
Jordan	X	—	—	X	—	—	X	—	—
Kuwait	X	—	—	X	—	—	X	—	—
Lebanon	X	—	—	X	—	—	X	—	—

AVAILABILITY OF NORDISK INSULINS IN HIGHLY PURIFIED PORK QUALITY

COUNTRY	VELOSULIN			INSULATARD (NPH)			MIXTARD		
	40	80	100	40	80	100	40	80	100
Libya	X	X	—	X	X	—	X	X	—
Malaysia	—	X	—	—	X	—	—	X	—
Malta	X	—	—	X	—	—	X	—	—
Netherlands	X	—	—	X	—	—	X	—	—
New Zealand	X	X	—	X	X	—	X	X	—
North Yemen	X	—	—	X	—	—	—	—	—
Norway	X	—	—	X	—	—	X	—	—
Peru	X	X	—	X	X	—	X	X	—
Poland	X	—	—	X	—	—	—	—	—
Spain	X	—	—	X	—	—	X	—	—
Sweden	X	—	—	X	—	—	X	—	—
Switzerland	X	—	—	X	—	—	X	—	—
Turkey	X	—	—	X	—	—	X	—	—
United Arab Emirates	X	—	—	X	—	—	—	—	—
United Kingdom	X	X	X	X	X	X	X	X	X
United States of America	—	—	X	—	—	X	—	—	X
Uruguay	X	—	—	X	—	—	—	—	—

Information made available by Nordisk-USA, 1982

INTERNATIONAL AVAILABILITY OF NOVO INSULINS — MAY 1, 1982

COUNTRY	ACTRAPID MC			SEMILENTE MC			RAPITARD MC			MONOTARD MC			LENTE MC			ULTRALENTE MC			PROTAPHANE MC 100	ISOPHANE MC 100
	40	80	100	40	80	100	40	80	100	40	80	100	40	80	100	40	80	100		
Albania																				
Algeria																				
Argentina																				
Australia			x			x			x			x			x			x	x	x
Austria	x			x			x			x			x			x				
Bahamas	x	x					x			x						x				
Bangladesh	x			x						x			x							
Barbados	x	x					x	x		x	x		x	x						
Belgium	x			x			x			x			x			x				
Bermuda										x										
Bolivia																				
Brazil	x	x		x	x					x	x									
Bulgaria	x			x						x			x							
Chile	x			x						x										
Czechoslovakia	x			x						x			x							
Cuba		x									x									
Cyprus	x			x			x			x			x			x				
Denmark	x			x			x			x			x	x		x				
Dominican Rep.	x	x		x						x			x	x						
Ecuador	x			x						x										
Egypt	x			x						x										
Ethiopia																				

INTERNATIONAL AVAILABILITY OF NOVO INSULINS — MAY 1, 1982

COUNTRY	ACTRAPID MC 40	80	100	SEMILENTE MC 40	80	100	RAPITARD MC 40	80	100	MONOTARD MC 40	80	100	LENTE MC 40	80	100	ULTRALENTE MC 40	80	100	PROTAPHANE MC 100	ISOPHANE MC 100
Finland	x			x			x			x			x			x				
France	x			x			x			x			x			x				
Germany. E.	x			x			x			x			x							
Germany. W.	x			x			x			x			x	x		x				
Ghana																	x			
Gibraltar																				
Greece	x			x			x			x			x			x				
Guyana	x	x											x	x						
Haiti	x									x	x	x								
Hong Kong	x	x		x	x		x	x		x	x		x	x		x	x			
Hungary	x	x		x						x	x					x				
Iceland	x			x			x			x			x	x						
India	x	x		x	x					x	x									
Indonesia	x			x						x										
Iran																				
Iraq	x			x						x			x							
Ireland	x	x		x	x		x	x		x	x		x	x		x	x			
Israel	x	x		x	x		x			x	x		x	x		x	x			
Italy	x			x						x										
Japan	x			x			x			x			x			x				
Jordan	x			x			x			x			x			x				
Kenya	x			x						x	x		x							

INTERNATIONAL AVAILABILITY OF NOVO INSULINS — MAY 1, 1982

COUNTRY	ACTRAPID MC			SEMILENTE MC			RAPITARD MC			MONOTARD MC			LENTE MC			ULTRALENTE MC			PROTAPHANE MC 100	ISOPHANE MC 100
	40	80	100	40	80	100	40	80	100	40	80	100	40	80	100	40	80	100	100	100
Kuwait	x	x		x			x			x	x		x			x				
Lebanon	x			x			x			x			x			x				
Malaysia		x	x		x	x		x	x		x	x		x	x					
Malta	x			x			x	x		x	x		x							
Mexico																				
Morocco	x			x			x			x	x	x	x			x				
Netherlands	x			x			x			x			x	x		x				
Neth. Antilles		x						x				x			x					
New Zealand		x	x			x			x			x			x			x	x	
Nigeria																				x
Norway	x			x			x			x			x			x				
Pakistan		x																		
Panama											x									
Paraguay	x									x										
Peru	x									x										
Philippines	x	x		x			x	x		x	x		x	x						
Poland	x	x		x	x		x	x		x	x		x	x			x			
Portugal	x			x			x			x			x			x	x			
Rumania				x						x			x							
Rwanda																				
Seychelles																				
Singapore		x	x		x	x			x			x			x					

INTERNATIONAL AVAILABILITY OF NOVO INSULINS — MAY 1, 1982

COUNTRY	ACTRAPID MC			SEMILENTE MC			RAPITARD MC			MONOTARD MC			LENTE MC			ULTRALENTE MC			PROTAPHANE MC 100	ISOPHANE MC 100
	40	80	100	40	80	100	40	80	100	40	80	100	40	80	100	40	80	100	100	100
South Africa	x	x		x	x		x	x		x	x		x	x		x	x			
South Korea																				
Spain	x			x			x			x			x			x				
Sri Lanka	x	x		x	x		x	x		x	x			x	x					
Sudan	x			x						x										
Suriname	x									x										
Sweden	x			x			x			x			x			x				
Switzerland	x			x			x			x			x	x		x				
Syria	x			x			x			x			x			x				
Taiwan	x	x					x			x	x									
Tanzania																				
Thailand	x	x	x	x	x	x	x	x	x	x	x	x	x	x	x					
Trinidad			x									x								
Tunisia																				
United Kingdom	x	x		x	x		x	x		x	x		x	x		x	x			
U.S.A.			x			x						x			x			x	x	
U.S.S.R.	x												x							
Venezuela	x	x		x	x					x	x									
Yugoslavia																				
Zaire	x			x						x										
Zimbabwe	x	x		x	x		x	x		x	x		x	x		x	x			

NOTE: "MC" is a Novo designation used in Europe and elsewhere to describe Novo purified insulins

(Information made available. Squibb-Novo. Inc., 1982.)

FAST-FOOD GUIDE

FOOD ITEM	BREAD	MEAT	FAT	OTHER	CALORIES	CHOLESTEROL (MG.)	SODIUM (MG.)
WENDY'S							
Single Hamburger	2	3	2		470	70	774
Double Hamburger	2	6	2		670	125	980
Triple Hamburger	2	9	2		850	205	1217
Single w/cheese	2	4	3		580	90	1085
Double w/cheese	2	7	3		800	155	1414
Triple w/cheese	2	10	4		1040	225	1848
Chili	1	2	0	1 v*	230	25	1065
French Fries	3	0	3		330	5	112
McDONALD'S							
Egg McMuffin	2	2	1		327	229	885
English Muffin (buttered)	2	0	1		186	13	318
Pork Sausage	0	1	3		206	43	615
Scrambled Eggs	0	2	1		180	349	205
Hashbrown Potatoes	1	0	1		125	7	325
Big Mac	3	3	3		563	86	1010
Cheeseburger	2	2	1		307	37	767
Hamburger	2	1	1		255	25	520
Quarter Pounder	2	3	2		424	67	735
Quarter Pounder (w/cheese)	2	4	2		524	96	1236
Filet-O-Fish	3	1	4		432	47	781
Regular Fries	2	0	2		220	9	109

*v = vegetable

FOOD ITEM	BREAD	MEAT	FAT	OTHER	CALORIES	CHOLESTEROL (MG.)	SODIUM (MG.)
KENTUCKY FRIED CHICKEN							
ORIGINAL RECIPE DINNER: two pieces of chicken, mashed potato, gravy, coleslaw and roll							
Wing & Rib	3	3	4	1 v*	603	133	Information
Wing & Thigh	3	3	5	1 v*	661	172	Unavailable
Drumstick & Thigh	3	4	3	1 v*	643	180	—
EXTRA CRISPY DINNER: two pieces of chicken, mashed potato, gravy, coleslaw and roll							
Wing & Rib	4	3	6	1 v*	755	132	—
Wing & Thigh	4	3	7	1 v*	812	176	—
Drumstick & Thigh	4	4	4	1 v*	765	183	—
Corn on the Cob	2	0	1	1 v*	169	—	—
TACO BELL							
Bean Burrito	3	1	2		343	Information	272
Beef Burrito	2	4	1		466	Unavailable	327
Burrito Supreme	3	2	2		457	—	367
Combination							
Burrito	3	2	1		404	—	300
Enchirito	3	3	1		454	—	1175
Pintos 'N Cheese	1	1	1		168	—	102
Taco	1	2	0		186	—	79
Tostado	2	1	0		179	—	101

*v = vegetable

FOOD ITEM	BREAD	MEAT	FAT	OTHER	CALORIES	CHOLESTEROL (MG.)	SODIUM (MG.)
ARBY'S							
Roast Beef	2	3	0		350	45	880
Beef & Cheddar	2	3	2		450	55	1220
Super Roast Beef	4	3	3		620	85	1420
Ham N Cheese	2	3	1		380	60	1350
Turkey Deluxe	2	3	3		510	70	1220
Club	2	4	3		560	100	1610
Junior Roast Beef	2	2	0		220	35	530
Potato Cake	1	0	2		155	Information	Information
Coleslaw	0	0	1	1 v*	60	Unavailable	Unavailable
Reg. French Fries	2	0	2		211	—	—
Large French Fries	3	0	3		343	—	—
Arby's Sauce (1 pkg.)				free	10	—	—
Horsey Sauce (1 pkg.)	0	0	1		45	—	—
BURGER KING							
Whopper	3	3	4		630	Information	990
Whopper w/cheese	3	4	5		740	Unavailable	1435
Double Beef Whopper	3	6	5		850	—	1080
Double Beef Whopper (w/cheese)	3	7	5		950	—	1535
Whopper Junior	2	2	2		370	—	560
Whopper Junior (w/cheese)	2	2	3		420	—	785
Hamburger	2	2	1		290	—	525
Cheeseburger	2	2	2		350	—	730
Double Cheeseburger	2	4	2		530	—	990
Reg. French Fries	2	0	2		210	—	230
Reg. Onion Rings	2	0	3	1 v	270	—	450

*v = vegetable

Adapted with permission: St. Francis Hospital Diabetes Center Tulsa, Oklahoma 1982

GOOD SOURCES OF POTASSIUM

Food	Amount	Potassium (mg.)
apricots, fresh, canned	2 medium	301
apricots, dried	4 halves	136
banana	½ medium	150
cantaloupe	¼ small melon	340
cherries, raw	10	129
grapefruit	½	432
grapefruit juice	4 oz.	177
honeydew	1 wedge, 2″ wide	374
orange	1 small	173
orange juice	4 oz.	250
peach	1 medium, 2½″ dia.	406
strawberries	1 cup	186
carrots	1 raw	246
cucumber	1 raw	272
mushrooms	1 cup	140
parsnips (cooked without salt)	½ cup	290
potato, baked	1 small	340
tomato	1 raw	222
spinach (cooked without salt)	½ cup	250
skim milk	8 oz.	406
plain low-fat yogurt	8 oz.	531
coffee	6 oz.	65

FIBER CONTENT OF COMMON FOODS

Food	Amount	Calories	Plant Fiber (g.)
apples	1 small	55	3.9
apricots	2 medium	39	1.3
banana	½ small	60	1.3
blackberries	½ cup	30	3.6

Food	Amount	Calories	Plant Fiber (g.)
cherries	10	44	0.9
grapefruit	½	41	1.3
grapes	10	34	0.4
muskmelon	½ cup	26	0.9
orange	1 small	45	2.1
peach	1 medium	33	1.0
pear	1 small	70	2.5
pineapple	½ cup	41	1.3
plums	2 medium	58	2.3
strawberries	¾ cup	36	2.4
tangerine	1 medium	34	1.8
beans, white	½ cup	91	4.2
beans, kidney	½ cup	94	4.5
beans, lima	½ cup	126	1.4
bran (100%), cereal	½ cup	66	10.0
bread, rye	1 slice	54	2.7
bread, whole-grain wheat	1 slice	63	2.7
corn, kernels	⅓ cup	41	2.1
corn, grits	½ cup	59	1.9
corn bread	1 square	151	2.7
corn flakes	¾ cup	64	2.1
crackers, graham	2 squares	53	1.4
oats, whole	½ cup	61	1.6
pancakes	1	61	0.4
parsnips	⅔ cup	72	5.9
peas	½ cup	44	5.2
potato, white	1 small	80	3.8
rice, brown	½ cup	83	1.3
rice, white	½ cup	79	0.5
roll, dinner	1	81	0.8
rye flour, dark	2½ tbs.	60	2.8
rye wafers	3 squares	64	2.3
spaghetti	½ cup	82	0.8
squash, winter	½ cup	43	3.6
sweet potato	¼ cup	72	2.9
wheat flour, whole-grain	2½ tbs.	60	1.8

Food	Amount	Calories	Plant Fiber (g.)
wheat cereal, flakes	¾ cup	75	3.0
wheat cereal, shredded	1 large	84	3.0
asparagus	½ cup	15	1.2
bean sprouts	½ cup	17	0.9
beans, string	½ cup	12	1.7
beets	½ cup	22	1.5
broccoli	½ cup	15	2.6
brussels sprouts	½ cup	24	1.8
cabbage	½ cup	11	1.6
carrots	½ cup	19	2.2
cauliflower	½ cup	12	0.9
celery	½ cup	5	1.7
cucumber	½ cup	7	0.8
eggplant	½ cup	17	1.2
kale	½ cup	16	1.4
lettuce	½ cup	3	0.5
onions	½ cup	25	1.6
radishes	½ cup	9	1.2
rutabaga	½ cup	26	1.6
squash, summer	½ cup	9	2.3
tomato	½ cup	27	2.0
turnip	½ cup	13	1.3
zucchini	½ cup	9	2.5

From James Anderson and Kyleen Ward, "Long-Term Effects of High-Carbohydrate, High-Fiber Diets on Glucose and Lipid Metabolism: A Preliminary Report in Patients with Diabetes," *Diabetes Care,* 1:77, 1978. Adapted with permission of Dr. James Anderson and the American Diabetes Association.

SODIUM CONTENT OF SOME FOODS

200–400 mg.	*400–800 mg.*	*Over 800 mg.*
hard cheese (1 oz.)	canned sardines	smoked herring (3 oz.)
evaporated milk (1 oz.)	(3 oz.)	canned shrimp (3 oz.)
non-fat dry milk	frankfurter (1)	ham (3 oz.)
(½–1 cup)	kielbasa (1 link)	fast foods

200–400 mg.

canned salmon (3 oz.)
shellfish, boiled (3 oz.)
bacon (1 slice)
bologna (1 oz.)
ham-and-cheese loaf
  (1 oz.)
salami (1 oz.)
sausage (1 link or 1 patty)
instant oatmeal
  or cream of wheat
  (1 serving)
ready-to-eat cereals
  (1 serving)
green olives (4)

400–800 mg.

dry roasted and salted nuts
  (1 cup)
canned vegetables
  (1 cup)

Over 800 mg.

prepared main dishes,
  i.e., macaroni and
  cheese, pizza, TV
  dinners, chow mein
canned soups
sauerkraut (1 cup)
tomato juice (1 cup)
tomato sauce (1 cup)
vegetable juice cocktail
  (1 cup)
baking soda (1 tsp.)
garlic salt (1 tsp.)
meat tenderizer
  (like Accent) (1 tsp.)
onion salt (1 tsp.)
dill pickle (1)
soy sauce (1 tbs.)
bouillon cubes
potato chips
corn chips
pretzels
salted popcorn
salted peanuts

CHOLESTEROL CONTENT OF FOODS

Food	Amount	Cholesterol (mg.)
CHEESE		
American	1 oz.	27
blue	1 oz.	21
cheddar	1 oz.	30
Cheezola	1 oz.	1
cottage (1% fat)	1 cup	9
cottage (creamed)	1 cup	34
cream	2 tbs.	34
mozzarella	1 oz.	22
mozzarella (part skim)	1 oz.	16

Food	Amount	Cholesterol (mg.)
Muenster	1 oz.	27
Parmesan (grated)	1 tbs.	4
Swiss	1 oz.	26
EGGS		
whole	1 medium	258
Egg Beaters	¼ cup	0
caviar, sturgeon	1 tbs.	>48
FATS, OILS, CREAMS, GRAVIES		
bacon fat	1 tbs.	1
vegetable oils and		
shortenings	1 tbs.	0
butter	1 tsp.	12
cream (heavy)	1 tbs.	20
cream (half-and-half)	1 tbs.	6
non-dairy creamer	1 tbs.	0
margarine (all veg. fat)	1 tbs.	0
mayonnaise	1 tbs.	10
mayonnaise (imitation)	1 tbs.	5
SALAD DRESSINGS		
blue cheese	1 tbs.	4
Russian	1 tbs.	10
FISH		
halibut	3 oz.	50
flounder	3 oz.	50
cod, raw	3½ oz.	50
fish sticks	4–5	70
haddock, raw	3½ oz.	60
salmon, raw	3½ oz.	35
sardines	8 medium	120
tuna, canned in		
oil or water	3½ oz.	63
SHELLFISH		
clams, raw	6 large	36
crab, steamed	½ cup	62

Food	Amount	Cholesterol (mg.)
lobster	½ cup	62
mussels	3½ oz.	150
oysters, raw	6	45
scallops, bay and		
sea, raw	3 oz.	45
shrimp	½ cup or 11 large	96

GRAIN PRODUCTS

biscuits, homemade	1 average	15
French toast	1 slice	111
muffins	1 average	21
noodles, egg,		
cooked	1 cup	50
pancakes	1 average	33
stuffing, bread	½ cup	16
waffles, homemade	1 medium	62

MEATS

lean beef, cuts	3 oz.	78
chicken, cuts	3 oz.	66
duck	3½ oz.	70
pork, cuts	3½ oz.	70

ORGAN MEATS

brains	3½ oz.	2100
gizzard, chicken	1 oz.	55
heart		
beef, lean, braised	3½ oz.	274
chicken, cooked	3½ oz.	231
turkey, simmered	3½ oz.	238
kidneys		
beef, braised	3½ oz.	375
calf, raw	3½ oz.	375
hog, raw	3½ oz.	375
lamb, raw	3½ oz.	375

Food	Amount	Cholesterol (mg.)
liver		
beef, cooked	3½ oz.	438
calf, raw	3 oz.	300
chicken, simmered	3 oz.	746
sweetbreads, cooked		
calf or lamb	3½ oz.	396
tongue, beef, smoked	3½ oz.	210
FAST FOODS		
McDonald's		
Big Mac	1 serving	86
Quarter Pounder w/cheese	1 serving	96
shake	1 serving	29
hamburger	1 serving	25
Filet-O-Fish	1 serving	47
Arthur Treacher's		
shrimp, fried	1 serving	93
chicken filet	1 serving	64
chips (french fries)	1 serving	1
Kentucky Fried Chicken		
chicken (Original Recipe)	3½ oz.	133
chicken (Extra Crispy)	3½ oz.	176
SALADS		
chicken, canned	1 oz.	8
ham, canned	1 oz.	6
macaroni	1 cup	84
potato	1 cup	65
SOUPS		
chicken noodle, canned, made with water	1 serving	6
tomato, canned, made with water	1 serving	4
vegetable beef, canned, made with water	1 serving	4
cauliflower, creamed, homemade	1 serving	38
chicken, creamed, canned, made with water	1 serving	22
Manhattan clam chowder, canned, made with water	1 serving	40

Food	*Amount*	*Cholesterol (mg.)*
LUNCHEON MEATS		
bologna	1 oz.	28
liverwurst	1 oz.	35
olive loaf	1 oz.	10
salami	1 oz.	10
Spam	1 oz.	15
SAUSAGES		
frankfurter	1 average	32
Italian	1 oz.	8
pork, links	3½ oz.	100
MEAT SUBSTITUTES MADE		
FROM SOY PRODUCTS		0
MILK AND		
MILK PRODUCTS		
buttermilk (skim)	1 cup	10
low-fat milk, 1%	1 cup	10
low-fat milk, 2%	1 cup	20
skim milk	1 cup	5
whole milk	1 cup	34
yogurt		
low-fat	1 cup	14
skim	1 cup	4
whole	1 cup	30
milk beverages		
chocolate milk	1 cup	33
chocolate milk, 1% fat	1 cup	8
chocolate milk, 2% fat	1 cup	18
eggnog	1 cup	149
COMBINATION FOODS		
chicken à la king	1 cup	186
cheese soufflé	1 serving	251
clam fritters	1 serving	129
chili con carne	1 serving	15
egg roll, shrimp	1 serving	12
fish creole	1 serving	31

ANALYSIS OF POPULAR DIETS

Diet	Purported Rationale	Comments
HIGH PROTEIN, LOW CARBOHYDRATE Atkins Scarsdale Stillman	Elimination of one entire food group will yield rapid weight reduction. Protein-containing foods require more calories to digest, thus weight reduction is faster.	Nutritionally unbalanced; hij in fat and cholesterol; cons pation due to lack of fiber; t tigue; ketones in blood and u ine; provides short-term weig loss; unappetizing.
PROTEIN-SPARING Liquid or powdered protein	Severe calorie restriction. Yields rapid weight reduction.	Nutritionally unbalanced; shor term weight loss; loss of fluic and electrolytes; low bloc pressure; some reported deatl due to abnormal heart rhythr loss of body fat and protein.
APPETITE SUPPRESSANTS Amphetamines	Severe calorie restriction. Yields rapid weight reduction.	Nervousness; dry mouth; ii somnia; drug abuse/depen ence.
SEMISTARVATION KETOGENIC REGIMES Protein-sparing modified fast	High-quality protein is provided to maintain nitrogen balance and lean body mass. Body fat is burned, ketones result; reduction in feelings of hunger.	Must be undertaken with mec ical supervision.
PRITIKIN	Change the quality of the diet so it is lower in fat, cholesterol and simple carbohydrates. This is done to prevent or treat chronic diseases, i.e., heart disease and diabetes.	Diet may be too low in fat an animal protein. May be def cient in iron and calcium. Fe scientific studies reported i medical literature.
BEVERLY HILLS	Lose weight due to a combination of enzymes in fruit, which is the mainstay of the diet.	Too high in simple carbohy drates for anyone with diabe tes. May cause diarrhea an excretion of sodium and potas sium. Not enough protein t maintain good health.

CALORIE-DEFICIT DIET Weight Watchers TOPS	Inclusion of carbohydrates to prevent ketosis. Calories are restricted but usually not less than 1,000, so a 2–3-pound weight loss per week may result.	Safe and nutritionally balanced; can protect from between-meal hunger; can be easily adapted to patient's lifestyle; some may find diets too rigid.
BEHAVIOR MODIFICATION Self-monitoring environmental changes	Observation of eating habits through record keeping, with subsequent changes made in eating behavior resulting in lifelong weight reduction.	Slow, steady weight loss; may cause some frustration.
STARCH BLOCKERS	Specific enzyme inhibitor will prevent absorption of starch calories.	Gastrointestinal upset. No longer approved for sale by the FDA.

COOKBOOK IDEAS

The ABC's of Diabetic Cooking
Jane Helse, R.D., and Elizabeth Lansing. New York: Dell Publishing Co., 1979. Chapters on travel, dining out, fast-food exchanges, alcohol, ideas for children. All recipes provide the number of food exchanges per serving.

Oriental Cooking for the Diabetic
Dorothy Revell, R.D. San Francisco: Japan Publications, 1981. Provides special Oriental foods in the exchange system. Appendix on sodium restriction, spices and herbs and low-sodium recipes. Recipes include those for tempura, soybean curd, sauces, dressings and many other Oriental specialties. Each serving is calculated for the appropriate exchange group.

The American Diabetes Association and American Dietetic Association Family Cookbook
Englewood Cliffs, N.J.: Prentice-Hall, 1980. Chapters on meal planning, fast foods, sick-day rules, alcohol, restaurant eating, menus for special occasions. Over 300 recipes. Recipes provide food exchanges per serving and estimated nutrients per serving, i.e., calories, carbohydrates, proteins, fat, sodium and potassium.

The American Heart Association Cookbook
    4th ed.; New York: David McKay, 1978. Provides over 200 recipes with
    calorie count of each. Charts included in text provide cholesterol and fat
    content of foods. Low-fat cooking ideas are presented.

The Art of Cooking for the Diabetic
    Katherine Middleton and Mary Abbott Hess. Chicago: Contemporary Books,
    1978. Chapters on the adult and child with diabetes, eating out, alcohol,
    exercise. Free foods, traveling, brown bagging, food labeling, sweeteners
    and over 300 recipes. Recipes provide food exchanges per serving and
    nutritive values per serving, i.e., calories, carbohydrates, proteins, fat and
    sodium.

The Fabulous Fiber Cookbook
    Jeanne Jones. San Francisco: 101 Productions, 1981. Exciting recipes
    provide a variety of high-fiber foods. Recipes are calculated for serving
    size and food exchanges. A fiber exchange list is also provided.

COMMUNITY RESOURCE DIRECTORY

Al-Anon Family Group
   Headquarters
P.O. Box 182
Madison Square Station
New York, NY 10010

Alcoholics Anonymous
World Services, Inc.
P.O. Box 459
Grand Central Station
New York, NY 10010

American Association
   of Diabetes Educators
North Woodbury Road
Box 56
Pitman, NJ 08071
(609) 589-4831

American Association
   of Ophthalmology
1100 17th Street, N.W.
Washington, DC 20036
(202) 883-3447

American Association
   of Sex Educators, Counselors
   and Therapists
P.O. Box 23294
Washington, DC 20004

American Cancer Society
777 Third Avenue
New York, NY 10017

American College
of Obstetricians and
Gynecologists
One East Whacker Drive
Chicago, IL 60601
(312) 222-1600

American Dental Association
Bureau of Dental Health
Education
211 East Chicago Avenue
Chicago, IL 60611

American Diabetes Association
2 Park Avenue
New York, NY 10016
(212) 683-7444

American Dietetic Association
430 North Michigan Avenue
Chicago, IL 60611
(312) 280-5000

American Foundation for the
Blind
15 West 16th Street
New York, NY 10011
(212) 620-2000

American Heart Association
44 East 23rd Street
New York, NY 10010
(212) 477-9170

American Kidney Fund
P.O. Box 975
Washington, DC 20044
(301) 986-1444

American Lung Association
1740 Broadway
New York, NY 10019
(212) 245-8000

American Medical Association
535 North Dearborn Street
Chicago, IL 60610
(312) 751-6166

American Nurses' Association
2420 Pershing Road
Kansas City, MO 64108
(816) 474-5720

American Pharmaceutical
Association
2215 Constitution Avenue, N.W.
Washington, DC 20037
(202) 628-4410

American Podiatry Association
20 Chevy Chase Circle, N.W.
Washington, DC 20015
(202) 537-4900

American Printing House
for the Blind
P.O. Box 6085
Louisville, KY 40206
(502) 895-2405

American Psychiatric Association
1700 18th Street, N.W.
Washington, DC 20009
(202) 232-7878

American Public Health
Association, Inc.
1015 18th Street, N.W.
Washington, DC 20036
(202) 467-5000

American Public Welfare
Association
1155 16th Street, N.W.
Washington, DC 20036

American Red Cross
17th and D Streets, N.W.
Washington, DC 20006
(202) 737-8300

Ames Company
Division of Miles Laboratories
1127 Myrtle Street
Elkhart, IN 46514
(219) 264-8901

Auto-Syringe, Inc.
(Model AS-6C-U-100)
Londonderry Turnpike
Hooksett, NH 03104

Association for the Advancement
of Health Education
1201 16th Street, S.W.
Washington, DC 20036

Becton Dickinson Consumer
Products
(insulin syringes)
365 West Passaic Street
Rochelle Park, NJ 07662
(201) 368-7312

Bio-Dynamics, Inc.
(Chemstrips)
9115 Hague Road
Indianapolis, IN 64250
(317) 845-2000

Blue Cross/Blue Shield
Director of Public Relations
425 North Michigan Avenue
Chicago, IL 60690

Braille Volunteers of Huntington
P.O. Box 9422
Huntington, WV 25704

Bureau of Health Education
Center for Disease Control
Atlanta, GA 30533

Calorie Control Council
c/o Robert H. Kellen Co.
64 Perimeter Center East
Atlanta, GA 30346
(404) 393-1340

Cardiac Pacemaker, Inc.
(CPI Model 9100)
Subsidiary of Eli Lilly and
Company
4100 North Hamline Avenue
P.O. Box 43079
St. Paul, MN 55164

Center for Research
for Mothers and Children
National Institute of Child Health
and Human Development
National Institutes of Health
Landow Building, Room C703
Bethesda, MD 20205

Char-Mag Company
of Glendale, Inc.
(Syringe Magnifier)
6026 North Apple Blossom Lane
Milwaukee, WI 53217
(414) 962-6059

Consumer Product Safety
Commission
Washington, DC 20207

Diabetes in the News
Ames Education Service
P.O. Box 3105
Elkhart, IN 46515
(312) 664-9782

Division of Metabolic and
Endocrine Drug Products
Bureau of Drugs
Food and Drug Administration
Parklawn Building, Room 14B04
Rockville, MD 20852

Division of Research Resources
National Institutes of Health
Building 31, Room 5B51
Bethesda, MD 20205

Eli Lilly and Company
  (insulin)
307 East McCarty Street
Indianapolis, IN 46285
(317) 261-2319

Eli Lilly and Company
Educational Resources Program
P.O. Box 100B
Indianapolis, IN 46206

Family Service Association of
  America
44 East 23rd Street
New York, NY 10010

Food and Drug Administration
5600 Fishers Lane
Rockville, MD 20852
(301) 443-3380

Health Care Financing
  Administration
East Highrise, Room 505
6325 Security Boulevard
Baltimore, MD 21207

Health Insurance Institute
Department H
277 Park Avenue
New York, NY 10017

International Diabetes Federation
10 Queen Anne Street
London, WIM OBD, England
London 01-637-3644

Jewish Family Service
Council of Jewish Federation
  and Welfare Funds
315 Park Avenue South
New York, NY 10010

John W. Hall and Associates,
  Inc.
P.O. Box 14868
Shawnee Mission, KS 66215

Juvenile Diabetes Foundation
  National Offices
23 East 26th Street
New York, NY 10010
(212) 889-7575

Library of Congress
Division of the Blind
  and Physically Handicapped
1291 Taylor Street, N.W.
Washington, DC 20542
(202) 882-3500

Medic Alert Foundation
  International
P.O. Box 1009
Turlock, CA 95381
(209) 632-2371

Medidisc Corporation
P.O. Box 14306
North Palm Beach, FL 33408

Mental Health Association, Inc.
1800 North Kent Street
Arlington, VA 22209
(703) 528-6405

Metropolitan Life Insurance
  Company
Health and Welfare Division
One Madison Avenue
New York, NY 10010

Microdesign Systems
  (Mediscope)
7400 Shore Front Parkway
P.O. Box 188
Arverne, NY 11692

Monoject
   (insulin syringes)
Division of Sherwood Medical
1831 Olive Street
St. Louis, MO 63103
(314) 621-7788

National Association for Mental
   Health
10 Columbus Circle
New York, NY 10019

National Association of Patients
   on Hemodialysis and
   Transplantation
156 Williams Street
New York, NY 10038
(212) 619-2727
24-hour hotline
   (516) 334-1041

National Association for the
   Visually Handicapped
305 East 24th Street
New York, NY 10010

National Center for Health
   Education
211 Sutter Street
San Francisco, CA 91404

National Center for Health
   Services Research
Center Building, Room 8-30
3700 East-West Highway
Hyattsville, MD 20782

National Center for Health
   Statistics
Center Building, Room 2-58
3700 East-West Highway
Hyattsville, MD 20782

National Conference of
   Catholic Charities
1346 Connecticut Avenue, N.W.
Washington, DC 20036
(202) 785-2757

National Home Caring Council in
   Homemaker Home Health Aid
   Services, Inc.
67 Irving Place
New York, NY 10003
(212) 674-4990

National Diabetes
   Information Clearinghouse
Box NDIC
Bethesda, MD 20205
(301) 468-2162

National Eye Institute
National Institutes of Health
Building 31, Room 6A-49
Bethesda, MD 20205

National Foundation–March
   of Dimes
622 Third Avenue
New York, NY 10016
(212) 922-1460

National Heart, Lung and Blood
   Institute
National Institutes of Health
Federal Building, Room 4C12
Bethesda, MD 20205

National Hospice Organization
1311A Dolly Madison Boulevard
McLean, VA 22101
(703) 356-6770

National Institute on Aging
National Institutes of Health
Building 31, Room 5C-21
Bethesda, MD 20205

National Institute of Allergy
and Infectious Diseases
National Institutes of Health
Building 31, Room 7A-49
Bethesda, MD 20205

National Institute of Arthritis,
Diabetes, Digestive
& Kidney Disease
National Institutes of Health
Building 31, Room 9A-16
Bethesda, MD 20205

National Institute of Dental
Research
National Institutes of Health
Westwood Building, Room 507
Bethesda, MD 20205

National Institute of
Environmental Health Service
P.O. Box 12233
Research Triangle Park, NC
27709

National Institute of General
Medical Sciences
National Institutes of Health
Westwood Building, Room 925
5333 Westbard Avenue
Bethesda, MD 20205

National Institute of Mental
Health
5600 Fishers Lane
Room 17C-20
Rockville, MD 20857

National Institute of Neurological
and Communicative Disorders
and Stroke
National Institutes of Health
Federal Building, Room 710
Bethesda, MD 20205

National Kidney Foundation
2 Park Avenue
New York, NY 10016
(212) 889-2210

National Naval Medical Center
Endocrinology Branch
Bethesda, MD 20814

National Society to Prevent
Blindness
79 Madison Avenue
New York, NY 10016
(212) 684-3505

New York Life Insurance
Company
Public Relations Department
51 Madison Avenue
New York, NY 10010

Nordisk-U.S.A.
(insulin)
7315 Wisconsin Avenue
Bethesda, MD 20014
(301) 656-5410

Paddock Laboratories, Inc.
(Instant Glutose)
2744 Lyndale Avenue
South Minneapolis, MN 55408

Pfizer Laboratories
235 East 42nd Street
New York, NY 10017
(212) 573-2422

Planned Parenthood Federation of
America
810 Seventh Avenue
New York, NY 10019
(212) 541-7800

Prudential Life Insurance
  Company of America
Prudential Plaza
Newark, NJ 07010

Recordings for the Blind
215 East 58th Street
New York, NY 10022
(212) 751-0860

Salvation Army
120 West 14th Street
New York, NY 10011
(212) 620-4900

Science and Education
  Administration
(Ext. SEA-A) South Building,
  Room 5404
U.S. Department of Agriculture
Washington, DC 20205

Searle Company
  (Nutrasweet)
P.O. Box 5110
Chicago, IL 60680

Squibb-Novo, Inc.
  (insulin)
120 Alexander Street
Princeton, NJ 08540
(609) 921-8989

Social Security Administration
Dickinson Building, Room 2400
1500 Woodlawn Drive
Baltimore, MD 21241

The Upjohn Company
7000 Portage Road
Kalamazoo, MI 49001
(616) 323-4000

Ulster Scientific, Inc.
  (Autolet)
P.O. Box 902
Highland, NY 12528
(914) 691-6226

U.S. Department of Agriculture
Agricultural Research Service
Washington, DC 20205

Veterans Administration
Box 11M
810 Vermont Avenue, N.W.
Washington, DC 20420
(202) 389-5117

INDEX

Page numbers in italics refer to illustrations.